Martin Wehling

Editor

Drug Therapy for the Elderly

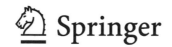 Springer

Editor
Martin Wehling
Institute of Experimental
    and Clinical Pharmacology and Toxicology
Director Clinical Pharmacology Mannheim
Medical Faculty Mannheim
University of Heidelberg
Mannheim
Germany

ISBN 978-3-7091-0911-3   ISBN 978-3-7091-0912-0 (eBook)
DOI 10.1007/978-3-7091-0912-0
Springer Wien Heidelberg New York Dordrecht London

Library of Congress Control Number: 2012945526

Drug Therapy for the Elderly

Foreword

> It is much easier to write upon a disease than upon a remedy.
> The former is in the hands of nature and a faithful observer
> with an eye of tolerable judgment cannot fail to delineate a likeness.
> The latter will ever be subject to the whim,
> the inaccuracies, and the blunder of mankind.
>
> William Withering (1741–1799)

When William Withering wrote these words, he never could have imagined that they would still be relevant to the practice of medicine into the next millennium. However, there remains a lingering truth to Withering's words that should humble all those who prescribe medications to older patients. There are many reasons that make geriatric pharmacotherapy especially challenging. Geriatric patients often have multiple coexisting illnesses, leading to the use of complex drug regimens. An increased burden of morbidity often results in polypharmacy; polypharmacy can lead to redundant drug effects and is the most important risk factor for serious drug-drug interactions and adverse drug events. Adverse drug events are often nonspecific and can go unrecognized in older patients. Sometimes, drug side effects lead to the prescription of additional medications, creating a prescribing cascade, and potentially increasing the risk of drug-related problems in older patients even more. Complicating these challenges are the many pharmacologic and physiologic changes that occur with aging, posing additional risks of drug-related injury for geriatric patients. Last but not least, errors in management are extraordinarily common in medication prescribing and monitoring in the elderly, resulting in dangerous near-misses, close calls, and preventable drug-related injuries. All of these challenges are even further complicated by the dearth of evidence that exists around the benefits, risks, and comparative effectiveness of the multitude of drug treatments that are commonly used in older patients.

There is universal recognition of the need to optimize and rationalize the medication regimens of older patients. The editor of this important contribution to the medical literature, Martin Wehling, is an eminent pharmacologist, and he has assembled a distinguished group of experts to create a textbook that should serve as an important reference for health care professionals across the disciplines who wish to provide the very best care to our growing geriatric population.

February 2012   Jerry H. Gurwitz M.D.
Chief, Division of Geriatric Medicine, Executive Director
Meyers Primary Care Institute
The Dr. John Meyers Professor of Primary Care Medicine
University of Massachusetts Medical School, Worcester, MA, USA

Preface

Drug therapy is the most important therapeutic intervention by any physician. Even surgeons prescribe numerically more drugs than making decisions on individual operations. The number of diagnoses increases with the age of patients, and so does the number of drugs: Men aged 80+ have 3.24, women of the same age have 3.57 diagnoses in average. As a guideline dealing with one of those diagnoses recommends three drugs on average, it is not difficult to understand why elderly patients often receive ten and more drugs. A U.S. study showed that patients aged 65+ consume five and more drugs in over 50 % of cases, and 10 % of elderly patients even used ten and more. This phenomenon of so-called polypharmacy has grave consequences: For the United States alone, it is estimated that each year about 100,000 patients die of serious adverse drug reactions. The potential of drug-drug interactions increases exponentially with the number of drugs; however, this is not the biggest problem of polypharmacy. Not mentioning costs, which in the light of the demographic revolution is a yet-increasing threat to all health care insurance systems, it reflects the generally insufficient quality of treatment in the elderly. This results—among other reasons—from the fact that most drug therapies have never been tested in the elderly; guidelines often simply extrapolate findings from younger to elder patients if the latter patient group is mentioned at all.

The lack of evidence is one of the major sources of suboptimal treatment in the elderly, and no drug has ever been tested in position 8 or 10 of a list of potentially outcome-relevant drugs. In clinical trials, patient selection aims at those without relevant concomitant diseases and thus medications; this almost automatically excludes most elderly patients from studies, and no drug will be tested on a background of more than four or five drugs. Polypharmacy thus results from extrapolations and simple additions of drugs—a process that often leads to a deadly cocktail. As a consequence, we need not only the systematic generation of data on drug efficacy and safety in the elderly but also an answer to the burning question of how to reduce polypharmacy rationally and consistently in the realm of non-evidence-based drug therapies in the elderly.

In this context, the book has two major aims: to compile the available knowledge on gerontopharmacology and to guide physicians to a rationalistic approach for successful drug therapy in the elderly. This includes the wide application of a novel classification of drugs relating to their *Fitness for the Aged* (FORTA; see chapter "Critical Extrapolation of Guidelines and Study Results: Risk-Benefit Assessment for Patients with Reduced Life Expectancy and a New Classification of Drugs According to Their Fitness for the Aged"), which not only assesses negative drug aspects such as the Beers' list, but also adds the emerging positive experiences in important therapeutic situations. It should be mentioned beforehand that the paucity of data and the yet-early days of an international discussion lead to limitations of this classification, which is only meant as proposal and inspirational attempt; in many instances, it still reflects author opinions only. It applies to chronic therapies for which data in the elderly are more prevalent than for those on acute interventions (e.g., in intensive care situations). This explains that, for example, for stroke as one of the most prevalent diseases in the elderly, only risk factors and preventive measures are addressed, but not the acute treatment, which is mainly done by specialists. In situations in which special knowledge and treatment modalities do not exist for the elderly in comparison to younger patients, we refer to standard books and training; thus, it is conceivable that chapters on gastrointestinal diseases or antibiotics are lacking. This book should concentrate on age-specific problems and not become diluted by the repetition of age-independent standard knowledge that can be found in reference works. Ideally, it should be received as a book supplementing those not devoted to the elderly; thus, the book volume could be restricted to less than 350 pages. Referencing is also very limited and by far not complete. Along this line, basic drug data contained in the *Physician's Desk Reference* or similar national drug listings (e.g., Rote Liste® in Germany) are not repeated unless they are important for age-related issues. Therefore, some chapters appear inadequately small compared to the importance of the clinical entities addressed. This results from the lack of data and reflection thereof in the book, but slim or lacking chapters should also inspire and encourage researchers to generate the data in clinical trials.

An important task for the authors was the thorough reflection of geriatric syndromes directly relating to drug therapy in the elderly, such as dementia, fall risk, and frailty. This includes both the induction of these syndromes by drugs and their treatment by drugs. In addition, more generic aspects of drug therapy in the elderly are addressed, including altered pharmacokinetics or compliance/adherence issues. These topics underlie the disease-oriented chapters (including the "missing" ones), and not notoriously repeated there; for example, it does not need to be reiterated in all chapters that kidney function is essential to the excretion of many drugs. To ease orientation, study acronyms are explained within and at the end some chapters.

The authors hope that this book may positively contribute to one of the most important therapeutic areas of the future: drug therapy in the elderly.

Mannheim   Martin Wehling
February 2012

Contents

About the Editor

Martin Wehling is full professor of clinical pharmacology at the University of Heidelberg. He is also an internist (cardiologist) and has long-standing experiences in basic science (cell physiology, steroid pharmacology, nongenomic steroid actions); clinical trials (translating basic science into human studies); and clinical medicine (invasive cardiology, endocrinology, geriatrics). In 2004, he was appointed by AstraZeneca as director of discovery (= translational) medicine. In 2007, he returned to his academic

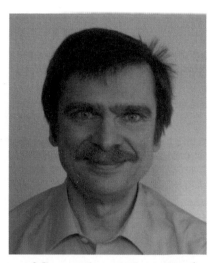

position. In 2000, he founded the Center of Gerontopharmacology (together with the head of the department of geriatric medicine, R. Gladisch), which supports the development of drug therapy in the elderly both scientifically and in daily practice. He has the only outpatient service for gerontopharmacology in Germany.

Potential Conflicts of Interest of the Editor

Martin Wehling was employed by AstraZeneca R&D, Mölndal, as director of discovery medicine (= translational medicine) from 2004 to 2006 while on sabbatical leave from his professorship at the University of Heidelberg. After return to this position in January 2007, he received lecturing and consulting fees from Sanofi-Aventis, Novartis, Takeda, Roche, Pfizer, Bristol-Myers, Daichii-Sankyo, Lilly, and Novo-Nordisk.

List of Contributors

Martin Wehling Medical Faculty Mannheim, University of Heidelberg, Mannheim, Germany

Heinrich Burkhardt IV. Medical Clinic, Geriatrics, University Clinics Mannheim, Mannheim, Germany

Donna M. Fick School of Nursing, Pennsylvania State University, University Park, PA, USA

Lutz Frölich Central Institute for Mental Health J 5, Mannheim, Germany

Joseph T. Hanlon University of Pittsburgh, Division of Geriatric Medicine, Pittsburgh, PA, USA

Stuart M. Lichtman 65+ Clinical Geriatric Program, Memorial Sloan-Kettering Cancer Center, Commack, NY, USA

Zachary A. Marcum University of Pittsburgh, Division of Geriatric Medicine, Pittsburgh, PA

Robert Lee Page 2nd School of Pharmacy, University of Colorado, Aurora, CO, USA

John Mark Ruscin Department of Internal Medicine, SIU School of Medicine, Springfield, IL, USA

Stefan Schwarz Central Institute for Mental Health J 5, Mannheim, Germany

Ulrich Wedding Division of Palliative Care, University Clinics Jena, Clinic for Internal Medicine II, Jena, Germany

General Aspects

Heterogeneity and Vulnerability of Older Patients

Heinrich Burkhardt

Pharmacotherapy Between Individualization and Standardization

Modern pharmacotherapy has to meet high-quality standards for the optimized treatment of every patient. On the one hand, standardization is indispensable for the determination of stable dosages and effect prediction and hereby is one of the major prerequisites for prescription safety and treatment efficacy. On the other hand, individualization of pharmacotherapy is mandatory because both patient-related and environmental factors lead to a wide variability of clinical phenotypes with critical relevance to drug treatment. Despite all standardization procedures and recommendations, pharmacotherapy is still characterized best as an individual experiment in daily practice; factors influencing the therapeutic response are never entirely known a priori, and the effect size cannot be securely calculated in advance. To minimize risks and maximize benefits, a careful estimation process for the risk-benefit ratio should take place at the beginning of every pharmacotherapeutic intervention. Today, information concerning the potential, and thus expected benefit, of a drug relies mainly on clinical studies in accordance with the principles of "evidence-based medicine" (EBM).

Randomized controlled trials (RCTs) represent the data source with the highest quality, and general validity is claimed for results derived from such studies. However, significant limitations of RCTs are often overlooked; RCTs are preferably performed in populations that are artificially homogeneous by virtue of narrow inclusion and wide exclusion criteria. They thus do not actually represent the entire population with a given disease but may even only be typical for a minority of patients within this population. This strict patient selection mainly reflects methodological considerations and limitations in that clear drug effects may become diluted by confounders such as concomitant diseases or relevant conditions (e.g., kidney impairment). As the selected study population does not represent all patients with the disease, results should not be automatically generalized to the treatment of all patients with a given disease. Serious concerns about the so-called external validity of trial data should be triggered when important subgroups are severely underrepresented, as is still true for most trials almost systematically excluding the elderly (Bugeja et al. 1997; Lee et al. 2001; Dodd et al. 2011; Witham and McMurdo 2007).

Evidence-derived recommendations on pharmacotherapy should never be rigorously applied without assessing a patient's individual clinical situation; a "cookbook-medicine"-type approach is strictly discouraged in the elderly. Modern pharmacotherapy has to be based on a comprehensive and differential process considering both standardized recommendations and individual arguments from the clinical situation to

H. Burkhardt (✉)
IVth Department of Medicine, Geriatrics, University Medical Centre Mannheim, Theodor-Kutzer-Ufer 1-3, Mannheim 68167, Germany
e-mail: heinrich.burkhardt@umm.de

M. Wehling (ed.), *Drug Therapy for the Elderly*,
DOI 10.1007/978-3-7091-0912-0_1, © Springer-Verlag Wien 2013

eventually deviate from recommendations or guidelines.

A differential pharmacotherapy in the elderly has to be based on clear and applicable arguments to realize a comprehensive individualization of the therapeutic approach.

In this context, the chronological age is certainly an insufficient argument, although still widely used. Rather than using the chronological age, clinical parameters like multimorbidity or frailty have been proposed to better describe the relevant biological vulnerability; these parameters meet the following demands:

– Sufficiently operationalized and applicable in the clinical setting
– Suitable to identify more vulnerable subgroups who are theoretically more likely to show a deviant risk-benefit ratio

Hereby, a reproducible input on comprehensive decision processes may be documented and discussed, thereby improving the transparency of individualized treatment decisions.

However, it should be discussed beforehand whether all elderly patients should be regarded as a special population in total for which particular issues and routines should be developed and applied, whether this is reasonable only for certain subgroups among the elderly, or finally, whether both options apply to this population. To answer this, the following points need to be addressed:

– How significant is the heterogeneity in the elderly in this context?
– How is this heterogeneity described?
– Which clinical consequences result from this heterogeneity?

Important Aspects of Differential Pharmacotherapy in the Elderly

From a clinical point of view, there is no doubt that elderly form a heterogeneous group compared with the relatively homogeneous groups of younger adults or adolescents. The heterogeneity of the elderly reflects both life-related and physiological aspects. Obviously, this not only results from genetic factors but also is mainly caused by accumulated risks and incidents during a long personal history. These influences reduce the physiological and psychological resources in a wide range of individual variation, so that some elderly stay fit or resilient and others become frail or vulnerable. Therefore, the remaining personal resources are central players in a concept to describe the age-related heterogeneity. Two major aspects are often stated to be important in this context that may describe this heterogeneity range in a practical way: multimorbidity and functionality. However, conceptual shortcomings still exist for both aspects (see the following discussion). Moreover, the features of heterogeneity are not static, and dynamic developments, including both improvement (recovering or compensation) and worsening (acceleration of impairment), may complicate the picture (Bengtson and Schaie 1999).

In this theoretical framework, two different approaches toward a differential pharmacotherapy in the elderly may be described. The first approach ("pharmacological approach") emphasizes age-related alterations of pharmacological aspects like pharmacokinetics and pharmacodynamics. The second approach is more clinically or geriatric oriented ("geriatric approach") and reflects changes in the risk-benefit ratio caused by impaired resources and increased and special geriatric risks and barriers. Both approaches may help to identify more vulnerable elderly patients for whom evidence for a defined pharmacotherapeutic approach may not simply be extrapolated from evidence obtained in younger adults.

Age-associated changes in pharmacokinetics and pharmacodynamics are generally outlined in chapter "Age-Associated General Pharmacological Aspects" and discussed for disease-related medication schemes in greater detail in part "Special Aspects with Respect to Organ Systems Based on Geriatric Clinical Importance." It has to be kept in mind that most of these changes are described as median changes for the entire elderly population, and a given patient may widely deviate from these medians. Therefore, the pattern of age-related changes and their significance for pharmacotherapy

Fig. 1 Framework of interacting contributors determining efficacy and safety of pharmacotherapy in the elderly. *ADR* adverse drug reaction

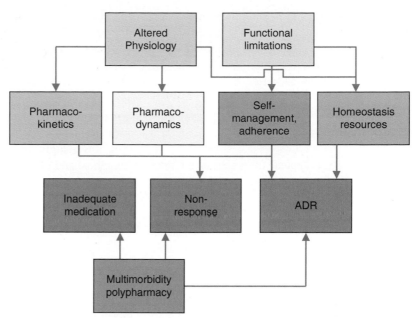

have to be examined and evaluated in every individual patient. Only by this can the individual risks and benefits of drug therapy be assessed. Nevertheless, median changes or risks found at a high prevalence in the elderly may support generalization and may render certain drugs as being critical or even inappropriate for the elderly. Such evaluations are the basis for labeling defined drugs according to the FORTA (Fit for the Aged) criteria (see chapter "Critical Extrapolation of Guidelines and Study Results: Risk-Benefit Assessment for Patients with Reduced Life Expectancy and a New Classification of Drugs According to Their Fitness for the Aged").

Age-related alterations are highly interactive and form a complex framework of interdependencies that determines the success of pharmacotherapy in the end (Fig. 1). Adverse drug reactions (ADRs), for example, may be determined by both changes in the patient's resources and changes in pharmacokinetics. Changes in an organ system (e.g., skeletal muscles) may influence both the patient's resources (locomotion, postural stability) and pharmacokinetic aspects (misinterpretation of creatinine values in the "normal" range).

The individual evaluation of the risk-benefit ratio prior to prescription not only allows for choosing and dosing a drug properly, but also critically defines subgroups of elderly at special risk or increased vulnerability. The most important factors involved in this regard are the following:

- Occurrence of age-specific ADRs (falls and delirium)
- Multimorbidity and polypharmacy
- Frailty
- Functional limitations
- Reduced life expectancy.

Adverse Drug Reactions

In general, the elderly are more likely to experience ADRs than younger adults and represent a particularly vulnerable population in this respect (Calis and Young 2001). Among the large number of ADRs are those that frequently occur in the elderly and are clinically much more serious than in younger adults. These are mainly falls and the confusional state. Both are discussed in more detail in chapters "Fall Risk and

Pharmacotherapy" and "Central Nervous System (CNS) Medications and Delirium." An increased risk for these particular ADRs associated with a particular drug may qualify this compound as inappropriate for the elderly.

Multimorbidity

Multimorbidity is typical for a significant share of the elderly population and as such is often seen as a marker of an increased ADR vulnerability as it is closely associated with polypharmacy. Polypharmacy is a frequent and critical issue in the elderly and represents a major challenge for optimized pharmacotherapy in the chronically ill elderly patient (see chapter "Polypharmacy" for more detail). There is no exact consented criterion for polypharmacy, although it is frequently defined by the simultaneous application of five and more drugs.

The simultaneous long-term prescription of five and more drugs is considered critical and often termed *polypharmacy* (McElnay and McCallion 1998).

In polypharmacy situations, possible drug interactions may no longer be calculable as they exponentially increase with medication numbers, as does the risk of ADRs. Unintended and ill-indicated prescribing cascades may be established to cope with avoidable ADRs, resulting in unfavorable risk-benefit ratios.

The definition of multimorbidity does not include age-associated changes in physiology and organ function (e.g., renal impairment), which also need to be considered for tailored, individualized drug therapies. It should be mentioned that multimorbidity may not always result in impaired functionality, although the term would suggest severe functional impairments as well. Furthermore, different patterns of multimorbidity (variation of concomitant diseases) may be the key for an understanding of treatment strategies and the therapeutic burden. In conclusion, multimorbidity varies substantially and is not well described and assessed just by the counting of diagnoses.

Frailty

The frailty syndrome has been defined as the age-associated decline of functionality in close relation to the aging phenotype and to the dynamics of aging processes that alter physiological responses (Fried et al. 2001). The phenotype of aging clearly associates with vulnerability and integrates significant physiologic aspects. The latter provide a theoretical and clinical basis of frailty. The main features of this syndrome are
- Reduced muscle mass
- Neurological or cognitive deficits
- Changes in energy metabolism (malnutrition)

The frailty syndrome is described in detail in chapter "Pharmacotherapy and the Frailty Syndrome" and is also discussed in the context of pharmacotherapy. Furthermore, frailty is a major aspect for the evaluation according to the FORTA criteria in part "Special Aspects with Respect to Organ Systems Based on Geriatric Clinical Importance." Recent developments clearly point to an increased future significance of the frailty syndrome and the frailty concept for the identification of the vulnerable elderly.

Functionality and the Concept of Activities of Daily Living

From a geriatric point of view, functionality and everyday competence are key issues for the stratification of the heterogeneous elderly population regarding the expected vulnerability. Functionality may allow for the direct description of barriers and impairment. The evaluation and quantification of basic and instrumental functionality follows the framework of daily activities (activities of daily living [ADLs] and instrumental activities of daily living [IADLs]; Table 1). These activities are translated into sum scores; one of the most prominent scores is the Barthel Index (Mahoney and Barthel 1965), which has been widely used over long periods of time. When handling such scores, their limitations and shortcomings have to be kept in mind. First, special barriers and impairments may not be well described as scores in

Table 1 The ADL/IADL framework of activities of daily living

ADLs (activities of daily living)	IADL (instrumental activities of daily living)
Feeding	Use of telephone
Grooming	Shopping
Bathing	Food preparation
Dressing	Housekeeping activities
Use of toilet	Ability to handle laundry
Fecal continence	Mode of transportation
Urinary continence	Self-management of medication
Transfer from bed to chair	Ability to handle finances
Walking	
Climbing stairs	

general are simplifying integrations of various domains and abilities.Second, scaling problems like ceiling and bottom effects may exist, and physicians and other users may not be aware of those limitations. For example, management of medication is an item of the IADL score, but a low score in this test does not necessarily indicate an impaired self-management of medication. Thus, it is still controversial how to identify vulnerable elderly best—by integral scores or the particular score items. The special items describing functional capabilities of importance for the self-management of pharmacotherapy are

– Reduced visual acuity
– Reduced dexterity
– Reduced cognition

For these functions, good predictability of future problems in the self-management of medication could be shown (Nikolaus et al. 1996). A simple and easily applicable method checking all three items simultaneously is the "timed test of money counting" (Nikolaus et al. 1995).

Reduced Life Expectancy

Another aspect important for the stratification with impact on differential pharmacotherapy is reduced life expectancy. Preventive pharmacotherapeutic strategies are clearly limited in their value if the horizon of the preventive effect is expected to exceed the remaining life expectancy. Some categories in which this may be regularly found are described by the following scenarios:

– Severe and advanced diseases (e.g., cardiac failure stage IV according to the New York Heart Association [NYHA])
– When palliative approaches are the leading therapeutic principles
– In the oldest old (80+ years; note that there is no generally accepted definition concerning this term, but 80 years and over is most frequently used)

Like all therapeutic strategies, pharmacotherapeutic schedules have to be reconsidered near the end of life as a true benefit for the patient may then be absent ("end-of-life debate"). Rather than automatically carrying on medication schedules, an early and repeated reassessment and discussion of the patient's individual wishes and needs should be sought. To guide this interactive process, criteria such as those proposed by Gillick may be helpful (1994).

Geriatric Syndromes

In many cases, the health status of the elderly is not sufficiently described if solely based on organ-oriented diagnoses as given in the *International Classification of Diseases* (*ICD*) manual. In addition, it is in the interest of the patient to consider and appropriately describe his or her functional status beforehand. This primarily functionality based assessment of the health status in the elderly frequently uncovers complex morbidity conditions not sufficiently described by organ-based diagnoses. These conditions are called *geriatric syndromes* and may represent both a significant contribution to the morbidity burden and of paramount importance for the treatment and intervention modalities in the elderly. Typically, these syndromes are caused by multiple factors and require a multidimensional therapeutic approach. However, even among geriatricians there is no clear consent about the systematics of geriatric syndromes; therefore, it is not surprising that these syndromes are not well represented in the *ICD* manual. According to Horan (1998), the geriatric syndromes that are most important and with the most consented are

- Immobility
- Falls
- Incontinence
- Cognitive decline and delirium.

These four are the classical geriatric syndromes, also termed the "geriatric giants." However, other, more symptom-oriented health problems are debated as well in this context (Inouye et al. 2007); some authors add the following syndromes to the list of geriatric syndromes:

- Iatrogenic health-related problems (e.g., ADRs)
- Depression
- Malnutrition
- Fluid and electrolyte imbalance.

The last four items are not discussed in this chapter in greater detail. ADRs are discussed for the major diseases in part "Special Aspects with Respect to Organ Systems Based on Geriatric Clinical Importance," and depression is discussed in chapter "Depression." Malnutrition and fluid-electrolyte imbalances are mentioned here to complete the list, but are not discussed in greater detail in this publication.

Focusing on the four accepted geriatric syndromes, part "Pharmacotherapy and Geriatric Syndromes" particularly considers their interrelation with pharmacotherapy. Three questions guide this discussion:

1. How does a pharmacotherapeutic strategy have an impact on the occurrence of a geriatric syndrome?
2. Are there pharmacotherapeutic approaches to treat a geriatric syndrome?

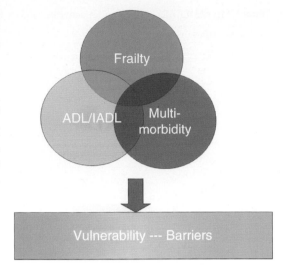

Fig. 2 Vulnerability as identified by different geriatric concepts. *ADL* activities of daily living, *IADL* instrumental activities of daily living

3. Does a geriatric syndrome contribute to the prediction of the success of pharmacotherapy in that it supports the identification of vulnerable patients?

In general, the therapeutic approach to geriatric syndromes may integrate pharmacotherapy as part of a multimodal strategy also comprising nonpharmacotherapeutic measures such as physiotherapy, occupational therapy, neuropsychological treatment, education, and others.

Evaluation of Different Approaches to Describe Heterogeneity and Vulnerability in the Elderly

The concepts mentioned allow an identification and description of the more vulnerable elderly at special risk. They also determine a differential pharmacotherapeutic approach reflecting essential patient-related aspects. These aspects are

- General vulnerability (frailty, impaired ADLs, geriatric syndromes) (Fig. 2)
- Barriers impeding successful self-management (special functional limitations)

Table 2 summarizes these aspects and comments on strengths and weaknesses.

Table 2 Arguments determining and modifying a differential pharmacotherapeutic schedule in the elderly

Argument	Primary aim	Strength	Weakness	Comment
Multimorbidity	Cumulative burden of morbidity	Allows an estimation of adequacy of polypharmacy; may suggest problems with adherence	Does not directly indicate vulnerability	Well operationalized but does not indicate real morbidity (functionality not included)
ADR	Special risk, such as delirium, falls	Describes a significant clinical problem	Does not indicate general vulnerability	Useful for special considerations concerning drug safety
Frailty	General and age-associated vulnerability	Pathophysiological links; describes phenotype of aging	Not yet optimized concerning measurement and assessment	Standardized criteria for diagnosis and assessment missing
ADL/IADL score	Global functionality	Indicates and describes need for help in daily living	Special barriers are not described; indicates general vulnerability only indirectly	Widely accepted and well standardized, but pure measure of functionality in daily living
Special functionality	Indicates special barriers with regard to pharmacotherapy	May describe individual problems along with self-management	Does not indicate general vulnerability; assessment tools not standardized	May help to identify self-management barriers prior to complex therapeutic strategies
Geriatric syndrome	Identifies complex clinical problems	Identifies typical and frequent geriatric issues	Describes neither general vulnerability nor special barriers; some entities not clearly defined	May identify subpopulation at risk, but not useful as general vulnerability index

ADR adverse drug reaction, *ADL* activity of daily living, *IADL* instrumental activity of daily living.

References

Bengtson VL, Schaie KW (eds) (1999) Handbook of theories of aging. Springer, Berlin

Bugeja G, Kumar A, Banerjee AK (1997) Exclusion of elderly people from clinical research: a descriptive study of published reports. BMJ 315:1059

Calis KA, Young LR (2001) Clinical analysis of adverse drug reactions. In: Atkinson AJ, Daniels CE, Dedrick RL, Grudzinskas CV, Markey SP (eds) Principles of clinical pharmacology. Academic, San Diego, pp 319–332

Dodd KS, Saczynski JS, Zhao Y, Goldberg RJ, Gurwitz JH (2011) Exclusion of older adults and women from recent trials of acute coronary syndromes. J Am Geriatr Soc 59:506–511

Fried LP, Tangen CM, Walston J, Cardiovascular Health Study Collaborative Research Group et al (2001) Frailty in older adults: evidence for a phenotype. J Gerontol A Biol Sci Med Sci 56:M146–M156

Gillick M (1994) Choosing medical care in old age: what kind, how much, when to stop. Harvard University Press, Cambridge

Horan MA (1998) Presentation of disease in old age. In: Tallis R, Fillit H, Brocklehurst JC (eds) Brockle- hurst's textbook of geriatric medicine and gerontol- ogy. Livingstone, Edinburgh, pp 201–206

Inouye SK, Studenski S, Tinetti ME, Kuchel GA (2007) Geriatric syndromes: clinical, research, and policy implications of a core geriatric concept. J Am Geriatr Soc 55:780–791

Lee PY, Alexander KP, Hammill BG, Pasquali SK, Peter- son ED (2001) Representation of elderly persons and women in published randomized trials of acute coro- nary syndromes. JAMA 286:708–713

Mahoney FI, Barthel DW (1965) Functional evaluation. The Barthel index. Maryland State Med J 14:61–65

McElnay JC, McCallion CR (1998) Adherence and the elderly. In: Myers LB, Midence K (eds) Adherence to treatment in medical conditions. Harwood Academic, Amsterdam, pp 223–253

Nikolaus T, Bach M, Specht-Leible N, Oster P, Schlierf G (1995) The timed test of money counting: a short physical performance test for manual dexterity and cognitive capacity. Age Aging 24:257–258

Nikolaus T, Kruse W, Bach M, Specht-Leible N, Oster P, Schlierf G (1996) Elderly patients' problems with medication. An inhospital and follow-up study. Eur J Clin Pharmacol 49:255–259

Witham MD, McMurdo ME (2007) How to get older people included in clinical studies. Drugs Aging 24:187–196

Epidemiologic Aspects

Heinrich Burkhardt

Definition of the Elderly

A common definition (World Health Organization 2011) describes elderly individuals as persons aged 65 and over. A previous definition given by the WHO even defined persons only 60 or more years old as elderly, but this cutoff is not generally accepted. In this context, it is necessary to discuss the definition of age. The definition of an calendarian cutoff for defined age groups merely depends on social consensus and not primarily on physiological changes that may occur even years before. Age-associated physiological changes in the endocrine system or in lens elasticity may start much earlier even in healthy subjects: between age 40 and age 45 for the endocrine system and during puberty for lens elasticity. A reliable and valid threshold value for significant changes in physiology cannot be calculated and applied due to a great variety of interindividual aging patterns and courses.

Within the large group of elderly individuals, persons at age 80 years and older may form a special subgroup presenting with increased prevalence rates of typical geriatric problems; for that reason, they may be defined as belonging to a separate age group—some call them the fourth

H. Burkhardt (✉)
IVth Department of Medicine, Geriatrics, University Medical Centre Mannheim, Theodor-Kutzer-Ufer 1-3, 68167 Mannheim, Germany
e-mail: heinrich.burkhardt@umm.de

age. Octogenarians (more so even older people) show a significant decline in key functionalities such as locomotion, continence, and cognition; therefore, functionality and impairment are a major topic when considering health-related aspects of high age.

Methodological Aspects

Epidemiologic data comprise a variety of data sources. Global trends mainly rely on national census data and international data platforms such as U.N. organizations or the WHO. For many countries, such data provide reliable information on the age distribution of the population, life expectancies, and regional and global trends for defined age groups.

Functionality and impairment data or descriptions of special barriers are often not sufficiently represented in census data; health insurance organizations or population-based large scale cohort studies may provide more sophisticated data sets. Remarkable regional differences due to the heterogeneity of health care systems and epidemiologic approaches need to be considered. Therefore, an international comparison of prevalence data has to utilize global surveys such as those by the WHO. The WHO provides data retrieved by the World Health Survey, which include entries on the prevalence of functional limitations among the elderly population in different countries. Unfortunately, not all countries are participating in this survey for a variety of reasons,

M. Wehling (ed.), *Drug Therapy for the Elderly*,
DOI 10.1007/978-3-7091-0912-0_2, © Springer-Verlag Wien 2013

and not all standardized questions are suitable for all regions, rendering a global comparison difficult to impossible. There is no global consensus how to measure functionality best, and frameworks developed in the United States and European countries will not fit situations in developing countries despite their wide acceptance in the scientific literature. This may also explain the paucity of regional data published from countries outside Europe and the United States.

Identifying data on general prescription rates of drugs in the elderly is even more challenging. In most countries, systematic drug surveys are lacking, and prescription rates can only be estimated from general consumption rates or total redeemed prescriptions, but the information is usually not stratified for defined age groups or individual diseases. Therefore, data on polypharmacy are often lacking or ambiguous. In some countries, national health surveys comprise medication data; however, these data are not published in an appropriate way to allow for calculation of prescription rates in the entire elderly population and are mostly restricted to subpopulations with defined diseases or health problems. For that reason, a global comparison of polypharmacy prevalence and prescription rates is even more challenging. Obviously, in developing countries access to pharmacotherapy is restricted due to financial and infrastructural limitations and a global and transcultural comparison of drug prescription patterns cannot be made with certainty. Finally, local and regional drug availability may be variable due to differences in licensing and adds to the complexity of drug analysis. Coding and grouping different drugs may also widely vary across different regions even if countries may be comparable for demographic, political, and sociocultural aspects.

In the European context, the Berlin Aging Study (BASE) appears as the most thorough population-based analysis concerning drug prescription in the elderly (Baltes and Mayer 2001). The BASE investigators not only performed a detailed analysis of prescription rates but also analyzed over-the-counter (OTC) drugs and evaluated appropriateness of individual prescriptions by reevaluating the individual disease patterns. Moreover, symptoms possibly associated with adverse drug reactions (ADR) were analyzed for each subject.

General Aspects

In Western countries and some developing countries (e.g., Brazil), the proportion of elderly in the population steadily increased over the past decades and the age group of people 80 years and older may even represent the most rapidly expanding subpopulation (e.g., Germany). Simultaneously, life expectancy of younger and middle-aged people is also increasing. Table 1 summarizes recent data from U.N. calculations and estimations. Although the current life expectancy at birth still differs markedly between the United States and a typical European country on the one hand and Brazil and India on the other, it is noteworthy that life expectancy of 65- or 80-year-old persons becomes similar for these countries.

As mentioned, a global perspective concerning drug prescription rates is rather complex and arbitrary. In Europe, prescription analysis consistently showed that most drugs are clearly prescribed to the elderly. In Germany, for example, a thorough analysis utilizing health insurance data found 64% of all drugs were prescribed to patients 60 years and older (Schwabe and Paffrath 2008). Also, individual prescription rates are increasing with advanced age and do not plateau up to age 80 and over. Table 2 summarizes prescription rates for different countries, with information retrieved from population-based studies. These studies are missing for India, and hospital-based data had to be given instead for comparison. Table 3 provides data on functionality, multimorbidity, and polypharmacy. Polypharmacy and multimorbidity prevalences are found to range from 12% to 25% of the elderly.

Functionality, Frailty, and Multimorbidity

Functionality is a significant constituent of well-being and an essential prerequisite for activities

Table 1 General demographic data

	United States	Brazil	India	Germany
Persons 65 and over (percentage of all, estimation 2010)[a] *expected 2020 data*	40.5 Mio	13.7 Mio	60.3 Mio	16.8 Mio
	(13.0%)	(7.0%)	(4.9%)	(20.4%)
	54.7 Mio	*20.3 Mio*	*87.5 Mio*	*18.6 Mio*
	(16.2%)	*(9.5%)*	*(6.2%)*	*(23.3%)*
Persons 80 and over (percentage of all, estimation 2010)[a] *expected 2020 data*	11.8 Mio	2.9 Mio	8.2 Mio	4.2 Mio
	(3.8%)	(1.5%)	(0.7%)	(5.1%)
	13.0 Mio	*4.4 Mio*	*12.6 Mio*	*6.0 Mio*
	(3.9%)	*(2.1%)*	*(0.9%)*	*(7.5%)*
Current life expectancy at birth[b]	Women: 81 1 years	Women: 82,1 years	Women: 64,2 years	Women: 18 years
	Men: 76.2 years	Men: 70,7 years	Men: 64.4 years	Men: 78.2 years
Current remaining life expectancy of 65-year-olds[b]	Women: 20 years	Women: 18 years	Women: 15 years	Women: 20 years
	Men: 16 years	Men: 16 years	Men: 14 years	Men: 16 years
Current remaining life expectancy of 80-year-olds[b]	Women: 10 years	Women: 10 years	Women: 7 years	Women: 9 years
	Men: 8 years	Men: 9 years	Men: 7 years	Men: 7 years

Mio: million

[a]Current data retrieved from the U.N. population estimation database for the year 2010, and the expected data for 2020 under constant fertility scenario given in *italics* (UNPD World Population Prospects 2006)

[b]Current estimation of the United Nations (UNPD World Population Prospects 2006; 2010–2015 constant fertility scenario for life expectancy at birth, 2000–2005 for life expectancy at given age); data from United Nations (2011)

and participation of the individual. The WHO acknowledges this in its framework of health and disease; functionality is addressed in a separate diagnostic manual that tries to assess this complex issue, the ICF (International Classification of Functioning, Disability and Health; WHO 2001). However, this framework is rather complicated; in daily practice and geriatrics, functionality as defined by self-competence in ADLs (activities of daily living) is assessed according to the ADL/IADL (instrumental activities of daily living) framework. Although rather simple, this framework is still not globally implemented in health surveys. Therefore, population-based data given in Table 3 concern several items and countries. As a common problem with the description and evaluation of complex concepts like functionality, data aggregation into a general index may mask individual and yet significant differences (Gupta 2008). Nevertheless, the general ADL index is widely applied to describe the level of general functionality in the elderly

(Stone et al. 1994; Sato et al. 2002). This index has limitations regarding the decision of whether self-management of pharmacotherapy still is feasible. For example, an individual with an ADL index of 70 of 100 points may still be able to manage medications properly as functional limitations are restricted to locomotion, but another patient with the same score may not be capable if the ADL limitation is mainly based on forgetfulness and low visual acuity.

Vulnerability of older persons is described not only by functional limitations or multimorbidity but also by the presence of the frailty syndrome as described in chapter "Pharmacotherapy and the Frailty Syndrome" in more detail. As the definition of the frailty syndrome by Fried's criteria (Fried et al. 2001) was published only in the early 2000s, the different aspects of this syndrome, like hand-grip strength or walking speed, are usually not assessed in population-based surveys dating further back, especially not outside Western countries. Nevertheless, to give some

Table 2 Drug prescription in elderly

Drugs	United States (%)	Brazil (%)	India (%)[a]	Germany (%)
Antihypertensives		8.9[b]		11.3[c]
Digoxin	9[d]			31.0[c]
β-blockers	7[d]	3.8[b]		5.5[c]
ACE inhibitors	7[d]	12.6[e]	25.2[f]	5.3[c]
Ca antagonists	8[d]	7.3[e]	28.3[f]	22.8[c]
Oral antidiabetics	3[d]	6.2[e]		11.4[c]
Analgesics	16[d, g]	3.6[b]		
NSAIDs	10[d]	4.3[b]		33.8[c]
Diuretics	20[d]	6.4–14.7[b, e]	28.3[f]	30.4[c]
Antipsychotics		3.9[e]		4.4[c]
Antidepressants	1[d]			3.3[c]
Corticosteroids				
Lipid-lowering drugs	15[d]	2.4[e]	26.9[f]	7.5[c]
Anticoagulants	8[d]			
Benzodiazepines	2%[d]			12.4[c, h]

NSAIDs nonsteroidal anti-inflammatory drugs

[a]No population-based survey in India concerning this topic; hospital data are given instead

[b]Population-based survey in an urban region in Brazil (Filhoa et al. 2004)

[c]Data from Berlin Aging Study (BASE), a population-based survey done between 1990 and 1993 among people 70 years and older people in an urban setting (Baltes and Mayer 2001)

[d]Population-based survey in the United States including over-the-counter drugs in elderly persons 65 years and older (Kaufman et al. 2002)

[e]Population-based survey in a defined region in Brazil among individuals 60 years and older (de Loyola Filho et al. 2006)

[f]A multicenter hospital survey in India done in 2008 and 2009 (Harugeri et al. 2010)

[g]In this survey, acetaminophen

[h]Labeled in the survey as hypnotics

impressions about the prevalence in the older population data from a population-based longitudinal study in the United States, the Cardiovascular Health Study may be cited. In this study, over 5,000 subjects older than 65 years were included. Based on body impedance analysis, prevalence data for the presence of sarcopenia could be retrieved (Janssen et al. 2004). These data revealed that 70.7% of men and 41.9% of women disclosed moderate sarcopenia, which was even severe in 17.2 % of men and 10.7% of women. In another population-based cohort (the New Mexico Elder Health Survey), the DXA (dual energy x-ray absorptiometry) method was applied to detect sarcopenia. Although the methodology differed from that used in the former cohort, prevalence rates for sarcopenia increased with advanced age from 13% to 24% in subjects aged below 70 to over 50% in octogenarians and older (Baumgartner et al. 1998). Applying the Fried criteria, the prevalence of the frailty syndrome was found between 15.5% and 31.3% in persons aged 85 years and over in the Cardiovascular Health

Study cohort. Some subgroups of elderly may disclose even higher prevalence rates. Purser et al. (2006) published 27% prevalence rates for frailty in a group of inpatients 70 years and older with coronary heart disease if assessed by Fried's criteria and exceeding 60% when the presence of any ADL impairment was taken as a criterion.

In Lawton and Brody's score of significant IADLs, "medication management" is listed among a total of eight items (Lawton and Brody 1969). This activity may be subdivided further:

– Recognizing the medication
– Correct dosing
– Managing the handling of the medication package with respect to dosing aid

Several studies clearly disclosed that elderly patients frequently fail to manage the handling of medication packages and correct dosing correctly (Atkin et al. 1994).

In another study by Nikolaus et al. (1996), 143 elderly patients without signs of cognitive decline were thoroughly analyzed concerning their ability to manage standard medication

Table 3 Functionality, multimorbidity, and polypharmacy in the elderly

Functional domain	United States (%)	Brazil (%)	India (%)	Germany (%)
Locomotion				
Unable to use public transportation				31.2[a]
Unable to take a walk	20.3–30.9[b]	6.2[c]	5.6–8.4[d]	10.6[a]
Unable to climb stairs	7.0–5.7[b]			11.4[a]
Unable to perform bed-chair transfer			1.3–1.7[d]	2.7[a]
Uses walking aid	10.9–12.9[b]			20.9[a]
Bound to wheelchair				3.1[a]
Postural stability impaired	18.7–66.0[e]			44.2[a]
Difficulty moving around[f]		44.7–63.6[g]	71.9–84.6[g]	52.3–75.0[g]
Self-care				
Unable to take shower/bath		2.0[c]		16.0[a]
Unable to go shopping[h]				33.7[a]
Difficulty in household activities[f]		54.6–63.8[g]	78.3–85.1[g]	
Needs help in clothing[h]	8.2–7.5[b]			5.9[a]
Needs help in grooming[h]	5.9–7.2[b]			1.3[a]
Difficulty in self-care[f]		16.2–39.5[g]	56.0–76.5[g]	18.8–45.8[g]
Needs help to use the toilet[h]				3.2[a]
Needs help in eating[h]	4.3–5.2[b]	4.5[c]		0.9[a]
Sensorium				
Uses visual aid				95.6[a]
Visual impairment	8.8–19.2[i]		25.3–27.5[j]	26.6[a]
Difficulty with seeing[f]		34.0–59.7[g]	66.6–61.4[g]	25.5–37.5[g]
Uses hearing aid				15.5[a]
Hearing impaired			15.4–19.5[j]	18.6[a]
Cognition				
Impaired cognition	2.7–27.4[k]	14.9[l]	9.8–11.0[j]	14.0[a]
Difficulty with remembering[f]		58.7–86.0[g]	70.2–80.3[g]	29.3–56.2[g]
Polypharmacy/multimorbidity				
Unable to manage medication[h]				2.6–14.8[m]
Five or more diagnoses			5.9[j,n]	28.0[a]
Five or more drugs prescribed	12.0–16.0[o]	25.2[p,q]		37.5[a]

[a]Data from Berlin Aging Study (BASE), a population based survey done between 1990 and 1993 among people 70 years or older in an urban setting (Baltes and Mayer 2001)

[b]Data from National Health and Nutrition Examination Survey (NHANES) III, a population-based survey in the United States, 1988–1994; data given as men-women (Ostchega et al. 2000)

[c]Data from population-based survey in Brazil. Pesquisa Nacional por Amostra de Domicílios (PNAD) 1998 (Lima-Costa et al. 2003)

[d]Population survey in India, NSS 60th Round Unit level data 2004; data differ between urban and rural regions (Prasad 2011)

[e]Same source as note b; data stratified to age and gender (Ostchega et al. 2000)

[f]Item used to qualify functionality in the World Health Survey (WHO 2011)

[g]Data from the World Health Survey 2003; data given for 60- to 80-year-old participants

[h]Item listed in activities of daily living/instrumental activities of daily living (ADLs/IADLs) framework

[i]Data from NHANES, a population-based survey in the United States, 1999–2002 (Vitale et al. 2006)

[j]Population survey in India NSS data 1995–1996; data differ to ethnic groups (Rajan 2007)

[k]Data from NHANES III, a population-based survey in the United States, 1988–1994; data stratified according to different age groups, 60–85 years (Zhang et al. 2001)

[l]Same source as note p (Tamanini et al. 2011)

[m]Population-based survey. Möglichkeiten und Grenzen einer selbstständigen Lebensführung hilfe- und pflegebedürftiger Menschen in Privathaushalten (MUG) 1990 (Wahl and Wetzler 1998)

[n]Three or more chronic conditions

[o]Same source as note b; data stratified to age 65–74 years and 75 years and over (Centers for Disease Control and Prevention 2011)

[p]Data from a population-based survey in Sao Paulo. Saúde, Bem-estar e Envelhecimento (SABE) among people 60 years or older (Secoli et al. 2010)

[q]In this cohort, six and more drugs

packages. Of these, 10.1% were unable to open a standard blister package, 44.5% were unable to open a flip top, and 16.8% were unable to open a standard medication container (dosette) as a frequently used predosing aid. These are surprisingly high rates, underlining that medication packages and dosing aids are far from easily manageable by the elderly; this may significantly contribute to dosing errors and treatment failures. To handle such a complex task, unimpaired functionality in at least three domains is required:

- Cognition
- Visual acuity
- Manual dexterity

To test for these three domains simultaneously, Nikolaus et al. (1996) recommended the timed test of money counting, which requires the patient to count a given set of coins and bank notes contained in a closed purse.

The prevalence of cognitive impairment is strongly increasing with advanced age beyond age 75. Table 3 compiles related data from different surveys. In addition, in the Cardiovascular Health Study the prevalence rate was 16% in women and 14% in men aged 75 years or older. Visual acuity may be impaired in the elderly due to a large number of diseases. The most significant ones are cataract, glaucoma, and maculopathy. In a population-based U.K. study, Van der Pols et al. (2000) found prevalence rates for impaired visual acuity up to 46–49%, with the highest rates seen among nursing home residents. However, in a significant portion of these elderly, even simple measures to correct visual acuity (adequate glasses) are not fully applied (Winter et al. 2004). Manual dexterity is less well analyzed in the elderly, and precise prevalence data are lacking. However, an increasing clinical significance in the elderly may be assumed from experimental data (Ranganathan et al. 2001).

Adverse Drug Reactions

Identification and analysis of ADRs utilize data from variable sources, thus creating a rather heterogeneous database. This covers anecdotal reports, monitoring studies, and cohort and case-control studies. These data are brought together by meta-analyses to recalculate real incidence rates, but this may be flawed by inherent methodological problems. Low-rate, but nevertheless serious, ADRs are often underreported in studies, and the association of symptoms of health-related problems with drug prescription may remain unclear or missed. Even in randomized controlled studies (RCTs) that are well controlled, monitoring of adverse effects and reporting of these is still often incomplete (Ioannidis and Lau 2001). Moreover, cohort studies and RCTs frequently do not represent daily practice ("real world") due to low external validity and exclusion of significant patient groups (Rothwell 2005). Therefore, pharmacovigilance often reveals serious adverse effects years after market introduction of newly developed drugs, and the risk-benefit ratio may shift significantly. This underlines the value of pharmacovigilance systems. Another problem in this context relates to the correct coding and categorization of the large variety of drugs available. This is especially seen in centrally acting drugs (e.g., neuroleptics), an issue that further flaws detailed analysis and comparison of different data sources. For example, a clear distinction between classic tricyclic antidepressants and modern selective serotonin reuptake inhibitors (SSRIs) is a prerequisite for an adequate evaluation of a proposed differential risk-benefit ratio; unfortunately, this is impossible in the majority of cohorts as differentiation of these drugs is lacking in the data matrix.

These aspects clearly explain the comparably large variance in reported incidence rates of ADRs. For elderly patients, alarmingly high prevalence rates for overall ADRs have been published. In a longitudinal population-based cohort, Schneeweiss et al. (2002) found higher incidence rates of ADRs with increasing age. In patients older than 70 years, 20 events per 10,000 patients were observed, and a U.S. survey among ambulatory elderly patients revealed an overall ADR incidence rate of 50.1 events per 1,000 patient years (Gurwitz et al. 2003). Among the elderly, nursing home residents represent a subgroup that is particularly vulnerable to ADRs, and the incidence rates even largely exceeded those values mentioned (Monette et al. 1995). Besides incidence rates in hospital-based cohorts, prevalence rates of ADRs during a hospital stay also may be calculated. A recent study from the European GIFA (Gruppo Italiano di Farmacoepidemiologia nell'Anziano) group analyzed data retrieved from such a hospital-based cohort of elderly inpatients. The authors found a 6.5% prevalence rate for ADRs and analyzed predictors of ADRs to build up a risk-scoring tool (Onder et al. 2010). Significant predictors were

– Reduced glomerular filtration rate (<60 ml/min)
– Multimorbidity (four and more comorbid conditions)
– Liver disease
– Five or more drugs prescribed
– Previous ADR

Similar to studies analyzing incidence rates, prevalence rates in hospital-based cohorts also were found to increase with advanced age and reach up to 24% in patients 70 years and older (Manesse et al. 1997). A more recent meta-analysis on this topic, however, found the considerable variability mainly depended on different methodologic approaches, thus confirming the mentioned issues (Kongkaew et al. 2008). Finally, Pirmohamed et al. (2004) performed a detailed analysis of hospital admissions associated with ADRs and found a considerable fraction to be preventable. This points to an unmet need in medical care and discloses a significant quality gap of drug prescribing and monitoring.

Drugs most frequently involved in ADRs are
– Cardiovascular agents
– Antibiotics
– Diuretics
– NSAIDs (nonsteroidal anti-inflammatory drugs)
– Anticoagulants
– Antidiabetics
Frequent symptoms caused by ADRs are
– Gastrointestinal symptoms (e.g., diarrhea, nausea, loss of appetite)
– Electrolyte imbalance
– Impaired renal function
– Bleeding

These lists apply to both younger adults and elderly alike. A few more symptoms have to be added to the list as these are of special significance in the elderly:
– Delirium
– Constipation
– Orthostatic hypotension
– Falls

These clinical problems show an increasing prevalence and incidence with advancing age, and it may be assumed that a considerable contribution to this gain may come from ADRs. Hence, a logical question in relation to these epidemiological results is whether these increasing incidence and prevalence rates are caused by age-related changes and increased vulnerability or just reflect polypharmacy and expanding drug prescriptions. To answer this, Field et al. (2004) performed a nested case-control analysis in a cohort of ambulatory elderly in the United States (New England). They found in 1,299 patients who experienced an ADR and 1,299 control subjects that indeed a significant association between ADR and comorbidity in relation to the number of prescribed drugs existed, but this was not so between ADR and age as such.

More frequent ADRs seen in the elderly not only are consequences of an increased vulnerability but are also significantly caused by polypharmacy and multimorbidity.

Table 3 compiles data on multimorbidity and polypharmacy in the elderly. The BASE investigators (see previous discussion) performed an extensive and individual analysis of prescribed drugs, thereby evaluating not only polypharmacy but also treatment errors due to unindicated drugs and both under- and overtreatment. They found unnecessary drugs prescribed to 13.7% of all persons and inappropriate drugs prescribed to 18.7% (Baltes and Mayer 2001). Among all inappropriate drugs, the most frequent ones were

– Reserpine
– Diazepam
– Amitriptyline
– Indomethacin

References

Atkin PA, Finnegan TP, Ogle SJ, Shenfield GM (1994) Functional ability of patients to manage medication packaging. A survey of geriatric inpatients. Age Ageing 23:113–116

Baltes PB, Mayer KU (eds) (2001) The Berlin aging study, aging from 70 to 100. Cambridge University Press, Cambridge

Baumgartner RN, Koehler KM, Gallagher D et al (1998) Epidemiology of sarcopenia among the elderly in New Mexico. Am J Epidemiol 147:755–763

Centers for Disease Control and Prevention (2011) National Health and Nutrition Examination Survey (NHANES) III. http://www.cdc.gov/nchs/data/nhanes/databriefs/preuse.pdf. Accessed 31 Oct 2011

de Loyola Filho AI, Uchoa E, Lima-Costa MF (2006) Estudo epidemiológico de base populacional sobre uso de medicamentos entre idosos na Região Metropolitana de Belo Horizonte, Minas Gerais, Brasil. Cad Saúde Pública Rio de Janeiro 22:2657–2667

de Winter LJM, Hoyng CB, Froeling PGAM, Meulendijks CFM, van der Wilt GJ (2004) Prevalence of remediable disability due to low vision among institutionalized elderly people. Gerontology 50:96–101

Field TS, Gurwitz JH, Harrold LR et al (2004) Risk factors for adverse drug events among older adults in the ambulatory setting. J Am Geriatr Soc 52:1349–1354

Filhoa JMC, Marcopitob LF, Castelob A (2004) Perfil de utilização de medicamentos por idosos em área urbana do Nordeste do Brasil. Rev Saude Publica 38:557–564

Fried LP, Tangen CM, Walston J, Cardiovascular Health Study Collaborative Research Group et al (2001) Frailty in older adults: evidence for a phenotype. J Gerontol A Biol Sci Med Sci 56:M146–M156

Gupta A (2008) Measurement scales used in elderly care. Radcliffe, Oxford

Gurwitz JH, Field TS, Harrold LR et al (2003) Incidence and preventability of adverse drug events among older persons in the ambulatory setting. JAMA 289:1107–1116

Harugeri A, Joseph J, Parthasarathi G, Ramesh M, Guido S (2010) Prescribing patterns and predictors of high-level polypharmacy in the elderly population: a prospective surveillance study from two teaching hospitals in India. Am J Geriatr Pharmacother 8:271–280

Ioannidis JP, Lau J (2001) Completeness of safety reporting in randomized trials: an evaluation of 7 medical areas. JAMA 285:437–443

Janssen I, Baumgartner RN, Ross R, Rosenberg IH, Roubenoff R (2004) Skeletal muscle cutpoints associated with elevated physical disability risk in older men and women. Am J Epidemiol 159:413–421

Kaufman DW, Kelly JP, Rosenberg L, Anderson TE, Mitchell AA (2002) Recent patterns of medication use in the ambulatory adult population of the United States: the Slone survey. JAMA 287:337–344

Kongkaew C, Noyce PR, Ashcroft DM (2008) Hospital admissions associated with adverse drug reactions: a systematic review of prospective observational studies. Ann Pharmacother 42:1017–1025

Lawton MP, Brody EM (1969) Assessment of older people: selfmaintaining and instrumental activities of daily living. Gerontologist 9:179–186

Lima-Costa MF, Barreto SM, Giatti L (2003) Condições de saúde, capacidade funcional, uso de serviços de saúde e gastos com medicamentos da população idosa brasileira: um estudo descritivo baseado na Pesquisa Nacional por Amostra de Domicílios. Cad Saúde Pública Rio de Janeiro 19:735–743

Manesse CK, Derkx FHM, de Ridder MAJ, Man in't Veld AJ, van der Cammen TJM (1997) Adverse drug reactions in elderly patients as contributing factor for hospital admission: cross sectional survey. BMJ 315:1057–1058

Monette J, Gurwitz JH, Avorn J (1995) Epidemiology of adverse drug events in the nursing home setting. Drugs Aging 7:203–211

Nikolaus T, Kruse W, Bach M, Specht-Leible N, Oster P, Schlierf G (1996) Elderly patients' problems with medication. An inhospital and follow-up study. Eur J Clin Pharmacol 49:255–259

Onder G, Petrovic M, Tangiisuran B et al (2010) Development and validation of a score to assess risk of adverse drug reactions among in-hospital patients 65 years or older: the GerontoNet ADR risk score. Arch Intern Med 170:1142–1148

Ostchega Y, Harris TB, Hirsch R, Parsons VL, Kington R (2000) The prevalence of functional limitations and disability in older persons in the US: data from the National Health and Nutrition Examination Survey III. J Am Geriatr Soc 48:1132–1135

Pirmohamed M, James S, Meakin S et al (2004) Adverse drug reactions as cause of admission to hospital: prospective analysis of 18.820 patients. BMJ 329:15–19

Prasad S (2011) Ailing and hospitalization in India—an analysis of NSS 52nd and 60th round. Vdm Verlag Dr. Müller Aktiengesellschaft, Saarbrücken

Purser JL, Kuchibhatla MN, Fillenbaum GG, Harding T, Peterson ED, Alexander KP (2006) Identifying frailty in hospitalized older adults with significant coronary artery disease. J Am Geriatr Soc 54:1674–1681

Rajan IS (2007) Population aging, health and social security in India. Center for Development Studies India. CREI, Osaka. http://www.econ.osaka-cu.ac.jp/CREI/discussion/2006/CREI_DP003.pdf. Accessed 15 Oct 2011

Ranganathan VK, Siemionow V, Sahgal V, Yue GH (2001) Effects of aging on hand function. J Am Geriatr Soc 49:1478–1484

Rothwell PM (2005) External validity of randomized controlled trials: to whom do the results of this trial apply? Lancet 365:82–93

Sato S, Demura S, Minami M, Kasuga K (2002) Longitudinal assessment of ADL ability of partially dependent elderly people: examining the utility of the index and characteristics of longitudinal change in ADL ability. J Physiol Anthropol Appl Human Sci 21:179–187

Schneeweiss S, Hasford J, Gottler M, Hoffmann A, Riethling AK, Avorn J (2002) Admissions by adverse drug events to internal medicine and emergency departments in hospitals: a longitudinal population-based study. Eur J Clin Pharmacol 58:285–291

Schwabe U, Paffrath D (eds) (2008) Arzneiverordnungs-report. Springer, Berlin

Secoli SR, Figueras A, Lebra ML, de Lima FD, Ferreira Santos JL (2010) Risk of potential drug-drug interactions among Brazilian elderly. Drugs Aging 27:759–770

Stone SP, Ali B, Auberleek I, Thompsell A, Young A (1994) The Barthel index in clinical practice: use on a rehabilitation ward for elderly people. J R Coll Physicians Lond 28:419–423

Tamanini JTN, Santos JLF, Lebrao ML, Duarte YAO, Laurenti R (2011) Association between urinary incontinence in elderly patients and caregiver burden in the city of Sao Paulo/Brazil: health, wellbeing, and ageing study. Neurourol Urodyn 30:1281–1285

United Nations, Department of Economic and Social Affairs, Population Division (2011) World population prospects: the 2010 revision, New York (comprehensive excel tables). http://data.un.org. Accessed 15 Oct 2011

Van der Pols JC, Bates CJ, Thompson JR, Reacher M, Prentice A, Finch S (2000) Visual acuity measurements in a national sample of British elderly people. Br J Ophthalmol 84:165–170

Vitale S, Cotch MF, Sperduto RD (2006) Prevalence of visual impairment in the United States. JAMA 295:2158–2163

Wahl HW, Wetzler R (1998) Moglichkeiten und Grenzen selbständiger Lebensführung in Privathaushalten. Integrierter Bericht zum gleichnamigen Forschungsverbundprojekt. Kohlhammer, Stuttgart

World Health Organization (2001) International classification of functioning, disability and health, Genf. http://www.who.int/classifications/icf/en/. Last accessed 25 Oct 2011

World Health Organization (2011) Definition of an older or elderly person. http://www.who.int/healthinfo/survey/ageingdefnolder/en/index.html. Accessed 13 Dec 2011

World Health Survey (2011) http://www.who.int/healthinfo/survey/en/. Accessed 15 Oct 2011

Zhang Y, Seshadri S, Ellison RC, Heeren T, Felson DT (2001) Bone mineral density and verbal memory impairment: third National Health and Nutrition Examination Survey. Am J Epidemiol 154:795–802

Age-Associated General Pharmacological Aspects

Martin Wehling

Pharmacokinetics

Pharmacokinetics describes the path of a drug in the body; its major constituents are

- *A*bsorption
- *D*istribution
- *M*etabolism and
- *E*limination (ADME rule)

The result of these subfunctions of pharmacokinetics is the course of the plasma (or cerebrospinal fluid [CSF]) concentration of a drug over time. Dose, dosage form, and administration route can be chosen; all other parameters are variably determined by the individual patient, and their impact is often difficult to predict. Utilizing the development of often-complex mathematical models, pharmacokinetics attempts to describe drug concentrations over time reproducibly with a high predictability.

Yet, a reliable prediction of adverse drug reactions (ADRs) cannot be achieved even by the molecular analysis of, for example, degrading enzymes as the variation of plasma drug concentrations is genetically determined only by 30–50%.

Therefore, despite all attempts to forecast outcomes (e.g., via genetic testing), any drug application remains an individual experiment that can only be successfully done on close observation (of the patient).

This means that despite the extensive knowledge of pharmacokinetics and pharmacogenetics, each drug application to humans represents an individual experiment that will only be meritorious if both wanted and unwanted effects are intensively searched for. This especially applies to elderly patients as they have altered functions of many organs, which are detailed here. The combination of drug concentration determinations and careful clinical observation will contribute to the increased safety of drug therapy. This includes history taking of typical side effects, such as muscle pain under statins or epigastric pain under nonsteroidal anti-inflammatory drugs (NSAIDs). However, this is an arduous and time-consuming task without a true alternative as many modern drugs (especially those with narrow therapeutic ranges) are like sharp knives: You need to learn how to use them, or they may cause more harm than good.

Special Aspects of Geriatric Pharmacokinetics

Physiological Alterations, with the Kidneys in Focus

Age-associated physiological alterations vary considerably between individuals. In addition, many chronic diseases are age dependent (such as Alzheimer's dementia, atherosclerotic disease in various vascular beds) and lead to an increasing

M. Wehling (✉)
University of Heidelberg, Maybachstr. 14, Mannheim 68169, Germany
e-mail: martin.wehling@medma.uni-heidelberg.de

M. Wehling (ed.), *Drug Therapy for the Elderly*,
DOI 10.1007/978-3-7091-0912-0_3, © Springer-Verlag Wien 2013

incidence of structural and functional deviations. These often directly contribute to incapacities and disabilities with direct impact on pharmacokinetics. Thus, it is often impossible to separate age-related alterations from those that depend on diseases with increasing incidence at higher age (such as diabetes mellitus type 2). As an example, there is a well-known decrease of glomerular function with age, reflecting a decreasing number of functional nephrons (Rowe et al. 1976). In the more detailed Baltimore Longitudinal Study, different patterns of time-dependent change of renal function were obvious (Lindeman 1993):

– Some patients had a constant filtration rate over long periods of time.
– Other patients exposed a slow, almost linear decay of function over decades.
– In a third group, a more rapid fall of renal function was observed that is more compatible with renal disease.

Yet, a controversy exists whether a true age-related process underlies this rapid decay or a disease component is relevant as the impact of diabetes mellitus or hypertension is hard to exclude. A similar situation exists for various physiological alterations that are typical for higher age. An overview is given in Table 1, which details implications of individual changes for pharmacotherapy.

Renal function in many elderly persons is compromised at both the glomerular and the tubular levels. Decreased kidney function thus is a typical and very important special feature of geriatric pharmacokinetics. Estimation of renal function by the formula of Cockcroft–Gault or the MDRD (modification of diet in renal disease) formula is an appropriate means to improve dosing of renally excreted drugs and does not require the determination of sophisticated parameters (e. g., 24-h collection of urine). As the Cockcroft–Gault formula can be implemented on slide rules only requiring the knowledge of age, body weight, serum creatinine, and sex and thus does not need to be calculated on a computer, it is preferable under practical aspects. Its accuracy is sufficient for drug dosing. The MDRD formula is more exact but requires computation. Both methods for estimation of renal function are only robust

for clearance values of greater than 10 ml/min. Below this limit, they become inaccurate and need to be replaced by direct measurement of clearance, most commonly by the collection of a 24-h urine sample.

Cockcroft–Gault formula (Cockcroft and Gault 1976):

$$C_{CR} \text{ (ml/min)} = (140 - \text{Age}) \times \text{Body weight (kg)}/[72 \times \text{serum creatinine (mg/dl)}]$$

(For women, the correction factor is 0.85, resulting in a reduction by 15%.)

MDRD formula (Levey et al. 1999):

$$\text{GFR (ml/min)} = 170 \times \text{Serum creatinine (mg/dl)}^{-0.999} \times \text{Age}^{-0.176} \times \text{Serum urea (mg/dl)}^{-0.293} \times \text{Serum albumin}^{0.318} \times \text{Body surface}/1.73$$

(For women, an additional correction factor is 0.762.)

The estimation formulas easily show that a "normal" serum creatinine of 1.0 mg/dl in an elderly patient does not necessarily indicate a normal kidney function, which would allow for full dosing of renally excreted drugs:

The Cockcroft–Gault-formula calculates a renal clearance of only 60 ml/min in a male patient (creatinine 1.0 mg/dl) who is 80 years old and weighs 72 kg, meaning that he has a renal function comparable to a young male with one kidney only.

This patient should receive only half the normal dose of a renally excreted drug to avoid overdosing and potential drug toxicity. This apparent paradox reflects the fact that at high age a reduced creatinine precursor production in skeletal muscles (sarcopenia) is offset by the equivalent reduction of kidney function; the resultant creatinine concentration remains unchanged. This situation may be compared with a bathtub in which water inflow (creatinine precursor production in skeletal muscle) is reduced to the same extent as is water outflow through the drain, resulting in no change of the water level. This linkage is depicted in Fig. 1. The lack of knowledge of the simple relation between creatinine production and excretion

Table 1 Selection of high age-associated changes of physiology and related impact on drug therapy

Change	Direct impact on pharmacokinetics	Direct impact on pharmacodynamics	Risk
Sleep-wake rhythm	No	Increased sensitivity for psychotropic drugs (especially benzodiazepines), often resulting in disorientation	Sleep disorder
Reduced accommodation capacity of the eye lens	No	No	Accident threat, compliance reduction, malnutrition
Clouding of the eye lens	No	No	Accident threat, compliance reduction, facilitation of anticholinergic ADRs
Reduction of total body water	Hydrophilic compounds	No	ADRs, e.g., increased toxicity of digoxin
Reduced liver blood flow	Risk of accumulation of drugs eliminated by the liver	No	Interactions, ADRs, e.g., beta-blockers, tricyclic antidepressants
Reduced glomerular filtration rate	Risk of accumulation of drugs eliminated by the kidneys	No	ADRs, e.g., increased toxicity of digoxin, aminoglycosides
Reduced sodium reabsorption	No	May result in increase of hyponatremic action of diuretics	Hyponatremia, delirium
Impaired reaction to β-adrenergic stimuli	No	Reduced sensitivity toward beta-blockers	Orthostatic reactions, fall risk increased
Bone calcification reduced (osteoporosis)	No	No	Fracture risk increased with falls, including those induced by drugs
Lower muscle mass (sarcopenia)	Yes	Yes	Fall risk increased, concealed reduction of kidney function as serum creatinine does not adequately increase due to lower production in skeletal muscle
Reduced production of saliva	No	No	Favors anticholinergic ADRs, "dry mouth" syndrome
Concentration of serum albumin reduced	Yes	No	Influence on drug plasma concentration if highly bound albumin, e.g., phenprocoumon or warfarin
Reduced nerve conduction velocity	No	Increased effect of muscle relaxants, including benzodiazepines	Fall risk increased

Source: Modified from Burkhardt et al. 2007.
ADRs adverse drug reactions.

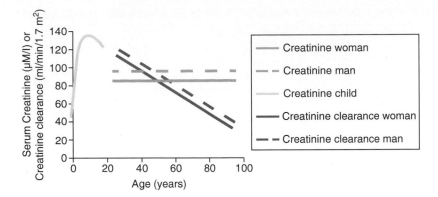

Fig. 1 Schematic course of serum creatinine and creatinine clearance in men, women, and children over age

changing concomitantly with age is the cause of many avoidable ADRs.

Further functionally relevant changes occurring at higher age relate to
- The gastrointestinal tract (reduced motility, delayed emptying of the stomach, higher pH due to reduced acid production)
- The liver (reduced first-pass metabolism at reduced liver mass, reduced perfusion especially by right heart failure)
- Plasmatic transport proteins (reduced albumin, increased α1-acid antitrypsin)

In general, body fat increases and body water decreases with age, resulting in reduced volumes of distribution. This leads to increased fractions of unbound drugs. In clinical practice, especially hydrophilic drugs such as digoxin should be started at lower loading and maintenance doses, and therapeutic drug monitoring should be performed if the therapeutic range is small. These facts (among other reasons) are the base for one of the most important generic recommendations in gerontopharmacology:

Start low, go slow. This means low starting doses, slow uptitration, but not ultimately to refrain from the full dose, which should be finally reached if tolerated and indicated.

It is important to note that the impairment of kidney function is by far the most important age-related alteration with impact on drug therapy in the elderly in daily practice. This functional deficit concerns about 40% of all drugs that are excreted predominantly by the kidneys, is vari-ably present in almost all elderly patients, but does not cause symptomatic illness by itself.

Thus, it is mandatory to estimate kidney function before any drug treatment is instituted in the elderly, a task that is easy to achieve (see previous discussion). Physicians must know how the drugs they prescribe leave their patients' body, via either the kidneys or the liver (or in some instances via both organs).

Knowing the route and modalities of drug excretion and estimation of kidney function in the elderly as indispensable prerequisites of drug therapy will enable the prescriber to adjust the dose accordingly and avoid unnecessary ADRs.

Even more trivial seems the fact that dosing of drugs requires an adjustment for body weight. In general, drug preparations are developed for younger patients with a mean body weight of around 75 kg (165 lbs), although regional differences are taken into account (e.g., lower average body weights in Japan); in addition, general trends in the development of weight averages by increasing obesity issues in Western societies are considered. These conditions determine the content of tablets, suppositories, or ampoules of marketed drugs. Obviously, elderly and especially very elderly patients expose reduced body weights; as detailed elsewhere, not only sarcopenia but also inappetence by dementia or teeth problems contribute to lower body weight. Thus, needless to say dose adjustments according to body weight are particularly important in elderly patients, who are often "nothing but skin and bones." This simple fact is often ignored as no adequate preparations with lower drug content or divisible design are available, resulting in overdosing by 30–80% (Campion et al. 1987); this source of inadequate dosing often meets other sources, such as impaired kidney function, and leads to easily avoidable complications of drug therapy.

Heterogeneity of Elderly Patients and Interactions of Various Aspects of Drug Therapy

Elderly patients are characterized by a dynamic process of aging that is not only limited to losses in functions or reduction of resources but also comprises compensatory and recovery processes. As these processes depend on both genetic and environmental determinants, it is conceivable that elderly people represent a very heterogeneous group of human beings. Some octogenarians are fit and largely free of chronic diseases, very active both physically and mentally, and others are frail and multimorbid, thus having lost their independence and entirely dependent on support by caregivers. This background of interindividual heterogeneity and consideration of the remaining life span and social and psychic aspects are major determinants of the choice of drugs for the elderly.

Here, only pharmacokinetic aspects are considered comprising all processes in the body that affect drug concentrations in various compartments (see previous discussion).

Alterations of pharmacokinetics in the elderly reflect those physiological and pathological changes of body functions and composition detailed previously. For the gastrointestinal tract, several deviations may affect the absorption of a drug:
- Reduced gastrointestinal motility
- Reduced splanchnic blood flow
- Reduced surface of intestinal mucous membranes
- Reduced gastric acid production

In general, these changes are small and may balance each other in that, for example, reduced motility results in increased contact times counteracting the impact of reduced membrane surfaces; thus, this aspect is of limited clinical relevance (exception: parenteral iron substitution may be necessary as iron absorption may be at its limits even in younger patients).

In addition to passive diffusion of drugs through the epithelial barriers, active transport may be important for drug absorption, and the single-most-important transport protein is p-glycoprotein. So far, no major or relevant changes in the expression of this protein have been described for elderly patients.

Distribution of a drug in the body depends on its physicochemical properties, mainly characterized by hydro- or lipophilicity. As body composition changes with age (increased fat, reduced water content of body compartments), volumes of distribution will change accordingly. Altered concentrations of plasma proteins, especially albumin reduction at higher age, may influence the drug distribution, at least theoretically. As a result, these changes may lead to increased serum levels of hydrophilic drugs and thus overdosing issues, with opposite effects on lipophilic drugs. Though more important (e.g., partially explaining increased digoxin levels in elderly patients compared to younger patients at the same dose) than age-related changes of absorption, these effects are relatively minor and mostly without clinical relevance.

The by far most important and clinically relevant functional changes of pharmacokinetics in the elderly relate to excretory organs, with the kidneys being the prominent culprit organs for hazardous drug therapy.

Drug elimination from the body is mainly ruled by its physicochemical properties and achieved by the liver or kidneys. Total drug clearance is simply the sum of the renal and hepatic clearances:

$$Clearance_{total} = Clearance_{hepatic} + Clearance_{renal}$$

As a rule of thumb, it may be assumed that lipophilic drugs are eliminated predominantly by the liver, hydrophilic drug by the kidneys. Hepatic clearance comprises two steps (phase 1 and phase 2): In phase 1, cytochrome P450 (CYP450) enzymes oxidize the molecule so that it becomes accessible to conjugation in phase 2 to increase water solubility. These processes are limited by hepatic blood flow (transport of parent drug into the liver) and the capacity of the degrading phase 1 enzymes. The CYP450 system comprises a large group of enzyme isoforms whose individual characteristics confer specificity for the metabolism of particular drugs. Thus, many drugs entirely depend on metabolism by only one enzyme, explaining the sensitivity of this process to enzyme inhibition, such as by competing drugs (drug-drug interaction), and its dependence on enzyme induction. Metabolizing enzymes may expose relevant polymorphisms that are important for nonresponse or overdosing issues with toxicity. Both aspects with relevance for pharmacokinetics in the elderly—hepatic blood flow and the capacity of phase 1 reactions—are slightly reduced in elderly people, resulting in a reduced hepatic clearance (Klotz 2009; Zeeh and Platt 2002). The dimension and impact of these age-related changes, however, are minor in comparison to the importance of genetic polymorphisms and related interindividual differences of enzyme phenotypes (see the following).

The most important determinant of renal function is the glomerular filtration rate, which decreases significantly with age (discussed previously). Alterations of tubular secretion and reabsorption are clearly less important for dosing in the aged. As this aspect was detailed previously, here only relevant aspects of drug metabolism are discussed further for which genetic variations are much more important than for the renal dimensions of drug elimination.

Pharmacogenetics and Drug Interactions

Consideration of individual parameters such as age, body weight, sex, liver and kidney function, and ethnicity has been the base of individualized, and thus optimized, drug therapy for decades. When more than one drug is applied, especially in polypharmacy (five or more drugs), not only the fiction of added wanted effects has to be considered, but also extreme augmentation of unwanted effects for which genetic factors may play a pivotal role. Metabolism of at least half of all drugs is catalyzed by CYP450 enzymes in the gut wall and especially the liver. These enzymes expose a wealth of genetic polymorphisms, resulting in impaired or increased capacities of metabolism compared to the majority of individuals.

Table 2 Enzymes important for biotransformation and examples for their substrates

Enzyme	Examples for drugs and other substrates
CYP1A1	Benzpyrene
CYP1A2	Caffeine
CYP2A6	Coumarines
CYP1B1	Estradiol
CYP2C9	NSAID
CYP2C19	Omeprazole, clopidogrel
CYP2D6	Neuroleptics, antiarrhythmics, beta-blockers
CYP2E1	Ethanol
CYP3A4	Nifedipine, simvastatin
Glutathion-S-transferase	Benzpyrene
N-Acetyl transferase (NAT2)	Isoniazide
Glucose-6-phosphate dehydrogenase	Antimalarials
UDP-glucuronosyl transferase	Bilirubin
Thiopurine methyl transferase	Mercaptopurine
Dihydropyrimidine dehydrogenase	5-Fluouracil

Source: Modified from Feuring et al. 2000
CYP cytochrome P, *NSAID* nonsteroidal anti-inflammatory drugs, *UDP* uridine diphosphate.

Enzymes (not only phase 1, but also phase 2 enzymes) with genetic relevance to drug metabolism are compiled in Table 2.

Pharmacogenetics describes hereditary variants of both enzymes and receptors underlying interindividual variabilities of pharmacokinetics and pharmacodynamics. Polymorphisms by definition are phenotypically recognizable variants in more than 1% of individuals. Phenotyping by test compounds (determination of metabolite concentrations in plasma) defined patient populations with regard to their hepatic metabolizing capacities, which are categorized into groups of rapid, intermediate, and poor metabolizers. Several studies showed that drug concentrations and effects consistently vary between patients with relevant polymorphisms especially in the CYP450 enzyme system.

CYP450 isoenzymes belong to an enzyme family of over 400 members, few of which are highly relevant for oxidative (and reductive) metabolism of drugs and xenobiotics such as insecticides (Goeptar et al. 1995). Based on homologies in the amino acid composition, the CYP450 system is classified into several subfamilies; they expose different substrate specificities and inducibilities. Important genetic polymorphisms have been identified, for example, for CYP1A1, CYP1A2, CYP2A6, CYP2C9, CYP2C19, and CYP2E1 (Lewis et al. 1998). The genetic polymorphism of CYP2D6 shall serve as an example. CYP2D6 (according to its primarily used substrate, also known as debrisoquine hydroxylase) metabolizes a large number of drugs, including neuroleptics (e.g., haloperidol, thioridazine) and antidepressants (tricyclic antidepressants, serotonin reuptake inhibitors); numerous antiarrhythmics (propafenone, flecainide, mexiletin); and beta-blockers (Bertilsson et al. 1995). CYP2D6 enzyme activity may be determined phenotypically by use of the test compounds debrisoquine or sparteine with subsequent determination of their metabolites and calculation of the metabolic ratio (MR) of test compound and metabolite in the urine. Thereby, three categories of phenotypes are formed:

1. Poor metabolizer (PM)
2. Extensive metabolizer (EM, normal phenotype)
3. Ultrarapid metabolizer (UM)

The prevalence of PMs in Europe and North America is at 7.5%; in China, Japan, and the African American population of North America it is at only 0–2% (Wormhoudt et al. 1999). As PMs may develop toxic drug levels more frequently than EMs, dosing has to be adjusted accordingly. The UM genotype is present in about 3–5% of Caucasians but in 15–20% of the Oriental population. Such individuals require very high drug doses to achieve adequate effects. In another situation, this polymorphism may be relevant: The antitussive drug codeine is partially metabolized to morphine. Studies found a positive correlation between the UM CYP2D6 genotype and the risk of addiction, as in these individuals a relatively high amount of morphine is produced compared to EMs. In general, a reduced or absent drug effect may be caused by

the UM status, as can be proven by the determination of drug concentrations in serum. This is particularly relevant for drugs with a narrow therapeutic range, which need to be dosed cautiously to hit the narrow margins of desired concentrations. Otherwise, either undertreatment (lack of effect at doses too low) or toxic effects (doses too high) will inevitably occur. Accordingly, in a study on tricyclic antidepressants, almost all PMs were nonresponders (Chen et al. 1996).

As a general note of caution, it appears that drugs with a narrow therapeutic range that are metabolized via polymorphic cytochromes (e.g., tricyclic antidepressants or antiarrhythmics) are more likely to be listed as drugs inappropriate for the elderly than other drugs.

Despite the lack of knowledge on the genetic background of the individual patient, genetic variations certainly contribute to adverse reactions in elderly patients. Genotyping is not done routinely (exceptions emerging), possibly relating to the fact that it could not yet prove its utility in outcomes research settings (improvement of clinical endpoints).

Competitive metabolism of different drugs by the same enzyme (CYP or other degrading/conjugating enzymes) may add to the problems inherent in genetic polymorphisms, especially those with low metabolic capacity.

Thus, an exponential increase of side effects, drug-drug interactions, correlates with increasing numbers of drugs applied to the same patient (Fig. 2). By simple math, one can calculate that the probability of a CYP450 3A4 drug-drug interaction in a patient on seven drugs is above 90%. Of all drugs, 30–40% are metabolized by this enzyme. Fortunately, most theoretically possible interactions are clinically irrelevant; such drug-drug interactions only cause around 10% of severe drug side effects, although calculations such as the one given previously and modern computer programs in practices highlight far too many of them. Thus, the clinical utility of a computer-assisted interaction search for "critical" interactions is very limited.

As mentioned, intensive observation and interrogation of the patient to detect side

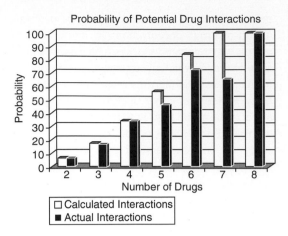

Probability of Potential Drug Interactions

☐ Calculated Interactions
■ Actual Interactions

Fig. 2 Correlation between the probability of calculated and measured drug-drug interactions and number of drugs applied (From Delafuente 2003 by kind permission of Elsevier)

Table 3 Important interactions of drugs in the elderly

Drug combination	Complication
Warfarin plus	
NSAID	Bleeding
Sulfonamide	Bleeding
Macrolide antibiotic	Bleeding
Fluorchinolone antibiotic	Bleeding
ACE inhibitor plus	
Spironolactone	Hyperkalemia
Potassium substitution	Hyperkalemia
NSAID	Hyperkalemia
Digoxin plus	
Amiodarone	Intoxication
Verapamil	Intoxication

ACE angiotensin-converting enzyme, *NSAID* nonsteroidal anti-inflammatory drug

effects or undertreatment are by far more effective than the "calculation" of interactions.

A classical example is the interaction between ciprofloxacin and theophylline. The latter drug has a very small therapeutic range; concomitant administration of ciprofloxacin—a strong inhibitor of CYP1A2—may increase the concentration of theophylline significantly, resulting in a classical overdosing syndrome characterized by tachycardia and delirium.

Important interactions of drugs in the elderly are shown in Table 3.

NSAID, digoxin, and oral anticoagulants (in the United States, warfarin; in Europe, phenprocoumon) are the leading drugs causing interactions in the elderly.

Other drugs may induce metabolizing enzymes, such as rifampicin (rifampin) or carbamazepine, resulting in ineffective therapies. This mechanism, however, is not a leading cause of concern in the elderly.

Drug-drug interactions may also be induced at the level of drug absorption in the gut. Intestinal absorption of many drugs is facilitated by ABC transporters, with the most prominent transporter being P-glycoprotein, the gene product of the MDR (multidrug resistant) 1 genes. As P-glycoprotein-mediated transport is limited in its capacity,

different substrates may interact at this level. Like hepatic cytochromes, P-glycoprotein may also be induced by rifampin. P-Glycoprotein acts as an efflux pump, and its induction may lower concentrations of substrates like digoxin. P-Glycoprotein also represents a permeator in the central nervous system (CNS); its induction there may critically lower drug levels in the CNS.

There are additional special risk situations, especially in polypharmacy, that need careful consideration. As mentioned, all drugs with a narrow therapeutic range or a particularly steep dose-effect curve are critical. Interactions may occur at all levels of pharmacokinetics. Drugs may chemically interact before or during absorption or compete for transporters. St. John's wort is an infamous example for the latter mechanism as it is a strong inductor of P-glycoprotein. It may thus reduce plasma levels of digoxin or cyclosporin, the latter with potentially deleterious consequences for heart transplant recipients. Interactions may also occur at the level of drug binding to plasma proteins. This applies to drugs with a high fraction bound to plasma proteins, such as amiodarone, phenytoin, ketoconazole, or warfarin/phenprocoumon. They compete for protein binding, resulting, for example, in high concentrations of oral anticoagulants (Podrazik and Schwartz 1999).

Drug-drug interactions are not restricted to pharmacokinetic interactions, but pharmacodynamic interactions also exist and may even be more important in general (see the following discussion). This type of interaction may occur if two drugs act on the same receptor system, and effects thus may be augmented. This applies to many psychotropic drugs, with low-potency neuroleptics from the phenothiazine group as an example that also occupy alpha-adrenergic and histaminic receptors. Concomitant administration of an antihistaminic or analgesic agent may strongly enhance its sedative effect. In addition, orthostatic dysregulation or delirium may be precipitated without the need for a pharmacokinetic interaction, meaning elevated drug concentrations. These considerations are the base for the classification of most low-potency neuroleptics as inappropriate for the elderly. The following discussion summarizes problematic properties of drugs leading to interactions in elderly patients and drug groups that are often involved in interactions.

Properties and Conditions of Drugs and Drug Combinations that Increase the Risk of Interactions

– Narrow therapeutic range or a particularly steep dose-effect curve
– Addition of analogous effects
– Long-term treatment
– Simultaneous prescribing by several doctors
– Self-medication by the patient

Drug Groups with a Strong Potential for Interactions

– Oral anticoagulants
– NSAIDs
– Digitalis glycosides
– Theophylline
– Antiepileptics
– Most psychotropic drugs
– Angiotensin-converting enzyme (ACE) inhibitors and other potassium-sparing drugs

Adverse Drug Reactions

Adverse drug reactions represent the most prominent and frequent adverse events in therapeutic interventions. Epidemiological studies consistently show a higher threat of elderly patients to suffer ADRs as multimorbidity and the resulting polypharmacy are inevitable risk factors for ADRs. Two particular entities of ADR should be mentioned here as they are typical for elderly patients, and their incidence steeply rises with age:
1. Falls
2. Delirium
   In addition to the high incidence of ADRs in the elderly, the situation is even more complicated by the fact that the presentation of ADRs is often atypical or only exposes weak symptoms. Inappetence and fatigue may be the only symptoms of a typical intoxication by digitalis glycosides. Parkinsonian symptoms are often misinterpreted as depression; weight loss may be the only sign for chronic drug intoxication. These ADRs that are typical for the elderly are discussed in detail elsewhere in this book and only mentioned here to underscore their tremendous importance.

Pharmacodynamics

Pharmacokinetics describes the course of a drug in the body, pharmacodynamics its clinical effects on the body. Typically, drugs act by binding to a specific receptor that expresses a binding site for the drug and signals on drug binding into the cell. Additional drug targets are enzymes (e.g., α-glucosidase for acarbose), but also catalytically active plasma proteins such as the coagulation factor X for heparins. Variations in pharmacodynamics result from individual differences in the genetic background and environmental impact on receptors and signaling cascades. In that, it resembles the determinants for the variation of drug plasma levels as described for pharmacokinetics. In this comparably young area of research, genetic differences for receptors such as the angiotensin II receptors have been demonstrated and correlated with clinically relevant differences in the effects of angiotensin receptor antagonists. In particular, such genetic variations are certainly important for the action of psychotropic drugs (e.g., neuroleptics). The detailed analysis of receptor polymorphisms and their contributions to clinical effects will become an important tool in this respect, although its final utility cannot be fully estimated today.

In addition to the genetic aspects as causes for effect variations, age-dependent alterations of the function and structure of drug target organs are of paramount importance. Aging processes are only partly dependent on genetic background, but also reflect environmental influences such as physical activity, nutrition, and mental activity/ education. Although principally applicable to all organs, such changes are notorious and clinically very relevant in the brain and cardiovascular system (see the following material).

In general, if a defined target structure ("receptor" in a wider sense) binds a drug, which is the standard situation of a drug-receptor interaction, the pharmacodynamic activity is described as drug-receptor interaction or dose–response curve. The dose–response curve typically exposes a sigmoidal shape in the log transformation, forming a plateau for the biological effect at higher concentrations.

Pharmacodynamic effects are much more difficult to analyze than pharmacokinetic changes as the direct in vivo measurement of the initial effect of a drug (e.g., its impact on intracellular second messengers) is often not possible. An example is the change of the beta-adrenergic system at high age. Elderly patients often show not only impaired responsiveness to beta-adrenergic drugs but also reduced effects of beta-blocking agents (Abernethy et al. 1987). This pharmacodynamic impairment of acute effects could result in decreased efficacy of long-term treatment with beta-blockers. However, in clinical practice no reduced efficacy of beta-blockers in elderly patients could be detected so far, although their tolerability decreases at higher age.

Pharmacodynamic effects are much harder to analyze in respect to age-related changes compared with pharmacokinetic changes, which are simply determined by the measurement of serum or plasma drug concentrations.

An example with much greater clinical relevance than the previous one is the increased sensitivity of elderly patients to the effects of psychotropic drugs. In contrast to the beta-blocker situation, the reasons for the very obvious and clinically relevant disadvantages of psychotropic drugs in the elderly are widely unknown. This particularly applies to the abundant use of benzodiazepines in elderly patients, in whom these drugs can elicit paradoxical reactions of excitation instead of sedation. Another important example of altered pharmacodynamics in the elderly is an increased sensitivity of renal function for the deleterious effect of NSAIDs. Not only does glomerular filtration rate decrease, but also renal blood flow. The latter effect results in a stronger dependence of renal function from vasodilatory prostaglandins, which becomes clinically apparent in particular in the presence of volume depletion (Clive and Stoff 1984). This explains the significantly higher risk of elderly patients to suffer renal damage from NSAIDs. Unfortunately, the newer cyclooxygenase II inhibitors are not better in this regard.

In Table 4, important changes of pharmacodynamics in the elderly are summarized.

Plasma Concentrations of Drugs and Clinical Effect

An increasing role in drug therapy is attributed to the so-called PK/PD modeling, which describes the relation between pharmacokinetics and pharmacodynamics. The coupling between plasma concentrations of a drug and its clinical effect may be very different for various drugs: In one case, there is an instant action that closely follows the plasma concentration; in another case, the effect only occurs after weeks of dosing. For a more detailed analysis, it would be essential to know the drug concentration at its receptor. To

Table 4 Examples for age-dependent changes of pharmacodynamics

Drug	Pharmacodynamic effect	Age-related change
Benzodiazepines	Sedation, increased fall risk, paradoxical excitation	Increased
Diltiazem	Blood pressure lowering effect	Increased
Levodopa	Dose-related adverse drug reactions (delirium, dyskinesia)	Increased
Morphine	Analgesia, respiratory depression (intensity and duration)	Increased
Warfarin/phenprocoumon	Anticoagulation	Increased
Theophylline	Bronchodilation	Reduced
NSAID, including COX-2 inhibitors	Renal impairment	Increased

Source: Modified from Feuring et al. 2000.
COX cyclooxygenase, *NSAID* nonsteroidal anti-inflammatory drug.

obtain this is either impossible or very challenging. Another factor obstructing a straightforward approach to describe the relation between plasma concentrations and related effects of a drug are compartments in the body that are only reached by the drug with a considerable delay (so-called deep compartments). The prototype of a deep compartment is the brain. The most important consequence is the phenomenon of "hysteresis," which describes the lag of drug action compared to plasma concentrations. This may be of great importance, as shown in the following example:

Carvedilol may be dosed once a day in hypertension treatment (in some European labels), but needs to be given twice a day in the treatment of heart failure. The antihypertensive action of a beta-blocker even today—35 years after the introduction of the first drug, propranolol—is not fully understood. After treatment initiation, the diastolic value remains constant or even increases. Weeks later, diastolic pressure starts to fall, and the final effect can only be assessed after 6–8 weeks of treatment. Although not known in detail, CNS actions seem to be responsible for these very delayed actions, which are considered an example for extensive hysteresis. This implies that blood pressure does not follow plasma drug concentrations closely and rapidly, but rather reflects an integral function of drug concentration over time. This is the reason for the once-daily dosing in hypertension treatment

in some countries, although the half-life of the compound would not be fully sufficient for this.

The situation is different if heart failure is being treated by the same drug. In this situation, peripheral effects are more important, especially those transmitted by beta-receptors in the heart, indicated by lower heart rates and antiarrhythmic control. This results in the cardioprotective effect of beta-blockers in heart failure. The peripheral effects closely follow plasma concentrations of the drug, as can be easily determined by heart rate readings.

This example of a beta-blocker underlines the fact that pharmacodynamics is often difficult to derive from pharmacokinetics. Thus, it is indispensable to measure clinical effects carefully. Due to the increased variability in elderly patients, this is particularly true for them; they also often have reduced compensatory reactions, such as the orthostatic reaction of the cardiovascular system. All drug therapies in elderly patients therefore require careful planning regarding the desirable effect size (e.g., blood pressure reduction to 140 mmHg systolic) and the time horizon (this blood pressure should not be reached too fast, and 3–6 months should be allowed for its full development), which need to be prespecified and explained to the patient. In this context, it is important to note that "slow" blood pressure medications (beta-blockers, discussed already, and diuretics) retard the onset of the effect, but the

Table 5 Typical drug-disease interactions in the elderly

Underlying disease	Drug	Adverse drug reaction
Dementia	Psychotropic drugs, levodopa, antiepileptics	Confusion, delirium
Chronic renal impairment	NSAID	Deterioration
Cardiac conduction abnormalities	Tricyclic antidepressants	Heart block
Arterial hypertension	NSAID	Worsening of hypertension
Diabetes mellitus	Diuretics, corticosteroids	Deterioration
Benign prostate hyperplasia	Antimuscarinergic drugs, e.g., disopyramide	Urinary retention
Depression	Beta-blockers, benzodiazepines, centrally acting antihypertensives, steroids, alcohol	Worsening, suicide
Hypokalemia	Digoxin, diuretics	Dangerous arrhythmias

NSAID nonsteroidal anti-inflammatory drug.

newer drugs (ACE inhibitors, angiotensin II antagonists, or dihydropyridine calcium channel blockers) may precipitate inadequately rapid effects.

Without adherence to the mentioned time frame, especially elderly patients will complain about symptoms such as dizziness, vertigo, or even syncopes; as the worst consequence, nocturnal hypotension may induce strokes.

Changes of Target Organs and Metabolism in the Elderly

Pharmacodynamics is dependent on disease- and age-related alterations of target organs. This dependence describes another type of drug-related interactions: drug-disease interactions (Table 5). The age-related alterations of target organs are addressed by the given contraindications for drug use but should be explicitly mentioned here. The fact that drugs requiring renal excretion may not be given or only given at reduced doses in patients with renal impairment belongs to the basic pharmacologic knowledge of every physician.

However, it is largely underrepresented in education and therefore in physicians' knowledge that numerous drugs may induce functional and even structural damage to the **kidneys. This may be the cause for subsequent intoxications.**

In this context, NSAIDs are the leading drugs again as they—often in combination with other drugs impairing renal function—may induce acute renal failure. Dangerous drug partners are ACE inhibitors and spironolactone; often a minor gastroenteritis aggravates the situation by dehydration, and as a consequence, even dialysis may become necessary.

Another important drug-disease interaction of NSAIDs (which appear most frequently as culprits of disaster in the elderly) relates to the treatment of arterial hypertension. On average, one antihypertensive drug needs to be added to current therapy if NSAIDs are added to treatment as they increase the drug demand for adequate control.

The following drug-disease interaction is also underestimated in its practical relevance: Various drugs induce diabetes mellitus or aggravate it. In this list, beta-blockers, diuretics (via hypokalemia), and glucocorticoids are the most frequently used drugs; cyclosporin A and HIV protease inhibitors are uncommon in the elderly. For this reason (among other reasons; see chapter "Arterial Hypertension"), the older antihypertensive drugs, beta-blockers, and diuretics are no longer first-line drugs in patients with uncomplicated hypertension.

The increased sensitivity of a damaged or simply old brain against sedatives/hypnotics is of concern as well: Not only opiates, but also benzodiazepines (paradoxical reaction, accelerated cognitive impairment, and depression) are involved in relevant drug-disease interactions.

A long list of drugs exists that aggravate preexisting dementia or may uncover subclinical stages of the disease by interference with compensatory mechanisms. Benzodiazepines, especially long-acting compounds such as bromazepam or nitrazepam (mean elimination half-life 26 h) in the European Union and chlordiazepoxide, diazepam, or lorazepam in the United States are notoriously involved and represent an extensive problem because of their abundant use.

Depression is very common in the elderly and may become worse in the presence of various drugs, including beta-blockers and psychotropic drugs; this is particularly problematic as depression is often underdiagnosed in the elderly.

Therapy Management

By itself, higher age is no contraindication for treatment with any drug. Yet, this patient group requires particularly careful consideration of the pros and cons of drug treatment, which has to reflect the symptoms, quality of life, and life expectancy before drugs are applied. Nonpharmacological interventions must be explored as they may represent valuable supportive means supplementing or even replacing drug therapy. Drugs with questionable benefit to the patient should be avoided in general as all drugs carry the risk of inducing new ADRs or augmenting existing ones. In particular, this applies to centrally active drugs in the elderly.

Drug treatment in the elderly represents a special challenge in that a critical assessment of potential individual benefits weighed against risk is even more demanding than in younger patients.

Before initiation of drug treatment, clinically meaningful therapeutic effects must be defined.

Important target endpoints of geriatric pharmacotherapy are
– Reduction of morbidity and—in many instances less important—mortality
– Improvement of quality of life

In general, starting doses should be lower than in younger adults and subsequently increased up to normal or even high final doses if no symptoms occur. For further individualization, genotype-based dose adjustments may become valuable adjunct modifications in the future, in addition to common dosing modifications in reflection of the kidney and liver functions. The special requirements and challenges of drug therapy in the elderly should not discourage physicians from granting the benefits of drug treatment to this highly relevant and pharmacologically challenging, but also rewarding, group of patients. It is important—and this not only applies to the elderly patient—to concentrate on the most effective and essential therapies and thereby attempt to reduce the number of drugs whenever possible. Finally, it should be emphasized again that every application of drugs to humans represents an individual experiment that may only be successful despite all pharmacokinetic and pharmacogenetic information if the clinical course of the patient is properly monitored.

The recommendations discussed next for drug treatment in the elderly compile a selection of basic rules that, however, cannot replace careful reasoning and observation in the individual patient (see overview). The selection aims at identifying the nine most important rules; many more could be given.

Physicians' Guiding Principles of Drug Therapy in the Elderly

– Use only a few drugs that you know well and feel comfortable with.
– In general, start drug therapy at low doses and titrate dose slowly up according to clinical effects (start low, go slow).
– CNS-active drugs are particularly dangerous for the elderly; try to avoid them whenever possible.

- Define endpoints and desired effects prospectively.
- Know and consider kidney function.
- Not all diseases are amenable to successful drug therapy.
- Keep treatment simple; prefer once-daily or—at maximum—twice-daily applications.
- Containers must be clearly labeled; no "childproof" containers please.
- Comprehensive information of patients, caregivers, and relatives/friends is essential.

References

Abernethy DR, Schwartz JB, Plachetka JR et al (1987) Comparison in young and elderly patients of pharmacodynamics and disposition of labetolol in systemic hypertension. Am J Cardiol 60:697–702

Bertilsson L, Dahl ML, Ingelman-Sundberg M, Johansson I, Sjoqvist F (1995) Interindividual and interethnic differences in polymorphic drug oxidation – implication for drug therapy with focus on psychoactive drugs. In: G Pacifici, GN Fracchia (Hrsg) Advances in drug metabolism in man. EUR 15439 EN, EC, DGXII-E-4. Office for Publication of the European Commission, Luxembourg, pp 85–136

Burkhardt H, Wehling M, Gladisch R (2007) Prevention of drug side effects in the elderly. Z Gerontol Geriatr 40:241–254, in German

Campion EW, Avorn J, Reder VA, Olins NJ (1987) Overmedication of the low-weight elderly. Arch Intern Med 147:945–947

Chen S, Chou WH, Blouin RA et al (1996) The cytochrome P450 2D6 (CYP2D6) enzyme polymorphism: screening costs and influence on clinical outcomes in psychiatry. Clin Pharmacol Ther 60:522–534

Clive DM, Stoff JS (1984) Renal syndromes associated with nonsteroidal antiinflammatory drugs. N Engl J Med 310:563–572

Cockcroft DW, Gault MH (1976) Prediction of creatinine clearance from serum creatinine. Nephron 16:31–41

Delafuente JC (2003) Understanding and preventing drug interactions in elderly patients. Crit Rev Oncol Hematol 48:133–143

Feuring M, Wehling M, Falkenstein E (2000) Impact of genetic factors and diseases on drug action. Internist 41:332–337, in German

Goeptar AR, Scheerens H, Vermeulen NP (1995) Oxygen and xenobiotic reductase activities of cytochrome P450. Crit Rev Toxicol 25:25–65

Klotz U (2009) Pharmacokinetics and drug metabolism in the elderly. Drug Metab Rev 41:67–76

Levey AS, Bosch JP, Lewis JB et al (1999) A more accurate method to estimate glomerular filtration rate from serum creatinine: a new prediction equation. Ann Intern Med 130:461–470

Lewis DF, Watson E, Lake BG (1998) Evolution of the cytochrome P450 superfamily: sequence alignments and pharmacogenetics. Mutat Res 410:245–270

Lindeman RD (1993) Assessment of renal function in the old: special considerations. Clin Lab Med 13:269–277

Podrazik PM, Schwartz JB (1999) Cardiovascular pharmacology of aging. Cardiol Clin 17:17–34

Rowe JW, Andres R, Tobin JD et al (1976) The effect of age on creatinine clearance in men: a cross-sectional and longitudinal study. J Gerontol 31:155–163

Wormhoudt LW, Commandeur JN, Vermeulen NP (1999) Genetic polymorphisms of human N-acetyltransferase, cytochrome P450, glutathione-S-transferase and epoxide hydrolase enzymes: relevance to xenobiotic metabolism and toxicity. Crit Rev Toxicol 29:59–124

Zeeh J, Platt D (2002) The aging liver: structural and functional changes and their consequences for drug treatment in old age. Gerontology 48:121–127

Critical Extrapolation of Guidelines and Study Results: Risk-Benefit Assessment for Patients with Reduced Life Expectancy and a New Classification of Drugs According to Their Fitness for the Aged

Martin Wehling

It is hard to understand that the largest group of drug consumers—elderly patients—is underrepresented in clinical trials. To avoid unclear results from patients with multimorbidity, elderly patients aged 65 or more years are almost routinely excluded from clinical trials. They obscure effect detection by events from concomitant diseases not addressed by the drug intervention, thereby diluting the "true" events under question. Only very recently, few exceptions from this rule have surfaced, with a study on arterial hypertension in the very elderly and several studies on new anticoagulants in the treatment of atrial fibrillation as signs of hope. In addition, regulatory authorities increasingly demand studies on pharmacokinetics in the elderly, although such studies are generally small and not powered to detect endpoint effects or assess safety in the elderly. Still, in the typical case of a newly developed drug, its clinical development was mainly restricted to younger adults, but it will be used predominantly in the group of elderly patients in whom it had never or only insufficiently been tested. This points to a large evidence gap in this context; as evidence-based medicine (EBM, defined by Sackett; Sackett et al. 2007) critically depends on evidence and guidelines almost automatically claim evidence as their major source of reasoning, we witness the critical absence of genuinely EBM-based guidelines for the elderly (Wehling 2011). For example, in the 2007 European guideline on arterial hypertension (Mancia et al. 2007), less than one page is devoted to treatment of the elderly although arterial hypertension represents one of the few therapeutic areas for which data in the elderly are emerging (see section "Positive Assessment of Drugs for the Elderly"). In the reappraisal of the guideline in 2009 (Mancia et al. 2009), also one page seemed sufficient for this. In the U.S. The Seventh Report of the Joint National Committee on Prevention, Detection, Evaluation, and Treatment of High Blood Pressure (JNC 7) guideline (Chobanian et al. 2003), hypertension in the elderly is presented on less than two pages. But, there is hope: Recently the first consensus statement on the treatment of hypertension in the elderly (Aronow et al. 2011) extensively and comprehensively described all major aspects of hypertension treatment in the elderly on 81 pages.

In this situation, with exceptions emerging, it is conceivable that in most cases drug therapy in the elderly is still merely based on the extrapolation of results obtained in younger patients, and evidence-based guidelines are missing. In many instances, even consensus-based guidelines do not exist. These extrapolations could at least

M. Wehling (✉)
University of Heidelberg, Maybachstr. 14, 68169 Mannheim, Germany
e-mail: martin.wehling@medma.uni-heidelberg.de

M. Wehling (ed.), *Drug Therapy for the Elderly*,
DOI 10.1007/978-3-7091-0912-0_4, © Springer-Verlag Wien 2013

trigger a consensus process (which only reflects the average opinion of experts without a database) on which an opinion guideline could be based. Such guidelines would have only a very limited level of evidence (expert opinion), and this is a dilemma that could be seen as a major reason for the nonexistence of even this inferior form of guidelines. Common guidelines always mix evidence and opinions, but clearly mark this divergent origin of input.

As evidence and even opinion-driven low-grade guidelines are mostly lacking for the elderly, physicians have no choice but to develop their own opinion in a structured and rationalistic way by adhering to criteria and rules for responsible extrapolation, interpolation, and judgment based on experience and observation.

This comprises the complete assessment of available data, including those from subgroups of elderly patients in the large trials, case studies, and previous experiences of the physician, which represent weak sources of evidence, but also the consideration of criteria for rationalistic extrapolation to be specified here.

In this book, general principles of drug treatment in the elderly are discussed in the first, third, and fourth parts, details of treatment modalities specific for the elderly in the second part.

Two principally different therapeutic approaches need to be separated:

– Symptomatic treatments, which are guided by symptoms such as pain, and
– Preventive treatments to reduce morbidity and mortality that have no instantly measurable benefit to the patient.

Extrapolation of Data from Younger to Elderly Patients in Reflection of a Reduced Life Expectancy

While symptom-driven therapy is both empirically and individually extrapolated and tailored to the patient, who needs to be carefully monitored (often neglected in practice), preventive therapy requires a completely different approach.

Prior to all preventive measures, life expectancy and quality of life need to be assessed to **place the necessary risk-benefit estimation into the individual context.**

The following, abstract estimation should exemplify this:

> Assuming that a drug reduces mortality by 30% or increases life expectancy by 8 years, these data are derived from one or more studies in younger adults. A life expectancy of around 20 years is expected if looking at 65-year-old women. The doctor is facing the following question: Will the same therapy be beneficial in patients at age 80 or 90?

It is astonishing how this important question is being dealt with in practice. Patients at age 80 and above will often be denied drug treatment without further analysis of individual conditions; for example, statin therapy is simply considered to be useless in this patient group. In Norway, where statins had been clinically "discovered," care in patients up to 80 years is excellent as over 70% of those who should ideally be treated receive it in practice. However, at this age limit, statin therapy is almost completely withdrawn, and treatment rates dramatically fall to only 11% (Kvan et al. 2006). This is an extreme form of ageism; it is ignored that a 75-year-old male still has an average mean life expectancy of 10.4 years and even a 90-year-old male has still 4.1 more years to go (Table 1).

Applied to the given sample (life prolongation by 8 years for a 65-year-old female, average life expectation 19.7 years), a linear extrapolation for an 80-year-old female (life expectancy 9.3 years) would yield in a prolongation of life by $8/19.7 = x/9.3$; $x = 3.8$ years. Fifteen years later, at age 95, this increase in life span drops to 1.3 years. A well-tolerated treatment would certainly still be useful in an 80-year-old, but probably not if initiated 15 years later. The increase of life expectancy drops to a few months in a 100-year-old patient.

This simplifying consideration needs to be corrected for the often large discrepancy between chronological and biological age in the elderly, and additional attention needs to be paid to contraindications and concomitant diseases. On top of this, the relative effect as measured in percentage change of a given endpoint may decline for the same treatment with age, which certainly is often overlooked or at least unknown or

Table 1 Average life expectancy (years) in the United States 2006 versus age

| | Average life expectancy | |
Age	Males	Females
60	20.7	23.8
65	17.0	19.7
80	7.8	9.3
95	2.9	3.3

Source: Centers for Disease Control and Prevention (2010)

unproven, but could render treatment useless in the very elderly.

In the following discussion, these considerations are applied to the role of 3-hydroxy-3-methylglutaryl-coenzyme A (HMG-CoA) reductase inhibitors, so-called statins, in cardiovascular prevention for the elderly. In numerous endpoint studies on statins (e.g., 4S, Scandinavian Simvastatin Survival Study), an average effect on mortality reduction of about 25% has been demonstrated. In a linear extrapolation model, it is assumed that this relative effect remains constant at higher age. As data for the very elderly and statins are yet missing, extrapolation is not only possible, but indispensable to avoid undertreatment of elderly patients against all medical experience "just" because of lacking data. Otherwise, one could ask the question whether red-haired people should receive the same treatment as patients with other hair colors, but there are no studies on red-haired patients, and even subgroup analyses from large trials do not yield sufficient data to answer this question. It is strikingly obvious that red-haired people should be treated like the others, though specific data concerning them are lacking. The necessary extrapolation will mainly take the reduced life expectancy into account and result in an estimate for the effect size at the given age. In the case of statin therapy, it is conceivable that the absolute effect size in life years saved will decrease at higher age, and a more restrictive approach needs to be installed for very elderly patients; Table 2 shows a recommendation for the use of statins in the elderly that is explained next.

The Heart Protection Study (HPS) and Prospective Study of Pravastatin in the Elderly at Risk (PROSPER) study (Shepherd et al. 2002) are the evidence base for current recommenda-tions for statin therapy in 65- to 80-year-old patients, such as the NCEP (National Cholesterol Education Program) recommendation. This guideline relies on the assessment of risk factors, and treatment initiation and target levels are chosen in reflection of the cardiovascular risk of a given patient. In patients with coronary heart disease (CHD) or a CHD risk equivalent (e.g., diabetes mellitus), who represent the high-risk group, an LDL (low-density lipoprotein) cholesterol of less than 100 mg/dl is the target level for statin treatment; at a lower risk level, which is defined by the number of accompanying risk factors, the target levels increase to 130 or even 160 mg/dl. The age limits employed in the studies mentioned restrict any direct application of evidence to patients under 80 years of age, and even for patients older than 75 years the small number of study subjects from this age group positions statin application into the framework of extrapolations.

Thus, estimating remaining life expectancy in not only the very elderly but also younger patients with severe concomitant diseases is an indispensable instrument and criterion for the indication of statin therapy; it is obvious that major aspects of this estimate must remain arbitrary and uncertain, but this limitation is inherently present in all estimates of this kind.

If in age category 1 (65–79 years; Table 2), life expectancy is under 10 years (e.g., due to accelerated aging and frailty or malign or life-span-reducing diseases such as collagenoses), increased target levels of LDL cholesterol would be accepted, such as the ones in category 2 or 3. Both categories of high age (80–89 and 90+ years) merely reflect consensus opinions, and the recommendations have been derived from estimates as given previously. In both cases, the levels of LDL cholesterol for both the initiation and the target of statin therapy have been increased (also reducing the number of treatment indications) by 30–60 mg/dl to increase the relative effect against the limitation by the reduced life expectancy. It is assumed that—as in younger patients—at higher cholesterol levels larger absolute effects (the same relative change means larger absolute effects if the initial concentration is higher) can be achieved as the

Table 2 Recommendations for statin therapy in the elderly

Therapeutic targets in different age categories	Starting LDL cholesterol/target LDL cholesterol
1. *Patients aged 65–79 years or mean life expectancy of ≥10 years*	
CHD and CHD equivalent	>/<100 mg/dl
Two or more risk factors	>/<130 mg/dl
One risk factor	>/<160 mg/dl (up to 190 mg/dl optional)
2. *Patients aged 80–89 years or mean life expectancy of ≥5 years*	
CHD and CHD equivalent	>/<130 mg/dl
Two or more risk factors	>/<160 mg/dl
3. *Patients aged ≥90 years or mean life expectancy of ≥3 years*	
Clinically active CHD in the past 3 years	>/<160 mg/dl
Clinically inactive CHD or CHD equivalent	>190 mg/dl/<160 mg/dl

Source: Modified from Döser et al. 2004.
Risk factors: age (always risk factor in this population); smoking; arterial hypertension; low HDL cholesterol (<40 mg/dl); family history for premature CHD; male sex. "Positive risk factor": very high HDL cholesterol (>60 mg/dl), so one risk factor may be deducted.
CHD equivalent: diabetes mellitus; symptomatic stenosis of a carotid artery; peripheral arterial occlusive disease; abdominal aneurysm of the aorta.
CHD coronary heart disease, *HDL* high-density lipoprotein, *LDL* low-density lipoprotein.

dose–response curve for statins and mortality becomes exponentially steeper at higher cholesterol levels. In contrast, reduced life expectancy at higher age antagonizes the larger effect at higher cholesterol levels. As in the example discussed, this relationship will become more conceivable if an extreme assumption is envisioned: For a 60-year-old patient with 20 or more years to live, a 25% change of mortality is a big gain, which shrinks to much smaller gains in the 90-year-old with a remaining life expectancy of about 4 years; the recommendation mentioned aims at balancing this lower effect by a larger drug effect at higher initial and target LDL cholesterol levels. Another extreme example would be the impact of traffic accident prevention: For a young, 20-year-old person, any prevented death means 60 life years gained, compared to only 4 in the 90-year-old.

In the second age category, primary prevention by statins requires starting LDL cholesterol levels of 130 mg/dl; in the third category, primary prevention is not recommended. In both categories, CHD is a treatment indication, in the third category at 160 or even 190 mg/dl LDL cholesterol, depending on the presence or absence of symptoms. If the estimated life expectancy is less than 3 years, statin therapy does not seem to be justified; this may apply not only to

elder patients but also to younger patients with malignancies. For this case, more intense ethical discussions are needed in general. All these recommendations are restricted to chronic treatment and do not concern acute interventions (e.g., by high-dose atorvastatin in acute myocardial infarction).

This example should demonstrate how the estimation of remaining lifetime depending on age should influence therapeutic decisions with respect to both indication and intensity. Such estimates seem mandatory in all prognostic therapeutic interventions, which are not restricted to drug therapy. The fact that such estimates remain arbitrary to a large extent and just better biomarkers for the determination of biological age are urgently needed should be mentioned here.

Categorization of Drugs with Regard to Their Fitness for the Aged

Polypharmacy has repeatedly been mentioned as the leading problem of pharmacotherapy in the elderly. It is known that the number of diagnoses increases with age, resulting in a rise in the number of drugs prescribed: Men aged more than 80 years have an average of 3.24 diagnoses; women of the same age have 3.57 diagnoses

(Van den Akker et al. 1998). In a U.S. study (Kaufman et al. 2002), over 50% of patients aged 65 years or more consumed five and more drugs, 10% even ten and more drugs.

This polypharmacy carries a considerable risk: In the United States, it is assumed that adverse drug reactions lead to 2.1 million hospitalizations and 100,000 drug-related deaths per year (Lazarou et al. 1998). These figures show that quality of drug treatment is suboptimal; lack of evidence in the elderly is one of the major reasons (as discussed previously). In addition, no drug has ever been tested at position 8 or 10 of the drug list of a patient. Polypharmacy is constructed by extrapolations and assumptions that are often vague and complex and thus may lead to a deadly cocktail. The pressing question thus is: How should a rationalistic approach to restrict polypharmacy be practically supported? Obviously, not everything needs to be given, and the next discussion deals with reduction by negative lists.

Aiding Rationalization by Negative Lists of Drugs for the Elderly

An obvious approach to drug regime compression is the compilation of negative lists. Such lists identify drugs that should generally not be given to the elderly (Beers 1997). Beers was among the first to publish a negative list of drugs that should not be given to elderly patients that contains, for example, benzodiazepines and some antihistaminics. During the course of continuous amendments, a subclassification was developed by Zhan et al. (2001) that contains three categories:
1. Drugs to be strictly avoided
2. Drugs for which an indication only rarely exists in the elderly
3. Drugs that are used too frequently in the elderly as the risk-benefit-ratio does not support their wide use.

The Beers list and its modifications were applied in pharmacoepidemiological studies to describe and analyze potentially inappropriate prescribing (PIPE). For example, in a U.S. study

of one million veterans, 19% of elderly men and 23% of elderly women received at least one drug listed in the Beers list (Pugh et al. 2006). So far, the utility of negative lists, including the Beers list, in that their application would lead to significant improvement of clinical endpoints is not proven. Limitations include the fact that excluding drugs from all elderly patients may be inappropriate in individual cases. Amiodarone should not be given at all, but some patients with ventricular arrhythmias or implantable cardioverter/defibrillators (ICDs) will have to receive it against all odds.

More epidemiological and interventional data are required to assess the utility of negative lists for drug treatment in the elderly. Ultimately, their contribution to improved drug safety is not sufficient to address the problem of polypharmacy in the elderly adequately.

Positive Assessment of Drugs for the Elderly

The assessment of drugs regarding the positive aspects of their use in the elderly is another potential means to increase the efficacy and safety of drug therapy in the elderly.

Not only overtreatment (too many drugs) is often present in polypharmacy situations, but also undertreatment. This means that drugs are missing for which data show a clearly positive risk-benefit ratio at the level of endpoints in the elderly. Steinman et al. (2006) demonstrated in 196 elderly patients receiving five or more drugs that 65% of patients consumed drugs contained in a negative list, but paradoxically clearly indicated drugs were also withheld from 64% of patients. The latter mainly applied to blood pressure-lowering drugs like thiazides or ACE inhibitors, for which conclusive data showed their benefit in the elderly, for example, in the HYVET (Hypertension in the Very Elderly Trial) study (Beckett et al. 2008). These thoughts reflect the fact that despite the lack of evidence in the majority of treatment areas, in some important areas evidence from interventional trials on the elderly are emerging. An important disease in this context is arterial hypertension in the elderly, especially systolic hypertension, which is the prevailing form in the elderly. Several studies demonstrated the positive effect of antihypertensive treatment in the elderly: the SYST-EUR (Systolic Hypertension in Europe Trial) study or HYVET, which is the first study on antihypertensive treatment in the very elderly (80+ years; Beckett et al. 2008).

Arterial hypertension is prevalent in up to 70–80 % of patients 75 years and older, and an insufficiently low control rate of only 20 % is medical reality; it thus must be emphasized that undertreatment of this condition is one of most pressing problems in medical care of the elderly.

The insufficient treatment of arterial hypertension in the elderly is possibly the most rewarding option to achieve reduction of morbidity (stroke) and mortality by drug therapy in the elderly. Similarly, preventive reduction of LDL cholesterol represents an evidence-based opportunity of beneficial drug treatment in the elderly as shown in the PROSPER trial.

Proposal of a New Drug Classification Reflecting Utility in the Elderly: Fit for the Aged, FORTA

A strategy for the improvement of drug therapy in the elderly should comprise both the negative and the positive aspects of the spectrum of drugs used in the elderly, reflecting both
- Inappropriate medications and
- Medications that are indispensable for the cure or prevention of disease in the elderly.

The latter aspect seems to be more important than the former as—unlike negative listing in most cases—it is based on *evidence* from the studies mentioned and others.

To rationalize and simplify drug therapy in the elderly, a classification of important drugs regarding their efficacy and tolerability in the elderly was proposed: FORTA (drugs fit for the aged; Wehling 2008, 2009). In this classification, drugs are grouped in four categories and labeled

from A through D. Schematically, this proposal is similar to the labeling by the Food and Drug Administration (FDA) of drugs for their toxicity in pregnancy (A–D, X for clearly teratogenic drugs), which has long been in use.

A: In category A, drugs are listed that have been tested in larger clinical trials in the elderly with clearly positive risk-benefit ratios. Examples are
- ACE inhibitors
- Angiotensin receptor antagonists
- Long-acting dihydropyridine calciumantagonists
  for hypertension treatment;
- Statins
  for lipid treatment (restrictions in the very elderly as mentioned);
- ACE inhibitors
- Angiotensin receptor antagonists
- Beta-blockers
  For heart failure treatment

B: The B drugs show evidence for utility in the elderly but have disadvantages regarding effect size or side effects. Examples are
- Diuretics
- Beta-blockers
  for hypertension treatment

These drugs are less advantageous than those in category A as they are associated with disturbances of compliance, electrolyte disorders (diuretics), or frequent contraindications (e.g., heart block, sick sinus syndrome) and a smaller effect size (beta-blockers).

C: Category C drugs expose an overall negative or neutral risk-benefit ratio in the elderly and should be the first to be deleted in polypharmacy situations; they require close monitoring of efficacy and side effects, and their indication should be very critical. Examples are
- Digoxin in heart failure treatment, which should be restricted to a few patients with symptoms despite optimal therapy (or atrial fibrillation; in this case, however, this diagnosis is leading, and assessment is guided by this diagnosis)
- Amiodarone for the treatment of atrial fibrillation or
- Spironolactone for hypertension (hyperkalemia).

In this category, drugs are labeled that should only be critically indicated and empirically controlled. Their use should be more an exception than the rule.

D: Drugs in category D are compounds that should be avoided in almost all patients and would be found in negative lists such as Beers list; these include

- Benzodiazepines
- Promethazine or
- Pentazocine (mod./translated from Wehling 2008)

It is important to find better alternatives for the treatment of the elderly, which is almost always feasible.

This labeling of drugs that are either "fit for the aged" or not (with gray zones in between) should be a help for the practitioner to prioritize drugs in a complex situation of multimorbidity and dependent polypharmacy. The use of the FORTA classification should be facilitated by the criteria discussed next.

Use Instructions for the FORTA Classification

- Evidence based, but also shaped to meet requirements of real life (compliance, age-dependent tolerability, relative frequency of contraindications)
- Classification depends on indication/disease to be treated and may differ between indications (e.g., beta-blockers labeled A in CHD, but B in hypertension treatment; diuretics in heart failure A, in hypertension treatment B)
- Contraindications overrun classification (e.g., in case of allergies, even A drugs are forbidden)
- Does not replace individualized therapeutic decisions; as with all simplifications, allows for exceptions (even for the extremes A and D)
- Is only meant to facilitate rapid orientation and to trigger inspiration

These labels would ideally be established in the drug development process for newly marketed drugs by health technology assessment institutions [such as the National Institute for Health and Clinical Excellence (NICE) in England or the Institut für Qualität und Wirtschaftlichkeit im Gesundheitswesen (IQWIG) in Germany]. The assessment indispensably needs to include experiences from practice in real life as compliance modalities, use, and application pitfalls are pivotal for efficacy and safety in "the wild" (Field et al. 2007); controlled clinical trials often do not mirror these problems and produce artificial results not applicable to daily medical practice. The support by the FORTA categorization to optimize drug therapy in polypharmacy situations should help the practitioner make the best use of limited time in a bird's-eye view approach. Another important aspect of a structured approach is the reduction of legal liability claims against the doctor who can prove a rationalistic approach and cite literature to share responsibilities. Thereby, the doctor acquires the authority necessary to stop and install medications even if not compatible with guidelines developed for younger patients that are often not applicable to elderly patients (see previous discussion). The validation of FORTA or an amended version will be a time-consuming process that has only started to date. At least, a broader discussion has been induced, and it is being tested in practice now.

The topics of this and the preceding chapter on extrapolation of guidelines to elderly patients and the categorization of drugs according to their fitness for the aged are just two measures among many to improve quality of drug treatment in the elderly. Other chapters of the book address general pharmacological approaches to critical areas (e.g., estimation of kidney function or compliance) and then discuss special aspects of diseases in the elderly. Coping with all these aspects represents an immense challenge and strain to the therapist, who tries to treat elderly multimorbid patients optimally under the conditions of daily practice and insane time restraints (5–8 min per patient). All in all, this problem demonstrates probably best that it is still (despite the tremendous technical progress in the past and at present) absolutely justified to consider medicine as an art based on science.

The art of practicing medicine certainly requires more than knowledge (which is

particularly sparse in the realm of geronto-pharmacology) and critically depends on intuitive components that comprise integration, creativity, experience, and certainly also knowledge.

References

Aronow WS, Fleg JL, Pepine CJ et al (2011) ACCF/AHA 2011 expert consensus document on hypertension in the elderly: a report of the American College of Cardiology Foundation Task Force on Clinical Expert Consensus documents developed in collaboration with the American Academy of Neurology, American Geriatrics Society, American Society for Preventive Cardiology, American Society of Hypertension, American Society of Nephrology, Association of Black Cardiologists, and European Society of Hypertension. J Am Coll Cardiol 57:2037–2114

Beckett NS, Peters R, Fletcher AE et al (2008) Treatment of hypertension in patients 80 years of age or older. N Engl J Med 358:1887–1898

Beers MH (1997) Explicit criteria for determining potentially inappropriate medication use by the elderly. Arch Intern Med 157:1531–1536

Centers for Disease Control and Prevention (2010) National vital statistics reports. 58(21), 28 Jun 2010

Chobanian AV, Bakris GL, Black HR et al (2003) Seventh report of the Joint National Committee on Prevention, Detection, Evaluation, and Treatment of High Blood Pressure. Hypertension 42:1206–1252

Döser S, März W, Reinecke MF et al (2004) Recommendations on statin therapy in the elderly, data and consensus. Internist 45:1053–1062, in German

Field TS, Mazor KM, Briesacher B, Debellis KR, Gurwitz JH (2007) Adverse drug events resulting from patient errors in older adults. J Am Geriatr Soc 55:271–276

Kaufman DW, Kelly JP, Rosenberg L, Anderson TE, Mitchell AA (2002) Recent patterns of medication use in the ambulatory adult population of the United States: the Slone survey. JAMA 287:337–344

Kvan E, Pettersen KI, Landmark K, Reikvam A, INPHARM Study Investigators (2006) Treatment with statins after acute myocardial infarction in patients > or = 80 years: underuse despite general acceptance of drug therapy for secondary prevention. Pharmacoepidemiol Drug Saf 15:261–267

Lazarou J, Pomeranz BH, Corey PN (1998) Incidence of adverse drug reactions in hospitalized patients: a meta-analysis of prospective studies. JAMA 279:1200–1205

Mancia G, De Backer G, Dominiczak A et al (2007) 2007 ESH-ESC practice guidelines for the management of arterial hypertension: ESH-ESC task force on the management of arterial hypertension. J Hypertens 25:1751–1762

Mancia G, Laurent S, Agabiti-Rosei E et al (2009) Reappraisal of European guidelines on hypertension management: a European Society of Hypertension Task Force document. J Hypertens 27:2121–2158

Pugh MJ, Hanlon JT, Zeber JE, Bierman A, Cornell J, Berlowitz DR (2006) Assessing potentially inappropriate prescribing in the elderly Veterans Affairs population using the HEDIS 2006 quality measure. J Manag Care Pharm 12:537–545

Sackett DL, Rosenberg WM, Gray JA, Haynes RB, Richardson WS (2007) Evidence based medicine: what it is and what it isn't, 1996. Clin Orthop Relat Res 455:3–5

Shepherd J, Blauw GJ, Murphy MB et al (2002) Pravastatin in elderly individuals at risk of vascular disease (PROSPER): a randomised controlled trial. Lancet 360:1623–1630

Steinman MA, Landefeld CS, Rosenthal GE, Berthental D, Sen S, Kaboli PJ (2006) Polypharmacy and prescribing quality in older people. J Am Geriatr Soc 54:1516–1523

Van den Akker M, Buntinx F, Metsemakers JF, Roos S, Knottnerus JA (1998) Multimorbidity in general practice: prevalence, incidence, and determinants of co-occurring chronic and recurrent diseases. J Clin Epidemiol 51:367–375

Wehling M (2008) Drug therapy in the aged: too much and too little. Dtsch Med Wochenschr 133:2289–2291, in German

Wehling M (2009) Multimorbidity and polypharmacy: how to reduce the harmful drug load and yet add needed drugs in the elderly? Proposal of a new drug classification: fit for the aged. J Am Geriatr Soc 57:560–561

Wehling M (2011) Guideline-driven polypharmacy in elderly, multimorbid patients is basically flawed: there are almost no guidelines for these patients. J Am Geriatr Soc 59:376–377

Zhan C, Sangl J, Bierman AS et al (2001) Potentially inappropriate medication use in the community-dwelling elderly: findings from the 1996 Medical Expenditure Panel Survey. JAMA 286:2823–2829

Inappropriate Medication Use and Medication Errors in the Elderly

Zachary A. Marcum and Joseph T. Hanlon

Introduction

Medications are commonly used by older adults. While medications can relieve symptoms and prevent further disease complications, they unfortunately can also cause adverse drug events (ADEs). An ADE can be defined as "an injury resulting from the use of a drug" (Aspden et al. 2007; Nebeker et al. 2004). The right side of Fig. 1 shows the three types of ADEs: (1) adverse drug reactions (ADRs) (i.e., a response to a drug that is noxious and unintended and occurs at doses normally used for the prophylaxis, diagnosis, or therapy of disease or for modification of physiological function); (2) therapeutic failures (TFs) (i.e., failure to accomplish the goals of treatment resulting from inadequate drug therapy and not related to the natural progression of disease); and (3) adverse drug withdrawal reactions (ADWEs) (i.e., a clinical set of symptoms or signs that are related to the removal of a drug) (Edwards and Aronson 2000; Hanlon et al. 2010). Besides death, which fortunately is rarely due to medications, one of the worst consequences of medication use in older adults is hospitalization. Studies have shown that up to 16% of hospital admissions are due to ADRs, up to 11% due to TFs, and approximately 1% due to ADWEs (Beijer and de Blaey 2002; Kaiser et al. 2006; Marcum et al. 2011). Taken together, these medication-related problems are a significant cause of morbidity and mortality as well as unnecessary healthcare costs in older adults.

While some ADEs are unavoidable (e.g., leukopenia from chemotherapy or allergic reaction to penicillin), many may be preventable because they are due to medication errors. A medication error is a mishap that occurs during the prescribing, order communication, dispensing, administering, adherence, or monitoring of a drug (Aspden et al. 2007; Nebeker et al. 2004; Lisby et al. 2010; National Coordinating Council for Medication Error Reporting and Prevention 1998). The relationship between medication errors and ADEs is shown in Fig. 1. For more information about potential monitoring errors in older adults, refer to a recent comprehensive review (Steinman et al. 2011). Moreover, there is limited information about pharmacy dispensing errors that is specific to older adults; therefore, the topic is not further discussed in this chapter (Flynn et al. 2009). In addition, chapter "Adherence to Pharmacotherapy in the Elderly" in this book covers the topic of medication adherence in older patients. Thus, this chapter focuses on specific aspects of suboptimal prescribing and medication administration errors.

Z.A. Marcum and J.T. Hanlon (✉)
University of Pittsburgh, Division of Geriatric Medicine
Pittsburgh, PA, 3471 Fifth Ave. Kaufmann Building,
Suite 500, Pittsburgh, PA 15213, USA
e-mail: jth14@pitt.edu

M. Wehling (ed.), *Drug Therapy for the Elderly*,
DOI 10.1007/978-3-7091-0912-0_5, © Springer-Verlag Wien 2013

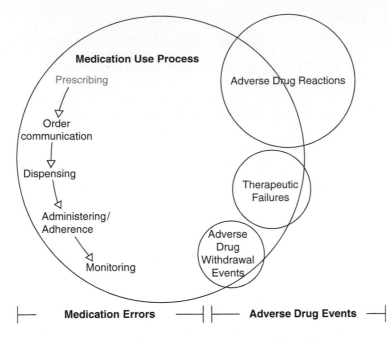

Fig. 1 A modified conceptual model for medication-related problems in older adults

Table 1 Methods to detect over-, under-, and inappropriate prescribing in older adults

Explicit measures	Implicit measures
Overprescribing: polypharmacy (e.g., 5+, 9+, 10+ medications)	Overprescribing: unnecessary use (i.e., lack of indication, effectiveness, or therapeutic duplication per the MAI)
Underprescribing (e.g., ACOVE; START)	Underprescribing (i.e., AOU)
Inappropriate prescribing: drugs that should be avoided (e.g., Beers criteria, STOPP); drug-disease interactions (e.g., Beers criteria, STOPP)	—

ACOVE Assessing Care of Vulnerable Elders, *AOU* Assessment of Underutilization, *MAI* Medication Appropriateness Index, *STOPP* Screening Tool of Older Person's Prescriptions, *START* Screening Tool to Alert Doctors to Right Treatment

Suboptimal Prescribing

There are three major types of suboptimal prescribing in older adults: (1) *overprescribing* (e.g., polypharmacy); (2) *underprescribing*; and (3) *inappropriate prescribing* (Dimitrow et al. 2011; Spinewine et al. 2007a). Table 1 summarizes some of the most widely studied explicit and implicit measures of suboptimal prescribing. The topics of polypharmacy and some aspects of inappropriate prescribing are covered in chapters "Polypharmacy," and "Inappropriate Prescribing

in the Hospitalized Elderly Patient" of this text. Next, we focus on underprescribing as well as other aspects of inappropriate prescribing not already covered in this text (i.e., dosing for renally cleared medications and drug-drug interactions [DDIs]).

Underprescribing

Evidence-based pharmacotherapy addressing the undertreatment of chronic conditions is summarized by two major sets of explicit criteria: (1)

Table 2 ACOVE-3 quality indicators for underuse of medications

Disease/medication	Pharmacotherapy
Atrial fibrillation	Anticoagulant
Heart failure	ACE-I, selective β-blocker
COPD	Inhaled long-acting bronchodilator/corticosteroid
CVA	Antithrombotic
Diabetes mellitus	ACE-I, aspirin
Hypertension and ischemic heart disease	β-Blocker
Hypertension and diabetes mellitus/heart failure/chronic kidney disease	ACE-I
Ischemic heart disease/myocardial infarction	Antiplatelet, β-blocker, statin
Osteoarthritis	Acetaminophen
Opioid therapy	Laxatives
Osteoporosis	Bisphosphonate
Peptic ulcer disease, high risk (i.e., 75+ years; NSAID, steroid, and/or warfarin use; or previous history of peptic ulcer disease)	PPI or misoprostol
Steroid use, systemic	Calcium/vitamin D/bisphosphonate

Source: Modified from Shrank et al. 2007

ACE-I angiotensin-converting enzyme inhibitor, *ACOVE* Assessing Care of Vulnerable Elders, *COPD* chronic obstructive pulmonary disease, *CVA* cerebrovascular accident, *NSAID* nonsteroidal anti-inflammatory drug, *PPI* proton pump inhibitor

Assessing Care of Vulnerable Elders (ACOVE) and (2) Screening Tool to Alert to Right Treatment (START) (Tables 2 and 3, respectively) (Shrank et al. 2007; Gallagher et al. 2008). Some potential advantages of using explicit criteria to measure underprescribing include the ability to apply them to computerized health care data and perhaps improve interrater reliability (Spinewine et al. 2007a). Alternatively, potential disadvantages include the need to use the consensus of an expert panel as opposed to an evidence base. In addition, explicit criteria may not apply to all patients (e.g., end-of-life care) and require regular updating (Spinewine et al. 2007a).

Application of the START criteria to hospitalized older adults found that 58–66% had evidence of underprescribing (Lang et al. 2010; Ryan et al. 2009). Moreover, application of the ACOVE criteria to another group of hospitalized elders detected that among the 78% of patients who were eligible for at least one indicator, more than half had at least one inappropriate rating for potential undertreatment (Spinewine et al. 2007b). This latter study also showed that a clinical pharmacist intervention resulted in these patients being six times as likely as control

patients to have at least one improvement in undertreatment (Spinewine et al. 2007b).

Implicit criteria in the form of the Assessment of Underutilization of Medication (AOU) can be used to assess potential undertreatment as well (Jeffrey et al. 1999). To make this assessment, one is required to match a patient's problem list and medication list and ask if there is an omission of a needed drug for an established active disease/condition. After review of the AOU's general and specific instructions, the health care professional is then required to give a rating between A (no drug omitted) to C (drug omitted) for each chronic condition. An advantage to the use of this implicit measure is that it is patient specific since it is based on medical record review. Conversely, a disadvantage is that it requires a skilled and trained health care professional to apply the measure (Spinewine et al. 2007a).

Two studies of interrater reliability with the AOU showed moderate-to-excellent agreement between pharmacist and physician pairs (Jeffrey et al. 1999; Gallagher et al. 2011). Application of the AOU to a group of hospitalized elders at discharge detected that 62% had a potential problem with medication undertreatment (Wright et al.

Table 3 START criteria for chronic conditions

Organ system/disease	Pharmacotherapy
Cardiovascular	
Atrial fibrillation	Aspirin/warfarin
Angina, stable	β-Blocker
ASCD, CVD, PVD	Aspirin/clopidogrel, statin
Heart failure	ACE-I
Myocardial infarction	ACE-I
Central Nervous System	
Depression symptoms >3 months	Antidepressant
Parkinson's disease	Levodopa
Endocrine	
Diabetes mellitus	ACE-I/ARB, antiplatelet, metformin, statin
Gastrointestinal	
Diverticular disease with constipation	Fiber supplement
GERD/stricture requiring dilation	PPI
Musculoskeletal	
Steroid use, maintenance	Bisphosphonate
Osteoporosis	Calcium with vitamin D
Rheumatoid arthritis	DMARD
Respiratory	
Asthma/COPD (mild/moderate)	Inhaled β-agonist or anticholinergic
Asthma/COPD (moderate/severe)	Inhaled corticosteroid

Source: Modified from Gallagher et al. 2008
ACE-I, angiotensin-converting enzyme inhibitor, *ARB* angiotensin II receptor blocker, *ASCD* atherosclerotic coronary disease, *COPD* chronic obstructive pulmonary disease, *CVD* cardiovascular disease, *DMARD* disease-modifying antirheumatic drug, *GERD* gastroesophageal reflux, *PPI* proton pump inhibitor, *PVD* peripheral vascular disease, *START* Screening Tool to Alert Doctors to Right Treatment

2009). Furthermore, two separate randomized studies that applied the AOU found that either a physician or a geriatric evaluation and management team intervention resulted in statistically significant improvements in underprescribing for hospitalized older adults (Gallagher et al. 2011; Schmader et al. 2004).

Dosing of Renally Cleared Medications

One of the most clinically important age-related physiological changes is a decline in renal function. It has been estimated that at least 30% of individuals in the United States have evidence of chronic kidney disease (CKD; defined as stage 3–5 with an estimated glomerular filtration rate [eGFR] < 60 ml/min/1.73 m^2) (Centers for Disease Control and Prevention 2007; Stevens and Levey 2005). Furthermore, it has been shown that prescribing errors with primarily renally cleared medications may occur in up to 52% of older nursing home patients with CKD (Hanlon et al. 2011; Papaioannou et al. 2000; Rahimi et al. 2008). Unfortunately, these studies all used different explicit criteria, and different pharmacotherapy sources have been shown to offer conflicting dosing information for primarily renally cleared medications (Vidal et al. 2005). Table 4 shows a list of 20 medications for which an expert panel reached consensus along with six drugs with a narrow therapeutic range whose dosing should be guided by serum drug levels (Hanlon et al. 2009). A number of randomized controlled trials (RCTs) have shown computerized physician order entry (CPOE) with decision support systems (DSSs) and pharmacist interventions to be successful in improving the prescribing of renally

Table 4 Consensus/guideline recommendations for renally cleared medications in older patients with chronic kidney disease

Medication/class	eCrCl (ml/min)	Maximum dosing recommendation (milligrams)
Acyclovir[a] (for zoster)	10–29	800 every 8 h
	<10	800 every 12 h
Amantadine[a]	30–59	100 daily
	15–29	100 every 48 h
	<15	100 every 7 days
Amikacin[b]	<60	Dose based on drug levels unless 1/kg dose for < 5 days
Chlorpropamide[a]	<50	Avoid use
Ciprofloxacin[a]	<30	500 every 24 h
Colchicine[a]	<10	Avoid use
Cotrimoxazole[a]	15–29	1 DS tablet daily
	<15	Avoid use
Digoxin	<60	Dose based on drug levels
Duloxetine	<30	Avoid use
Gabapentin (for pain)[a]	30–59	600 twice daily
	15–29	300 twice daily
	<15	300 daily
Gentamicin[b]	<60	Dose based on drug levels unless 1/kg dose for <5 days
Glyburide[a]	<50	Avoid use
Lithium	<60	Dose based on drug levels
Levetiracetam	50–80	500–1,000 every 12 h
	30–49	250–750 every 12 h
	<30	250–500 every 12 h
Memantine[a]	<30	5 twice daily
Meperidine[a]	<50	Avoid use
Nitrofurantoin[a]	<60	Avoid use
Probenecid[a]	<50	Avoid use
Procainamide	<60	Dose based on drug level
Ranitidine[a]	<50	150 daily
Rimantadine[a]	<50	100 daily
Spironolactone[a]	<30	Avoid use
Tobramycin[b]	<60	Dose based on drug levels unless 1/kg dose for <5 days
Tramadol	<30	50–100 every 12 h
Triamterene[a]	<30	Avoid use
Valacyclovir (for zoster)[a]	30–49	1,000 every 12 h
	10–29	1,000 every 24 h
	<10	500 every 24 h
Vancomycin[b]	<60	Dose based on drug level

Source: From Hanlon et al. 2009
DS double strength, *eCrCl* estimated creatinine clearance
[a]From two-stage Delphi survey (Hanlon et al. 2009)
[b]Parenteral dosage form. Others are oral dosage form

Table 5 Centers for Medicare and Medicaid Services drug-drug interactions

Drug affected	Precipitant drug(s)
Aspirin	NSAIDs
ACE-I	Potassium supplements, potassium-sparing diuretic
Anticholinergic	Anticholinergic
Antihypertensives	Levodopa, nitrates
Antiplatelet	NSAIDs
CNS medications	CNS medications
Digoxin	Amiodarone, verapamil
Lithium	ACE-I, thiazide diuretics, NSAIDs
Meperidine	MAOI
Phenytoin	Imidazoles
Quinolones	Type IA, IC, II antiarrhythmics
SSRIs	Tramadol, St. John's wort
Sulfonylureas	Imidazoles
Theophylline	Imidazoles, quinolones, barbiturates
Warfarin	Amiodarone, NSAIDs, sulfonamides, macrolides, quinolones, phenytoin, imidazoles

Source: From Centers for Medicare and Medicaid Services 2006
ACE-I angiotensin-converting enzyme-inhibitor, *CNS* central nervous system, *MAOI* monoamine oxidase inhibitor, *NSAID* nonsteroidal anti-inflammatory drug; *SSRI* selective serotonin reuptake inhibitor

cleared medications in adults, including those residing in nursing homes (Bhardwaja et al. 2011; Chertow et al. 2001; Field et al. 2009).

Drug-Drug Interactions

Given that older adults take more medications than other age groups, it is clinically sensible that the probability of one drug interfering with the pharmacokinetics or pharmacodynamics of another drug is higher in the elderly population (Mallet et al. 2007). Indeed, between 6% and 42% of elderly patients have been shown to have evidence of a DDI (Mallet et al. 2007). Similar to dosing of renally cleared medications, there is great discordance between pharmacotherapy texts and software references regarding what are considered to be clinically important DDIs. In part, to address this in U.S. nursing homes, the largest payer (i.e., the Centers for Medicare and Medicaid Services [CMS]) developed specific explicit guidelines for DDIs (Table 5) (CMS 2006). Specifically, 31 medication/classes that can affect 15 medication/classes are highlighted. It is important to note that one third of the affected medications are drugs with a narrow therapeutic range, and nearly one third of

the DDIs are due to a pharmacodynamic mechanism. Recently, there have been more research activities focusing on the impact of multiple anticholinergics or central nervous system drugs in older adults (Campbell et al. 2009; Taipale et al. 2010). Also, there has been greater attention toward examining potential DDIs as determined by studies using observational designs (Hines and Murphy 2011). Finally, an innovative study was recently published that examined the combined effects of a pharmacokinetic DDI with benzodiazepines in which older adults experience enhanced pharmacodynamic sensitivity (Zint et al. 2010). Importantly, there is a great need for consensus to be reached by expert panels to guide the development of CPOE/DSS and pharmacy software incorporating these standardized DDIs while avoiding alert fatigue (i.e., health care professionals ignoring these potential DDIs due to the receipt of multiple alerts).

Medication Administration Errors

In institutional settings (i.e., hospitals, nursing homes, and assisted living facilities), nurses and trained laypersons are responsible for making sure that the right patient gets the right drug at the right dose by the right route at the right time. Nearly 25 years ago in the United States, CMS adopted an observation method developed by Barker et al. for application in nursing homes (Barker et al. 2002a). CMS further declared that error rates of greater than 5% would classify an institution as not eligible for reimbursement. In one study of 36 health care facilities (12 nursing homes, 24 hospitals), 19% of doses (605/3,216) were administered in error, with the most common problems involving wrong time (43%), omission (30%), wrong dose (17%), and wrong drug (4%) (Barker et al. 2002b). However, only 7% of errors were considered to be potentially clinically important. This same rate of potentially clinically important errors was found in a recent study of medication administration errors by trained laypersons in 11 assisted living facilities (Zimmerman et al. 2011). Common problems found involve crushing or altering medications such as time-release or enteric-coated dosage forms and incorrect measurement of liquid dosage forms (e.g., insulin); these practices can lead to increased medication toxicity. It is hoped that greater attention to this issue, combined with more training for laypersons, the future use of bar-coded unit dose medications, electronic medication administration records, and scanning patient identification bracelets will further reduce these medication administration errors.

Conclusion

Medications are commonly used in older adults and can cause ADEs, including ADRs, TFs, and ADWEs. While some ADEs are unavoidable, many may be preventable because they are due to medication errors. This chapter reviewed specific aspects of medication errors, including suboptimal prescribing (underprescribing and inappropriate prescribing due to primarily renally cleared medications and DDIs) as well as medication administration errors. Understanding medication use and its effects in older adults across care settings will aid in designing future interventions for the improvement of health care for this population.

References

Aspden P, Wolcott J, Bootman L, Cronenwett LR, for the IOM Committee on Identifying and Preventing Medication Errors (eds) (2007) Preventing medication errors: quality chasm series. National Academies Press, Washington, DC

Barker KN, Flynn EA, Pepper GA (2002a) Observation method of detecting medication errors. Am J Health Syst Pharm 59:2314–2316

Barker KN, Flynn EA, Pepper GA et al (2002b) Medication errors observed in 36 health care facilities. Arch Intern Med 162:1897–1903

Beijer HJ, de Blaey CJ (2002) Hospitalisations caused by adverse drug reactions (ADR): a meta-analysis of observational studies. Pharm World Sci 24:46–54

Bhardwaja B, Carroll NM, Raebel MA et al (2011) Improving prescribing safety in patients with renal insufficiency in the ambulatory setting: the Drug Renal Alert Pharmacy (DRAP) program. Pharmacotherapy 31:346–356

Campbell N, Boustani M, Limbil T et al (2009) The cognitive impact of anticholinergics: a clinical review. Clin Interv Aging 4:225–233

Centers for Disease Control and Prevention (2007) Prevalence of chronic kidney disease and associated risk factors—United States, 1999–2004. MMWR Morb Mortal Wkly Rep 56:161–165

Centers for Medicare and Medicaid Services (2006) State operations manual: surveyor guidance for unnecessary medications (F329). http://www.cms.hhs.gov/transmittals/downloads/R22SOMA.pdf. Accessed 2 Oct 2011

Chertow GM, Lee J, Kuperman GJ et al (2001) Guided medication dosing for inpatients with renal insufficiency. JAMA 286:2839–2844

Dimitrow MS, Airaksinen MS, Kivelä SL et al (2011) Comparison of prescribing criteria to evaluate the appropriateness of drug treatment in individuals aged 65 and older: a systematic review. J Am Geriatr Soc 59:1521–1530

Edwards IR, Aronson JK (2000) Adverse drug reactions: definitions, diagnosis, and management. Lancet 356:1255–1259

Field TS, Rochon P, Lee M et al (2009) Computerized clinical decision support during medication ordering for long-term care residents with renal insufficiency. J Am Med Inform Assoc 16:480–485

Flynn EA, Barker KN, Berger BA et al (2009) Dispensing errors and counseling quality in 100 pharmacies. J Am Pharm Assoc 49:171–180

Gallagher P, Ryan C, Byrne S et al (2008) STOPP (Screening Tool of Older Person's Prescriptions) and START (Screening Tool to Alert Doctors to Right Treatment). Consensus validation. Int J Clin Pharmacol Ther 46:72–83

Gallagher PF, O'Connor MN, O'Mahony D (2011) Prevention of potentially inappropriate prescribing for elderly patients: a randomized controlled trial using STOPP/START criteria. Clin Pharmacol Ther 89:845–854

Hanlon JT, Aspinall S, Semla T et al (2009) Consensus guidelines for oral dosing of primarily renally cleared medications in older adults. J Am Geriatr Soc 57:335–340

Hanlon JT, Handler S, Maher R et al (2010) Geriatric pharmacotherapy and polypharmacy. In: Fillit H, Rockwood K, Woodhouse K (eds) Brocklehurst's textbook of geriatric medicine, 7th edn. Churchill Livingstone, London, pp 880–885

Hanlon JT, Wang X, Handler SM et al (2011) Potentially inappropriate prescribing of primarily renally cleared medications for older Veterans affairs nursing home patients. J Am Med Dir Assoc 12:377–383

Hines LE, Murphy JE (2011) A review of potentially harmful drug-drug interactions in the elderly: a review. Am J Geriatr Pharmacother 9:364–377

Jeffrey S, Ruby CM, Twersky J, Hanlon JT (1999) Effect of an interdisciplinary team on suboptimal prescribing in a long term care facility. Consult Pharm 14:1386–1391

Kaiser RM, Schmader KE, Pieper CF et al (2006) Therapeutic failure-related hospitalisations in the frail elderly. Drugs Aging 23:579–586

Lang PO, Hasso Y, Dramé M et al (2010) Potentially inappropriate prescribing including under-use amongst older patients with cognitive or psychiatric co-morbidities. Age Ageing 39:373–381

Lisby M, Nielsen LP, Brock B, Mainz J (2010) How are medication errors defined? A systematic literature review of definitions and characteristics. Int J Qual Health Care 22:507–518

Mallet L, Spinewine A, Huang A (2007) The challenge of managing drug interactions in elderly people. Lancet 370:185–191

Marcum ZA, Amuan ME, Hanlon JT et al (2011) Therapeutic failures and adverse drug withdrawal events leading to hospitalization among older outpatient veterans. In: Proceedings of international society for pharmacoepidemiology international conference on pharmacoepidemiology and therapeutic risk management, Chicago

National Coordinating Council for Medication Error Reporting and Prevention (1998) What is a medication error? Rockville. http://www.nccmerp.org. Accessed 30 Dec 2011

Nebeker JR, Barach P, Samore MH (2004) Clarifying adverse drug events: a clinician's guide to terminology, documentation, and reporting. Ann Intern Med 140:795–801

Papaioannou A, Clarke JA, Campbell G, Bédard M (2000) Assessment of adherence to renal dosing guidelines in long-term care facilities. J Am Geriatr Soc 48:1470–1473

Rahimi AR, Kennedy K, Thomason M et al (2008) Improper renal dosing in long-term care facilities. South Med J 101:802–805

Ryan C, O'Mahony D, Kennedy J et al (2009) Potentially inappropriate prescribing in an Irish elderly population in primary care. Br J Clin Pharmacol 68:936–947

Schmader KE, Hanlon JT, Pieper CF et al (2004) Effects of geriatric evaluation and management on adverse drug reactions and suboptimal prescribing in the frail elderly. Am J Med 116:394–401

Shrank WH, Polinski JM, Avorn J (2007) Quality indicators for medication use in vulnerable elders. J Am Geriatr Soc 55:S373–S382

Spinewine A, Schmader KE, Barber N et al (2007a) Appropriate prescribing in elderly people: how can it be measured and optimised? Lancet 370:173–184

Spinewine A, Swine C, Dhillon S et al (2007b) Effect of a collaborative approach on the quality of prescribing for geriatric inpatients: a randomized, controlled trial. J Am Geriatr Soc 55:658–665

Steinman MA, Handler SM, Gurwitz JH et al (2011) Beyond the prescription: medication monitoring and adverse drug events in older adults. J Am Geriatr Soc 59:1513–1520

Stevens LA, Levey AS (2005) Chronic kidney disease in the elderly—how to assess risk. N Engl J Med 352:2122–2124

Taipale HT, Hartikainen S, Bell JS (2010) A comparison of four methods to quantify the cumulative effect of taking multiple drugs with sedative properties. Am J Geriatr Pharmacother 8:460–471

Vidal L, Shavit M, Fraser A et al (2005) Systematic comparison of four sources of drug information regarding adjustment of dose for renal function. BMJ 331:263

Wright RM, Sloane R, Pieper CM et al (2009) Underuse of indicated medications among physically frail older U.S. Veterans at time of hospital discharge: results of a cross-sectional analysis of data from the Geriatric Evaluation and Management Drug Study. Am J Geriatr Pharmacother 7:271–280

Zimmerman S, Love K, Sloane PD et al (2011) Medication administration errors in assisted living: scope, characteristics, and the importance of staff training. J Am Geriatr Soc 59:1060–1068

Zint K, Haefeli WE, Glynn RJ et al (2010) Impact of drug interactions, dosage, and duration of therapy on the risk of hip fracture associated with benzodiazepine use in older adults. Pharmacoepidemiol Drug Saf 19:1248–1255

Special Aspects with Respect to Organ Systems Based on Geriatric Clinical Importance

Arterial Hypertension

Martin Wehling

Relevance for Elderly Patients, Epidemiology

Arterial hypertension is the most frequent cardiovascular disease and is one of the very important age-related diseases. Elderly people (65+ years) represent the most rapidly growing population cohort in industrialized countries. This development is termed *demographic revolution*, and it is obvious that it will dramatically increase the prevalence of this disease. In 70+-year-old patients, the prevalence of arterial (in particular systolic hypertension >140 mmHg) hypertension is at 70% compared to only 30–50% in younger adults, and it is still on the rise (Plouin et al. 2006). The deleterious effects of hypertension are well known—stroke, myocardial infarction, heart failure, renal failure—all of which massively contribute to morbidity and mortality of aging societies. Of all deaths, 13%, in countries with high income even 18%, are attributable to hypertension (Lawes et al. 2008). In 2001, disability-adjusted life years (DALYs) due to hypertension were most frequent in countries with high income in women aged 60+ years and in men aged 70+ years (Fig. 1).

The success of sufficient control of arterial hypertension in terms of morbidity and mortality reduction is without any reasonable doubt, and this evidence is at least 25 years old. The famous Framingham study was one of the earliest to detect a highly relevant 60% difference of cardiovascular mortality and a 31% difference of total mortality between treated and untreated hypertensives (Sytkowski et al. 1996). Meanwhile, studies have extended evidence for the impressively positive treatment effects into patients of higher age, such as the SYST-EUR study, which demonstrated a 42% reduction of stroke after 4 years of treatment by nitrendipine and enalapril in 60+-year-old patients (Staessen et al. 1999). More recently, HYVET showed a relevant, positive endpoint effect of blood pressure lowering even in 80+-year-old hypertensives (Beckett et al. 2008).

The large epidemiological impact of arterial hypertension, especially in the elderly population, and the benefits of drug treatment in terms of relevant endpoint effects demonstrated in controlled clinical trials are not debatable and consistently shown. Arterial hypertension is likely to be the disease whose sufficient treatment results in the biggest gains of QALYs (quality adjusted life years) and preventable deaths. Unfortunately, reality shows a dramatic underutilization of care for this highly prevalent treatable condition. In the United States, the latest Centers for Disease Control and Prevention (CDC) report (Keenan et al. 2011) showed an overall prevalence of hypertension of 29.9% in persons aged 18+ years. This analysis was based on National Health and Nutrition Examination Survey

M. Wehling (✉)
University of Heidelberg, Maybachstr. 14, Mannheim 68169, Germany
e-mail: martin.wehling@medma.uni-heidelberg.de

M. Wehling (ed.), *Drug Therapy for the Elderly*,
DOI 10.1007/978-3-7091-0912-0_6, © Springer-Verlag Wien 2013

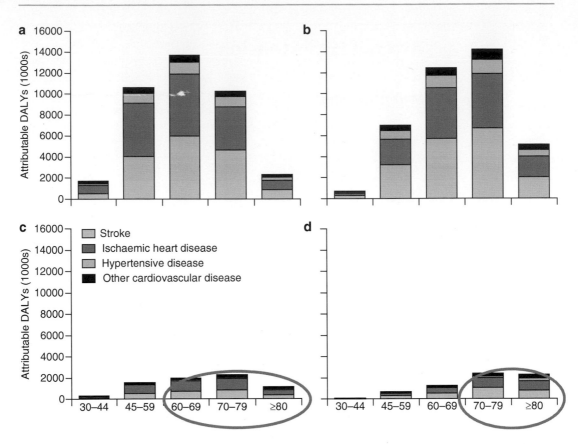

Fig. 1 (**a–d**) Absolute DALYs attributable to arterial hypertension in men (**a, c**) and women (**b, d**) in countries with low and intermediate (**a, b**) and high income (**d, c**) in relation to age groups. The predominant contribution of elderly patients in industrialized countries is annotated by the *circles* in (**c**) and (**d**). The decline of DALYs in men aged 80+ reflects their smaller absolute number; the relative number of DALYs/population size even increases further (not shown). *DALYs* disability-adjusted life years (From Lawes et al. 2008 by kind permission of Elsevier)

(NHANES) data from two survey periods: 2005–2006 and 2007–2008. The age-adjusted prevalence in elderly patients (65+ years) increased to 70.3%. The control rate was 43.7 in patients aged 18+ years and 45.6 in those 65+ years. For comparison, the EUROASPIRE-II Study (Boersma et al. 2003) demonstrated that Germany was "leading" in that the prevalence of hypertension (>140/90 mmHg) in the working population exceeded 50%. The control rate was only 6% (Hense 2000). In a newer study, the control rate in the elderly was even worse than in the younger adults (Milchak et al. 2008).

These facts show that the therapeutic situation of hypertensive patients, especially at higher age, is not satisfactory, and less than half of the patient population is well controlled (for therapeutic goals, see chapter "Coronary Heart Disease and Stroke"). In the United States, hypertension seems to be treated more efficiently than in many European countries; still, one cannot be content.

Like in younger patients, undertreatment results from many causes, including lack of awareness and—probably most important—adherence problems. The latter involve both patients and doctors.

In the elderly, nonadherence (or noncompliance in the older literature) is particularly problematic as age-related factors tend to augment it; this includes polypharmacy and especially all aspects of frailty, including visual and motoric disturbances and dementia. An inverse correlation exists between the number of medications/pills and adherence (Düsing 2001): Adherence was determined to be 86% for one pill/day and dramatically dropped to 25% for four pills/day. As shown in chapter "Critical Extrapolation of Guidelines and Study Results: Risk-Benefit Assessment for Patients with Reduced Life Expectancy and a New Classification of Drugs According to Their Fitness for the Aged", even four is a comparably small number of pills for elderly patients. In a 3-year cohort study in hypertensives, persistence was reduced to 15%, with diuretics exposing the worst persistence (Hasford et al. 2007). According to Conlin et al. (2001), persistence for diuretics drops to 21% after 1 year and to only 16% after 4 years.

In conclusion, arterial hypertension in the elderly is an important, if not the most important, disease regarding mortality and morbidity that can be efficaciously treated even in the very elderly. Unfortunately, one of the biggest inherent problems is the undertreatment of this condition in medical reality.

Therapeutically Relevant Special Features of Elderly Patients

Systolic Hypertension

In elderly patients, aging of the vasculature and other physiological alterations results in characteristics of arterial hypertension that are therapeutically relevant. The leading alteration is the increase of pulse pressure at higher age, which is characterized by a large difference between systolic and diastolic blood pressure. This change reflects the increased stiffness of large arteries in the central parts of circulation, mainly the aorta and proximal arteries (femoral and carotid arteries). The related impairment of the *Windkessel* function describes the reduced capacity of central arteries to take up a portion of the systolic stroke volume and push it back into circulation during diastole. The vessels are expanded by the stroke volume and regain their dimensions passively during cardiac relaxation by elastic forces. A younger person absorbs some of the systolic energy, thereby reducing the systolic increase of blood pressure and maintaining the diastolic pressure by the passive volume contribution. This mechanism prevents

a large pulse amplitude (resembles the water hammer or Corrigan's pulse, mainly used to describe the pulse phenomenon of aortic regurgitation) and helps to maintain the mean arterial pressure at sufficient levels. In the elderly, the reduced Windkessel function thus results in a higher systolic blood pressure, often exceeding 140 mmHg, as the diastolic values even tend to decrease. As systolic blood pressure only contributes 1/3 of the mean pressure, systolic pressure needs to increase twice as much as diastolic pressure decreases to maintain mean arterial pressure.

Figure 2 demonstrates the course of systolic and diastolic blood pressure over age in the United States, and Fig. 3 shows the pronounced rise in the prevalence of systolic hypertension at higher age.

For long it was debated whether isolated systolic hypertension represents a cardiovascular risk factor as in many cases it seems balanced by lower diastolic values at higher age, and mean arterial pressure (=1/3 systolic +2/3 diastolic blood pressure) thus does not necessarily increase. The pivotal question, therefore, concerned the treatment indication in isolated systolic hypertension to prevent clinical endpoints of the disease (stroke, myocardial infarction, heart failure, renal failure).

Meanwhile, there is a clear answer, and not many other areas in medicine are based on a comparable wealth of data: Isolated systolic hypertension is a very relevant risk factor for cardiovascular complications. Large epidemiological trials clearly showed that this condition was of paramount importance for the prognosis of patients, and in particular, this was true for elderly patients. Systolic blood pressure and pulse pressure (=difference between systolic and diastolic blood pressure) are strictly correlated with an age-adapted rate of cardiovascular events, as opposed to the diastolic values, which do not correlate with endpoints (Alderman 1999).

This situation creates a problem that is relevant to the elderly patients: An 80-year-old patient with an initial blood pressure of 160/60 mmHg, which should have the systolic pressure lowered to 140 mmHg, could face a further reduction of the diastolic value. As mean arterial pressure particularly reflects diastolic pressure,

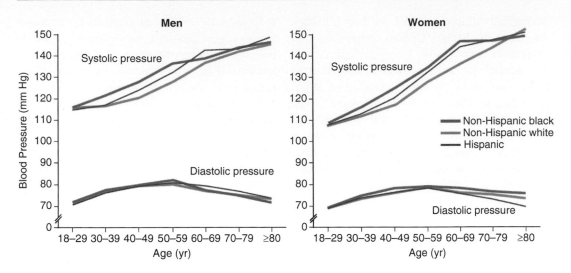

Fig. 2 Systolic and diastolic blood pressure over age in the United States (From Chobanian 2007 by kind permission of the Massachusetts Medical Society)

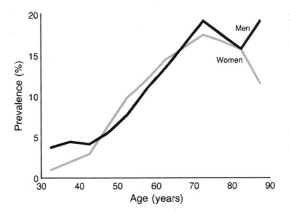

Fig. 3 Prevalence of systolic hypertension (>140 mmHg) sharply rises with increasing age (From Sagie et al. 1993 by kind permission of the Massachusetts Medical Society)

vascular perfusion may deteriorate, and the patient could become symptomatic for cerebral hypoperfusion (dizziness, loss of consciousness) or even develop thromboembolic disease (e.g., myocardial infarction or stroke). This means that those endpoints that should be prevented by anti-hypertensive therapy may be precipitated by it, and the outcome is negative rather than beneficial. This fact is commonly termed the J-curve phenomenon as there is an optimal therapeutic range of blood pressure, with higher endpoint rates both at blood pressure values too high *and* too low. The simple interpretation is that blood pressure lowering may be overdone, particularly in the elderly. This "Scylla-and-Charybdis" situation requires compromises regarding the therapeutic goal, and the desired systolic goal value of 140 mmHg (see below) may not be achievable if diastolic pressure drops too low. Heart rate should not be lowered as this results in an increased pulse pressure (increased stroke volume: fewer beats need to pump larger volumes per beat); beta-blockers are not advantageous for this (and other) reason(s). By no means is it justified to demand an elevated ("compensatory") blood pressure at higher age as it was reflected in former days by the lethal formula: Target systolic blood pressure (mmHg) = 100 + age (years).

The target for systolic blood pressure is 140 mmHg (maybe 140–145 at age 80+ years) at all ages; there is no demand for higher values at high age per se. However, should diastolic values decrease below 60 mmHg, higher systolic values should be accepted to avoid complications. The same holds true if orthostatic symptoms occur or a fall in systolic blood pressure by more than 15 mmHg is detected on standing.

Additional Age-Related Alterations of Relevance for Antihypertensive Therapy

The age-related impairment of *kidney function* (see chapter "Age-Associated General Pharmacological Aspects") is relevant not only for the dosing of renally excreted antihypertensives such as atenolol and has definitely to be considered in this context. It is also very important for the choice of compounds that precipitate hyperkalemia or induce renal impairment (ACE [angiotensin-converting enzyme] inhibitors, angiotensin receptor antagonists, mineralocorticoid antagonists) or for thiazide diuretics, which become ineffective at renal clearance rates of less than 50 ml/min.

Cardiovascular aging or cardiac diseases such as myocardial infarction or heart failure, which often occurred long ago, render the heart vulnerable to arrhythmias. This is important in relation to antihypertensive diuretic therapy, which may increase this vulnerability due to electrolyte disturbances, especially hypokalemia. The proarrhythmic effect of these drugs is especially pronounced at high age. This aspect has to be considered in the long-term treatment of arterial hypertension, and diagnostic measures such as Holter monitoring need to be taken. Unfortunately, the topic of arrhythmia induction by diuretics in the elderly is not well covered by research, but these drugs are under strong suspicion to cause excess mortality in this patient population.

In this context of cardiac diseases interacting with drug therapy, it is important to note that disturbances of cardiac conductance and triggering of heart actions need to be considered as well in the choice of antihypertensive drugs, especially the sick sinus syndrome or atrioventricular heart block situations. Absolute contraindications of beta-blockers or calcium channel blockers of the verapamil or diltiazem type have to be carefully respected and relative contraindications weighed against net benefits. Resting electrocardiogram (ECG) recording is mandatory prior to initiation of antihypertensive therapy, especially in the elderly. In the presence of bradycardia, it may be necessary to implant a simple pacemaker system that increases resting pulse rate and thereby improves systolic "hammer pulse" hypertension (discussed previously in this chapter).

Heart failure is a frequent condition of elderly patients and requires special care regarding negative inotropes in antihypertensive therapy, such as beta-blockers, which however have a dual indication in these patients. They treat not only hypertension but also heart failure. Beta-blockers need to be started at low doses to avoid transitory cardiac depression. Calcium channel blockers of the verapamil and diltiazem types are strictly forbidden, and this is expressed by the well-known contraindication in the labeling.

Dementia and vascular cerebral lesions are further important diseases or conditions potentially interacting with antihypertensive therapy. Cognitive impairment may occur if effective antihypertensive treatment is installed; confusion and dizziness are particularly frequent if the blood pressure is rapidly lowered to "normal." This was one of the main observations leading to the long-standing fiction of *compensatory hypertension*. There is the general rule to reduce blood pressure from critical values (>160 mmHg) rapidly (within a few days), while the fine-tuning into the range of treatment goals should be done slowly. This fine-tuning (to reach the general treatment goal of systolic pressure <140 mmHg) may easily require half a year. Impaired organ perfusion should recover during this time of slowly stepped-up therapy, and lower blood pressure readings will be better tolerated by the patient with fewer symptoms such as confusion, vertigo, or hypotension.

The decreased capacity of cardiovascular regulatory compensation in elderly patients often results in orthostatic or persistent hypotensive problems, especially during initiation of therapy.

The impact of the reduced compensatory mechanisms to maintain hemodynamic homeostasis in the elderly is widely underestimated. It is a major threat to these patients as it increases fall risk, and thereby morbidity and even mortality. This fact demands careful attention and special caution in the treatment of arterial hypertension in the elderly. Long-acting compounds with only small fluctuations of their pharmacokinetics are mandatory. Nifedipine serves as an example of a drug to be avoided as even in slow-release preparations rapid uptake and degradation of the compound destabilize blood pressure regulation and may be deleterious. Unfortunately, it needs to be pointed out that all antihypertensive therapies may precipitate hypotension and related problems, including hypoperfusion syndromes. This can only be addressed by intense monitoring of blood pressure effects; therefore, it is mandatory to take readings not only in the sitting but also in the standing positions. Orthostasis testing may show surprising reactions to standing in that significant decreases of systolic blood pressure below 100 mmHg without an adequate response of heart rate will be measured. Normal values in the sitting position do not exclude these hypotensive reactions in the elderly, which are the detectable correlates of clinically relevant orthostatic problems as side effects of antihypertensive therapy.

Other age-related alterations, such as the reduced gastrointestinal absorption of drugs or adherence problems, are generic, but particularly relevant in hypertension treatment as this condition is very common in the elderly.

In conclusion, organ alterations in elderly patients that are most relevant in the cardiovascular system, the kidneys, and the brain need to be reflected in the choice and dosing of antihypertensive drugs in the elderly.

Evidence-Based, Rationalistic Drug Therapy and Classification of Drugs According to Their Fitness for the Aged (FORTA)

Successful antihypertensive therapy has various dimensions that are only efficacious in their balanced combination, and this also applies to elderly patients.
- Lifestyle changes (weight reduction, low-salt diet without "social drugs" like caffeine or alcohol, smoking cessation, physical exercise, relaxation therapy, treatment of sleep disorders and others),

- Exclusion of secondary, thus treatable forms of arterial hypertension (e.g., endocrine disorders like Morbus Cushing or pheochromocytoma; sleep apnea, which causes or aggravates hypertension in as many as 30% of patients) and, finally,
- Drug therapy

are the major components of a complex strategy.

It should be mentioned that drugs may not only lower but some may even increase blood pressure. In the elderly, nonsteroidal anti-inflammatory drugs (NSAIDs) are the major culprits in this context as the prevalence of degenerative diseases of joints and other skeletal structures is sharply rising with age; hip, knee, and spinal joint problems are the key drivers for excessive NSAID consumption in 80+-year-old persons. Often, the family doctor does not even know about this medication, which is obtained over the counter (OTC) in the United States. In Europe, without OTC availability of NSAIDs, the problem is not much less severe. Someone will give the drug to suffering patients: friends, relatives, or doctors who gave up fighting NSAIDs.

As a rule of thumb, one can assume that in the presence of an NSAID medication
- One antihypertensive drug in excess of former drugs is required to control blood pressure, or
- Hypertension will become overt in those few elderly patients without former disease.

There is no significant difference between nonspecific cyclooxygenase (COX) inhibitors and specific COX-II inhibitors. In essence, the application of an NSAID leads to the requirement to readjust blood pressure control, which normally means intensify therapy, and the cessation of this medication (which is much rarer) requires the same (mostly reduction of therapy).

Systemic glucocorticoids (to treat, e.g., collagenoses, especially vascular forms such as arteriitis temporalis, or chronic obstructive pulmonary disease [COPD], which is highly prevalent in the elderly) represent another drug class leading to arterial hypertension, which has to be treated accordingly.

Epidemiologic data clearly demonstrate that drug therapy of arterial hypertension is highly efficacious even in the elderly. This fact is encouraging, and the data situation is comparably positive (meaning that clinical data exist for this condition in the elderly as opposed to many other therapeutic situations in gerontopharmacology). In the United States, the Joint National Committee on Prevention, Detection, Evaluation, and Treatment of High Blood Pressure Report (JNC) 7 (Chobanian et al. 2003) urgently needs updating and devotes just two pages to the elderly; the European ESC (European Society of Cardiology) and ESH (European Society of Hypertension) guideline (Mancia et al. 2007, 2009) devotes only one (see chapter "Critical Extrapolation of Guidelines and Study Results: Risk-Benefit Assessment for Patients with Reduced Life Expectancy and a New Classification of Drugs According to Their Fitness for the Aged"). Fortunately, on May 17, 2011, the first consensus document on the treatment of hypertension in the elderly was published (Aronow et al. 2011) that extensively and comprehensively detailed all major aspects of hypertension treatment in the elderly in 81 pages.

In practice, treatment strategies for the elderly are not principally different from those for younger adults, and in accordance with the aims of this book (not to repeat what is written in standard textbooks), they are outlined here only briefly. Indication for drugs follows these guidelines; first-line therapies are chosen from the five main groups of antihypertensives:
– Diuretics
– Beta-blockers
– Renin-angiotensin system (RAS) blockers:
  – ACE inhibitors
  – Angiotensin receptor antagonists
– Dihydropyridine calcium channel blockers

As in younger patients, only a few elderly hypertensives will be sufficiently treated by monotherapy; combination therapy is the rule rather than the exception (>80% of patients).

Antihypertensive drugs expose effects beyond blood pressure lowering; these additional properties and clinical data (if available) guide the choice of the right drug for the individual elderly patient. This may result in a deviation from therapy in younger adults. Fortunately, there is a comparably large set of studies on treatment of hypertension in the elderly, probably the largest

data set in this age group. The major studies in this context are SHEP, STOP-2, SYST-EUR, LIFE, ACCOMPLISH, and recently HYVET. While SHEP showed in principle that treatment of hypertension by beta-blockers/diuretics significantly lowers the rate of stroke compared with placebo in 60+-year-old patients, HYVET demonstrated this for the diuretic indapamide plus the ACE inhibitor perindopril in the very elderly (80+ years) for the first time. STOP-2 was the first study to compare old and new antihypertensives in the elderly; the new (at that time) antihypertensives ACE inhibitors and calcium channel blockers were not inferior to the old drugs, diuretics and beta-blockers. Results from SYST-EUR were impressive as a combination therapy of a calcium channel blocker plus an ACE inhibitor significantly decreased the incidence of stroke in elderly patients by 42%. In LIFE, the beta-blocker atenolol and the angiotensin receptor antagonist losartan were compared in elderly patients; losartan was significantly more efficacious in preventing clinical endpoints than atenolol. ACCOMPLISH had to be terminated prematurely as the fixed combination of benazepril and hydrochlorothiazide resulted in significantly more clinical endpoints (+20%) than the fixed combination of amlodipine and benazepril. As an example, the pivotal data from HYVET are shown in Fig. 4.

These studies and other evidence support a differentiation of antihypertensive drugs that is discussed for the different drug classes in the following chapters.

Diuretics

Relevant data are available only for thiazide diuretics, mainly for hydrochlorothiazide and indapamid, which should be employed at low doses only (e.g., 12.5–25 mg/day hydrochlorothiazide). Impaired kidney function (estimated creatinine clearance below 50 ml/min, Cockcroft-Gault formula as an example, see chapter "Age-Associated General Pharmacological Aspects") renders thiazides ineffective; in this case, they should be replaced by loop diuretics, especially by torsemide, which is pharmacokinetically preferable

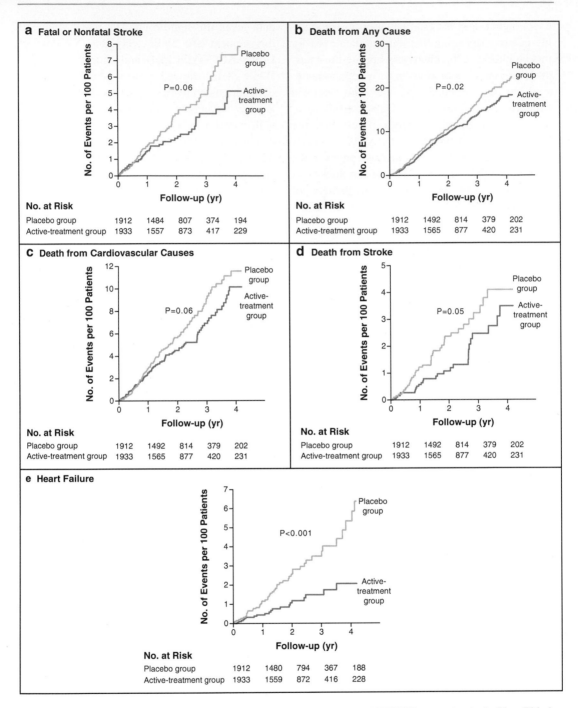

Fig. 4 Endpoint data of HYVET: antihypertensive treatment is successful even in 80+-year-old patients. The diuretic indapamide and the ACE inhibitor perindopril as additional antihypertensive if needed were tested versus placebo. *HYVET* Hypertension in the Very Elderly Trial (From Beckett et al. 2008 by kind permission of the Massachusetts Medical Society)

to frusemide (longer half-life, stable absorption as advantages). Potassium-sparing diuretics (e.g., triamterene) are dangerous in aged patients as hyperkalemia may occur rapidly and unforeseeably in particular if kidney function is reduced. Spironolactone (see chapter on "Heart Failure") is just mentioned here as a second-line drug for refractory hypertension, which is dangerous to elderly patients with compromised renal function also because of the hyperkalemia risk. Its indication should be limited to a few refractory patients in whom serum potassium is frequently measured.

Pros (thiazide diuretics):
– Data from several (old) studies, for indapamide even in 80+-year-old patients.
– In the subgroup of elderly patients from ALL-HAT equally effective for endpoint compared to ACE inhibitors or calcium channel blockers.
– Also treats heart failure as concomitant disease.
– Low costs.

Cons:
– Increases incidence of diabetes mellitus; aggravates existing diabetes mellitus.
– Electrolyte disorders are critical in the elderly, especially because of cardiac complications (arrhythmias triggered by hypokalemia); hyponatremia may induce delirium, confusion, irreversible cerebral damage.
– In ACCOMPLISH inferior to a calcium channel blocker (amlodipine) at endpoint level.
– Worst adherence data within all antihypertensive drug classes; will be the first to be thrown away by patient; to recommend diuretics is almost like recommending nontreatment.

The last point is particularly critical in elderly patients as they often suffer from incontinence or urinary retention (men with benign prostate hyperplasia); thus, diuretic-induced polyuria in the morning results in patients' rejection of these drugs. As a consequence, the use of diuretics in elderly patients should be handled in a more restrictive way than in current practice. The low price of diuretics is seducing doctors to overuse them.

Problems are severely augmented if the unintentional and irrational combination of loop plus thiazide diuretic is considered, causing the so-called sequential nephron blockade.

This condition blocks the ability of the kidneys to compensate for an excessive natriuresis by loop diuretics in the distal tubulus. If that nephron segment is also blocked by a thiazide, massive electrolyte disturbances may be rapidly induced. This most powerful diuretic combination is reserved for the most severe states of heart or renal failure and should only be instituted when dose escalation of loop diuretics (e.g., torsemide up to 200 mg/day) is not sufficient to correct fluid retention. Unfortunately, the combination is often prescribed unintentionally when a combination preparation containing hydrochlorothiazide remains in the drug cocktail despite addition of a loop diuretic. The thiazide component may be overlooked as in trade names its presence may not be explicitly stated (e.g., in Hyzaar® or Avalide®). The consequences of accidental sequential blockade of the nephron may be grave; in the best scenario, just dehydration may occur, which causes symptoms and urges the patient to stop all medications, including the culprit ones. In the worst scenario, dramatic electrolyte disorders (hypokalemia, hyponatremia) or dehydration thromboses in the deep venous system may develop. As a major downside, this problem has not yet been well studied in medical science; it should become a major focus of clinical research in the future. Unfortunately, almost all diuretics are off patent; thus, no interest in developing them further can be expected from the pharmaceutical industry. Diuretic therapy represents one of the few cardiovascular therapy areas in which overtreatment in terms of both indication and dosing is common, while in almost all other areas undertreatment is the main problem.

Beta-Blockers

Beta-blockers are major pillars of cardiovascular therapy but have lost ground in antihypertensive treatment strategies in recent years. The LIFE study has been mentioned; it showed a superiority of losartan over atenolol regarding clinical endpoints (25% fewer strokes under losartan). In an attempt to explain the difference, the CAFÉ

Study demonstrated that atenolol has an inferior effect on blood pressure in the central circulation if compared to amlodipine. Both compounds lower peripheral blood pressure equipotently, but pressures in the aorta were higher in the presence of atenolol. The beta-blocker does not decrease arterial wall stiffness as opposed to the comparator in CAFÉ, amlodipine, causing an augmented pulse wave reflection in the periphery. This "whiplash" effect and the impaired Windkessel function (see previous discussion) in elderly patients are considered reasons for increased central blood pressure values.

Pros (beta-blockers):
- Positive data (mainly from older studies).
- Concomitant treatment of cardiac diseases, especially coronary heart disease (CHD), atrial fibrillation, heart failure, for which controlled trials clearly demonstrated endpoint benefits, including mortality reduction.
- Low costs.

Cons:
- Increases incidence of diabetes mellitus; aggravates existing diabetes mellitus.
- In recent studies inferior to angiotensin receptor antagonists (losartan) and calcium channel blockers (amlodipine) regarding clinical endpoints.
- Many elderly patients do not tolerate beta-blockers, especially because of increasing incidences of relative and absolute contraindications, such as heart block, pulmonary diseases (COPD), and diabetes/metabolic syndrome.
- Erectile dysfunction is a problem with relevance not only to younger, but also to elderly patients.

In antihypertensive treatment, beta-blockers will still be frequently used despite their disadvantages, as cardiac diseases mandate their prescription, and the combination of hypertension and CHD is very common. In elderly hypertensives without cardiac indications for beta-blockers, their use should be restrictive within the first-line therapy, even in the absence of contraindications, and only be used as a third or fourth antihypertensive drug. As an important feature concerning the choice of beta-blockers, only those that efficiently lower heart rate should be prescribed. This requires a full antagonistic activity (see the following discussion and chapter "Coronary Heart Disease and Stroke") and thus the absence of an intrinsic sympathomimetic activity (ISA). Examples for "good" heart-rate-lowering beta-blockers are metoprolol, bisoprolol, and carvedilol.

Though principally belonging to this group, atenolol is disadvantageous in the elderly; they often have reduced renal function (see chapter "Age-Associated General Pharmacological Aspects"), and this drug has to be renally excreted. It cannot be metabolized in the liver like the aforementioned lipophilic compounds. Beta-blockers with ISA (e.g., pindolol or in Europe celiprolol) should not be used in the elderly. Nebivolol does not reduce heart rate efficiently due to additional vasodilatory effects; its benefits for elderly hypertensive patients are not clearly shown.

ACE Inhibitors/Angiotensin Receptor Antagonists

The ACE inhibitors and angiotensin receptor antagonists are discussed together as they interfere with the same hormone system, the RAS. They thus expose similar effects. Differential effects are still a matter of debate (e.g., on one hand effects on bradykinin only by ACE inhibitors, on the other hand a more complete blockade of the RAS by angiotensin receptor antagonists). Without reasonable doubt, members from either group were successful in clinical trials on elderly hypertensives (such as STOP-2, SYST-EUR, LIFE, SCOPE, ACCOMPLISH, HYVET). In reflection of their outstanding tolerability, they are in the first line of antihypertensive treatment in the elderly. About 5% of patients develop clinically relevant *coughing* under ACE inhibitors, which then should be replaced by angiotensin receptor antagonists. They were the first drugs with a "placebo-like" incidence of side effects. The clear-cut benefits at the endpoint level have been attributed to effects exceeding blood pressure lowering, in particular organ protection in the kidneys and the heart ("remodeling" as a key term). Regarding metabolism, these compounds are at least neutral, and even a reduction of the incidence of diabetes mellitus by these drugs is being discussed. As for all antihypertensives, there are clear differential indications for RAS inhibitors as they are also indicated in heart failure and, partly, CHD. The cost argument often stressed as a disadvantage of angiotensin receptor antagonists representing the almost-last high-price antihypertensives is no longer valid; more and more compounds lose their patent protection, with losartan starting this series in 2010.

In spite of these favorable features, a few cautions need to be mentioned:

– For hemodynamic reasons, pressure in the Bowman's capsules of the nephron is reduced in reflection of a preferential dilation of the vas efferens. Although therapeutically beneficial for renal protection, this effect leads to an acute reduction of glomerular filtration by an average of 8%. Much larger effects may be seen, especially in the elderly, as interindividual scattering is considerable and seems to widen at higher age. Thus, at creatinine clearance levels below 30 ml/min (which in elderly sarcopenic patients may be indicated by a minimally elevated serum creatinine level of only 1.3 mg/dl), initiation of therapy should not be done in the ambulatory setting. Otherwise, the patient may develop acute renal failure, rapidly require dialysis, or even die of hyperkalemia. It is thus recommended to start RAS inhibition in these patients in the hospital under close surveillance of renal parameters; this effort is justified as the initiation of RAS blockade will beneficially alter the course of renal failure even in moderate and severe renal failure. The break-even point for patients with acute deterioration, but less progress of renal impairment, by the initiation of RAS inhibition compared to those without

RAS inhibition is reached within a few months; from then, patients on RAS inhibition show a benefit regarding kidney function.

– Proteinuria is particularly sensitive to amendment by RAS inhibition, and recommendations reflect this fact by a therapeutic goal for systolic blood pressure of only 125 mmHg; unfortunately, this target level is hard to achieve in the elderly as hypotensive side effects (see previous discussion) will limit therapy in a fraction of patients, which sharply increases with age.

– If renal impairment exceeds 30–50% of initial levels after the start of RAS inhibition, renal artery stenoses (one sided and two sided) should be suspected.

RAS inhibitors are frequently involved in drug-drug interactions, which are mainly caused at the pharmacodynamic level; the classical pharmacokinetic drug-drug interactions are by far less relevant. In this context, interactions with NSAIDs are prominent (see previous discussion), especially in conjunction with dehydration (in the elderly often induced by gastrointestinal infections, but also hot weather or—sadly—care neglect). This combination (dehydration, RAS inhibition, NSAID) may rapidly lead to acute, severe renal failure, and dialysis often necessitated by hyperkalemia is the only adequate treatment. Spironolactone aggravates this situation.

Though principally possible, the combination of ACE inhibitors and angiotensin receptor antagonists does not lead to adequate effect augmentation as the same system is interfered with. Combination therapy should address different systems to optimize gains. In addition, the combination of both RAS inhibition principles seems to be associated with complications. The large ONTARGET study showed (although not explicitly for elderly patients) that ACE inhibitor and angiotensin receptor antagonist were equipotent, and the combination was not more effective than the individual compounds. Unfortunately, the incidence of hypotension was increased for the combination, and this effect is expected to be even more pronounced in the elderly (see previous discussion).

Pros (ACE inhibitor/angiotensin receptor antagonist):

- Excellent background of clinical data, including those from elderly patients
- Concomitant therapy of heart failure, CHD, comorbidities for which clear mortality data exist
- Compelling mechanistic evidence for organ protective effects, especially in the kidneys (diabetic and nondiabetic nephropathy) and the heart (remodelling in atrial fibrillation and heart failure)
- Metabolically neutral or even protective against diabetes mellitus
- Low costs, also beginning to apply for angiotensin receptor antagonists

Cons:

- Caution: renal failure, especially at start of therapy
- Caution: NSAID/dehydration

From my point of view, RAS blockers are the best drugs for the initiation of antihypertensive treatment in the elderly.

Dihydropyridine Calcium Channel Blockers

Dihydropyridine calcium channel blockers had an eventful history. The first drug in this group, nifedipine, was problematic and devaluated the principle as it has unfavorable pharmacokinetics with short half-life and extreme maximum plasma levels. These extremes lead to adrenergic counterregulation detectable by tachycardia and arrhythmias, which were lethal for some patients with unstable angina. All these disadvantages are invalid for the newer long-acting members of the group, with amlodipine as the prototype (half-life time 35 h). For longer-acting dihydropyridines, impressive data on beneficial effects even in elderly hypertensives are available (e.g., in SYST-EUR for nitrendipine or ACCOMPLISH for amlodipine). As there are only a few contraindications and tolerability is excellent in the absence of the unfavorable pharmacokinetics of

nifedipine, this group of antihypertensives has moved into the first line of treatment in the elderly. Relevant problems relate to the induction of local ankle edema in up to 20% of patients, though the incidence should be lower with newer compounds like lercanidipine (not available in the United States). Ankle edema is pathophysiologically different from edema in heart failure and rather reflects a local mismatch of vascular tone in the arterial and venous vasculature. Resistance arterioles are preferentially dilated by these drugs, resulting in an increased blood flow into the tissue, while venules are not affected. They thus do not allow for the increased outflow, which would be necessary to match increased inflow. In the lower parts of the body, gravity adds to this mismatch, and ankle edema develops. The mechanism explains why this form of edema does not reflect heart failure and does not respond to diuretics, which should be avoided in this situation. As an option with clinical relevance, the combination with RAS inhibitors significantly reduces the incidence of ankle edema as these compounds dilate not only arterioles but also venules and thus amend the mismatch.

Pros (dihydropyridine calcium channel blockers):

- Excellent background of clinical data, including those from elderly patients with systolic hypertension
- Metabolically neutral
- Low costs

Cons:

- Caution: hypotension on initiation of therapy
- Ankle edema, causing ineffective therapy with diuretics

These considerations support the following order of escalating drug therapy for elderly "uncomplicated hypertensives" (as those uncomplicated hypertensives represent only 10–15% of the hypertensive population, this is a rule for the exception rather than a general rule):

- Start with RAS inhibitor: ACE inhibitor or angiotensin receptor antagonist.

– If not sufficient, add long-acting dihydropyridine calcium channel blocker.
– Add beta-blocker.
– Add diuretic.

The two final positions are interchangeable. As said previously, in rare cases only this order is not disturbed by concomitant diseases or conditions in the elderly patient, and a more extensive elaboration does not seem justified.

Therapy with second-line drugs (as opposed to first-line drugs mentioned with the fine-tuning indicating differentiated levels within the first line) should only be briefly mentioned here. If first-line drugs are not sufficient to control blood pressure, the most frequent cause of "resistant hypertension" should be excluded: noncompliance. Only then second-line drugs in hypertension treatment should be considered, which inevitably also means that side effects are frequent and data in the elderly scarce or absent.

– Alpha-blockers (e.g., doxazosin) may be preferable in elder men with benign prostate hyperplasia.
– Clonidine is tolerated by elderly even less than by younger patients as problems with mucous membranes ("dry eye, dry mouth"), impaired vision, and orthostasis are often pre-existing and will be aggravated by this drug. Delirium, dizziness, and syncopes are other problems rendering this drug almost absolutely contraindicated in the elderly. If therapy is stopped, caution should be exercised, and stepwise dose reduction is mandatory to prevent hypertensive crises.
– Hydralazine should be reserved to treat end-stage renal failure patients as it is fraught by side effects, caused by arterial dilation, such as reflex tachycardia and arrhythmias. In addition, risk of allergic complications is not small.
– The adventure of applying minoxidil to elderly patients should be ultimately avoided if possible as side effects such as adrenergic activation with tachycardia and fluid retention are common and need to be treated by beta-blockers and diuretics; stimulated hair growth is another problem especially for women.

General Rules for the Antihypertensive Treatment of Elderly Patients

The main rule for antihypertensive treatment of elderly patients is described by the slogan "start low, go slow" meaning that the initiation of treatment, at least at systolic values below 170 mmHg, should be instituted at low starting doses. Treatment needs to be frequently monitored by blood pressure readings. As a rule of thumb, half of the normal starting dose is recommended, and for low-weight patients with sarcopenia, even only one fourth Monotherapy is the obvious initial choice in many patients, but combination therapy with small doses of the components may be advisable from the beginning if initial systolic pressure is greater than 180 mmHg. An algorithm from JNC 7 is depicted in Fig. 5.

A dilemma in the treatment of patients with systolic hypertension, thus the majority of elderly hypertensives, is the induction of a hypoperfusion syndrome in reflection of diastolic values falling too low. Several studies and epidemiological evidence showed that clinical endpoints, especially in patients with pre-existing cardiovascular disease, increase at diastolic values below 60 mmHg, thus representing the lower end of a J-curve. This is noted in JNC 7, and the ESC/ESH guidelines recommend 60 mmHg as a lower therapeutic limit. In SYST-EUR, however, values of 55 mmHg were not associated with increased endpoint rates. Apart from that, the occurrence of orthostatic or confusion complaints should limit actions to lower blood pressure even if systolic pressure is not a goal. A second attempt to intensify treatment may be undertaken at a later time when the patient has achieved better tolerability of low values. As an additional option, bradycardia may cause hypoperfusion symptoms, and pacemaker therapy is a definite cure.

In the assessment of side effects by antihypertensive treatment, major focuses should be the detection of cognitive impairment by rapid lowering of blood pressure; the potential increase of fall risk, especially in frail patients;

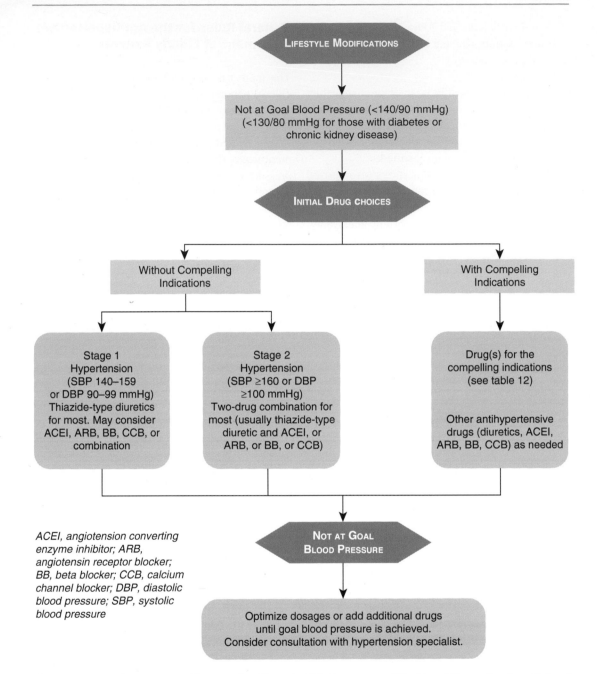

Fig. 5 Algorithm for treatment of hypertension (From the U.S. Department of Health and Human Services, National Institutes of Health National Heart, Lung, and Blood Institute National High Blood Pressure Education Program 2004)

and in particular electrolyte disorders and deterioration of renal function.

To detect orthostatic reactions, blood pressure readings should be taken in the standing position in all elderly hypertensives; a decrease of systolic pressure by 15–20 mmHg immediately after the postural change from sitting to standing should be taken as an indicator of overtreatment. Ambulatory 24-h measurement of blood pressure is a valuable instrument, mainly to detect nocturnal hypotension. It should be performed when readings at home and in the practice are acceptable, but patients are complaining about dizziness, disorientation, or headaches in the morning.

The right choice of antihypertensive drugs requires the diagnosis of concomitant diseases and preexisting conditions of relevance for the therapy, such as kidney function. In the elderly patient, the number of additional diagnoses, and thus therapy-modifying conditions, sharply increases with age.

Thus, the therapeutic goal for an elderly hypertensive is to lower systolic blood pressure to 140 mmHg if diastolic blood pressure does not fall below 60 mmHg or orthostatic reactions are shown in the postural maneuver. The last conditions are increasingly met at higher age, so that a systolic pressure of 140 mmHg cannot be reached in an increasing fraction of elderly patients, especially in those aged 80+ years. The new consensus guideline (Aronow et al. 2011) **recommends a systolic pressure of 140–145 mmHg in patients 80+ years of age.**

Important measures to improve drug adherence in elderly hypertensives:
- Use of fixed combination products to reduce pill numbers
- Give profound information to patients, relatives, and caregivers
- Establishment of a clear therapeutic plan
- Use of containers that can easily be opened by the elderly, not only children ("childproof" containers are a true obstacle mainly to elderly patients, in many instances not to children)
- Sufficient letter size for presbyopic patients
- Therapeutic guidance of patients
- Use of drug dispensers or blister containers with individual treatments

A socioeconomic approach to elderly patients should help to gain an overview of the patient's situation; it should help to avoid handing extensive therapeutic plans to a person with dementia who only occasionally finds the way to the doctor's office. The involvement of relatives, friends, or caregivers is essential, but this trivial requirement is often not met in practice. Blister packs containing the weekly or monthly individual medication have proven helpful and should be utilized.

Classification of Antihypertensive Drugs According to Their Fitness for the Aged (FORTA)

In this classification of antihypertensive drugs according to their Fitness for the Aged (FORTA), the same compounds may receive alternative marks if applied in different indications (see chapter "Critical Extrapolation of Guidelines and Study Results: Risk-Benefit Assessment for Patients with Reduced Life Expectancy and a New Classification of Drugs According to Their Fitness for the Aged")

Diuretics	B
Beta-blockers	B
RAS blockers	
ACE-inhibitors	A
Angiotensin receptor antagonist	A
Long-acting dihydropyridine calcium channel blockers	A
Calcium channel blockers, verapamil type	D
Spironolactone	C
Alpha-blockers	C
Clonidine	D
Minoxidil	D

This classification denominating even three groups of antihypertensives in class A demonstrates that treatment of arterial hypertension in the elderly has the advantage of access to highly efficient and safe drugs. As a consequence, given the high prevalence of this disease in this age group, the undertreatment problem, and the availability of these excellent and low-cost drugs, this condition is the most important situation in practice in which a drug has to be added rather than removed. This fact appears as an important token of the positive impact of this classification.

Study Acronyms

ACCOMPLISH Avoiding Cardiovascular Events Through Combination Therapy in Patients Living With Systolic Hypertension Study

ALLHAT Antihypertensive and Lipid-Lowering Treatment to Prevent Heart Attack Trial

CAFE Conduit Artery Function Evaluation Study

EUROASPIRE-II European Action on Secondary and Primary Prevention by Intervention to Reduce Events II Study

HYVET Hypertension in the Very Elderly Trial

LIFE Losartan Intervention for Endpoint Reduction in Hypertension Study

ONTARGET Ongoing Telmisartan Alone and in Combination with Ramipril Global Endpoint Trial

SCOPE Study on Cognition and Prognosis in the Elderly

SHEP Systolic Hypertension in the Elderly Program Study

STOP-2 Swedish Trial in Old Patients 2 Study

SYST-EUR Systolic Hypertension in Europe Trial

References

Alderman MH (1999) A new model of risk: implications of increasing pulse pressure and systolic blood pressure on cardiovascular disease. J Hypertens Suppl 17 (5):S25–S28

Aronow WS, Fleg JL, Pepine CJ et al (2011) ACCF/AHA 2011 expert consensus document on hypertension in the elderly: a report of the American College of Cardiology Foundation Task Force on Clinical Expert Consensus documents developed in collaboration with the American Academy of Neurology, American Geriatrics Society, American Society for Preventive Cardiology, American Society of Hypertension, American Society of Nephrology, Association of Black Cardiologists, and European Society of Hypertension. J Am Coll Cardiol 57:2037–2114

Beckett NS, Peters R, Fletcher AE et al (2008) Treatment of hypertension in patients 80 years of age or older. N Engl J Med 358:1887–1898

Boersma E, Keil U, De Bacquer D et al (2003) Blood pressure is insufficiently controlled in European patients with established coronary heart disease. J Hypertens 21:1831–1840

Chobanian A (2007) Isolated systolic hypertension in the elderly. N Engl J Med 357:789–796

Chobanian AV, Bakris GL, Black HR et al (2003) Seventh report of the Joint National Committee on Prevention, Detection, Evaluation, and Treatment of High Blood Pressure. Hypertension 42:1206–1252

Conlin PR, Gerth WC, Fox J, Roehm JB, Boccuzzi SJ (2001) Four year persistence patterns among patients initiating therapy with the angiotensin II receptor antagonist losartan versus other antihypertensive drug classes. Clin Ther 23:1999–2010

Düsing R (2001) Adverse events, compliance, and changes in therapy. Curr Hypertens Rep 3:488–492

Hasford J, Schroder-Bernhardi D, Rottenkolber M, Kostev K, Dietlein G (2007) Persistence with antihypertensive treatments: results of a 3-year follow-up cohort study. Eur J Clin Pharmacol 63:1055–1061

Hense HW (2000) MONICA study: epidemiology of arterial hypertension and implications for its prevention. 10-year results of the MONICA Study Augsburg. Dtsch Med Wochenschr 125:1397–1402

Keenan NL, Rosendorf KA, Centers for Disease Control and Prevention (CDC) (2011) Prevalence of hypertension and controlled hypertension—United States, 2005–2008. MMWR Surveill Summ 60(Suppl):94–97

Lawes C, Vander Hoorn S, Rodgers A, for the International Society of Hypertension (2008) Global burden of blood-pressure related disease, 2001. Lancet 371:1513–1518

Mancia G, De Backer G, Dominiczak A et al (2007) Guidelines for the management of arterial hypertension. Eur Heart J 28:1462–1536

Mancia G, Laurent S, Agabiti-Rosei E et al (2009) Reappraisal of European guidelines on hypertension management: a European Society of Hypertension Task Force document. J Hypertens 27:2121–2158

Milchak JL, Carter BL, Ardery G, Dawson JD, Harmston M, Franciscus CL (2008) Physician adherence to blood pressure guidelines and its effect on seniors. Pharmacotherapy 28(7):843–851

Plouin PF, Rossignol P, Bobrie G (2006) Hypertension in the elderly. Bull Acad Natl Med 190:793–805

Sagie A, Larson MG, Levy D (1993) The natural history of borderline isolated systolic hypertension. N Engl J Med 329(26):1912–1917

Staessen JA, Thijs L, Fagard R et al (1999) Predicting cardiovascular risk using conventional vs ambulatory blood pressure in older patients with systolic hypertension. Systolic Hypertension in Europe Trial Investigators. JAMA 282:539–546

Sytkowski PA, D'Agostino RB, Belanger AJ, Kannel WB (1996) Secular trends in long-term sustained hypertension, long-term treatment, and cardiovascular mortality. The Framingham Heart Study 1950 to 1990. Circulation 93:697–703

U.S. Department of Health and Human Services, National Institutes of Health, National Heart, Lung, and Blood Institute, National High Blood Pressure Education Program (2004) The seventh report of the Joint National Committee on Prevention, Detection, Evaluation, and Treatment of High Blood Pressure, NIH publication no 04-5230. National Heart, Lung and Blood Institute in cooperation with the National High Blood Pressure Education Program, Bethesda

Heart Failure

Martin Wehling and Robert Lee Page 2nd

Relevance for Elderly Patients, Epidemiology

Heart failure is a frequent disease in the elderly cohort. In most cases, coronary artery disease and myocardial infarction or arterial hypertension that had remained uncontrolled for years, resulting in diffuse myocardial damage (fibrosis, hypertrophy) and systolic failure, are the culprits. Heart failure can be considered as a progressive disorder that is superimposed on the aging process in a disease continuum (Fig. 1; Jugdutt 2010). The high prevalence of both conditions in elderly patients frequently results in mixed etiologies. While hospitalization and 1-year mortality rates for heart failure appear to be decreasing, the incidence of this syndrome continues to increase due to the aging of the population (Chen et al. 2011). The incidence of heart failure increases from 0.02/1,000 inhabitants at age 24–39 years to 11.6/1,000 inhabitants aged 85+, with a clear dominance of men (Fig. 2; Cowie et al. 1999). In the general population, about 1% of all people suffer from heart failure; in persons aged 85+, this figure rises to greater than 30% (Roger et al. 2011; data from Framingham, Fig. 3).

The immense impact of this disease on human health and well-being is underlined by the following data on prognosis: Depending on the stage of heart failure (classification according to the New York Heart Association [NYHA], stages I–IV), 1-year mortality increases from 10% in stage I to almost 50% in stage IV. Thus, this disease has a higher mortality than many malign diseases. Mortality at all stages is 50% in 5 years. The Framingham study showed that age is a strong risk predictor in that mortality increases by 27% in males and even 61% in females per decade (Ho et al. 1993). The latter figure shows that heart failure is no "male" disease in the elderly, but females catch up and may even take the lead at very high age. Concomitant diseases are frequent, and treatment of heart failure in the aged thus is a bigger challenge than in the young (Table 1). In particular, arterial hypertension, which showed a prevalence of 79% in patients over 75 years (Brunner-La Rocca et al. 2006); kidney failure (59%); stroke; and the presence of two and more diseases sharply rise with age. In an analysis of the National Health and Nutritional Examination Survey (NHANES), the proportion of patients with heart failure who had five or more comorbidities increased from 42.1% in 1988–1994 to 58.0% in 2003–2008 (Wong et al. 2011). These concomitant diseases need to be considered in the treatment regimen of elderly patients with heart failure.

M. Wehling (✉)
University of Heidelberg, Maybachstr. 14, Mannheim 68169, Germany
e-mail: martin.wehling@medma.uni-heidelberg.de

R.L. Page 2nd
School of Pharmacy, University of Colorado, Mail Stop C238, 12850 E Montview Blvd. V20-4125, Aurora, CO 80045, USA
e-mail: robert.page@ucdenver.edu

M. Wehling (ed.), *Drug Therapy for the Elderly*,
DOI 10.1007/978-3-7091-0912-0_7, © Springer-Verlag Wien 2013

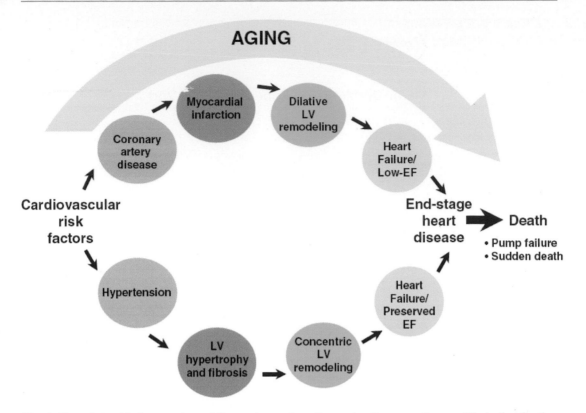

Fig. 1 The relationship between heart failure, aging, and cardiovascular disease continuum. *EF* ejection fraction, *LV* left ventricle (From Jugdutt 2010 with kind permission of Springer Science)

Therapeutically Relevant Special Features of Elderly Patients

Elderly patients are still underrepresented in clinical trials on heart failure; one of the few studies in this patient cohort (SENIORS) is discussed in the chapter on beta-blockers. Apart from this, only post hoc analyses on elderly subgroups of larger trials are available. Therefore, evidence-based guidelines on heart failure treatment in the elderly do not exist, and treatment recommendations have to be based on pathophysiological assumptions and extrapolations.

In this context, the following relevant conditions of therapeutic strategies need to be considered (modified from Bulpitt 2005; von Leibundgut et al. 2007):

– Elderly patients expose altered hemodynamic characteristics if compared to younger patients, in particular lower heart rates, even after

exercise, and reduced blood pressure values after hypertensive episodes.

– Orthostatic symptoms (see chapter "Arterial Hypertension" on general rules for the antihypertensive treatment of elderly patients) are more frequent as compensatory mechanisms, such as the increase of heart rate after postural change or exercise, become less competent at higher age.

– Overweight (mainly less-severe forms) and arterial hypertension in the very elderly (80+ years of age) are indicators of cardiac health ("force") and vitality, good and healthy nutrition, and fitness/physical activities. Classical risk factors (including low-density lipoprotein [LDL] cholesterol) lose predictive power at higher age, and treatment becomes more symptom oriented and guided by hemodynamic parameters.

– Alterations of organs, especially of the kidneys, multimorbidity, and polypharmacy

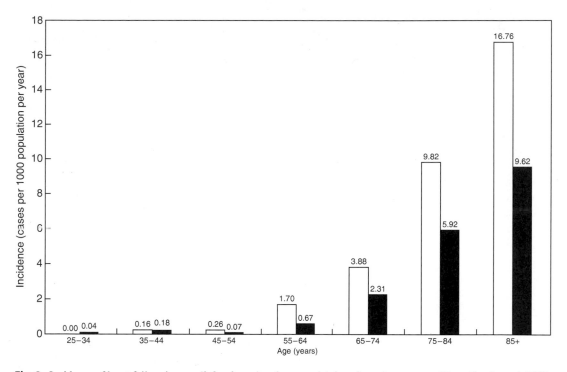

Fig. 2 Incidence of heart failure in men (*left columns*) and women (*right columns*) versus age (From Cowie et al. 1999 by kind permission of Oxford University Press/European Society of Cardiology)

and related problems of drug retention and higher rates of adverse drug reactions (ADRs) have been mentioned (in chapter "Arterial Hypertension") both generically and exemplary for arterial hypertension.

Important changes also concern brain function and psychology of elderly patients, not only if overt dementia is present, and are relevant to treatment modalities and concepts.

The life-prolonging aspects of drug treatment, which are equally important as symptomatic effects are in younger patients with a critical prognosis, lose weight in the overall treatment concept. Alike, major changes of lifestyle seem less promising at high age.

Adding to this, major changes of cardiac structures and function need to be recognized and embedded in the therapeutic regimen. In particular, the vulnerability of the aged heart renders it very susceptible for the induction of arrhythmias (e.g., proarrhythmic effects of diuretics via electrolyte disorders, or digitalis preparations, or even antiarrhythmics such as dofetilide). As mentioned in chapter "Arterial Hypertension,"

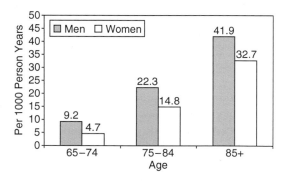

Fig. 3 Prevalence of heart failure versus age, data from the Framingham study (From Roger et al. 2011 with kind permission of Elsevier)

heart block situations or pacemaker disturbances (sick sinus syndrome) more frequently represent contraindications against beta-blockers compared to use in younger adults. The negative impact of nonsteroidal anti-inflammatory drugs (NSAIDs), including COX (cyclooxygenase) II inhibitors on the cardiovascular system via sodium retention and blood pressure elevation has been mentioned.

Dementia as a frequent concomitant disease may interfere with drug adherence; oppositely, it

Table 1 Comorbidities of patients with heart failure at age 60–74 years and at age 75+ years

	60–74 years ($n = 123$)	≥ 75 years ($n = 174$)
Women (%)	28	47
Age (years)	69 ± 4	82 ± 4
LVEF (%)	31 ± 11	38 ± 13
Systolic dysfunction (%)	90	74
Hypertension (%)	63	79
Diabetes (%)	43	32
COPD (%)	18	15
PAOD (%)	24	24
Renal failure (%)	48	59
Stroke/TIA (%)	11	20
Malignant disease (%)	4	14
Liver disease (%)	14	9
Osteoporosis (%)	4	15
Arthritis (%)	14	26

Source: From Brunner-La Rocca et al. 2006. With kind permission of Elsevier
COPD chronic obstructive pulmonary disease, *LVEF* left ventricular ejection fraction, *PAOD* peripheral arterial occlusive disease, *TIA* transient ischemic attack

may be improved by sufficient therapy of heart failure if hypoperfusion contributes to the cognitive impairment (Zuccala et al. 2005).

Life prolongation by all means is not the leading goal of heart failure treatment at high age; improvement of quality of life gains more weight and is achievable.

Evidence-Based, Rationalistic Drug Therapy and Classification of Drugs According to Their Fitness for the Aged (FORTA)

Severity of chronic heart failure has to be graded prior to any treatment, including drug therapy according to the FORTA classification. Although more recent classifications are available, the NYHA classification is still widely used. The following grading descriptions are the same for younger and elderly patients:

1. Cardiac disease without symptoms. Normal daily stress or exercise does not cause exhaustion, arrhythmias, dyspnea, or angina pectoris.
2. Cardiac disease with mild restriction of exercise capacity but no symptoms at rest. Normal daily stress or exercise causes exhaustion, arrhythmias, dyspnea, or angina pectoris.
3. Cardiac disease with moderate restriction of exercise capacity at normal stress and exercise but no symptoms at rest. Low levels of stress or exercise causes exhaustion, arrhythmias, dyspnea, or angina pectoris.
4. Cardiac disease with symptoms at all levels of exercise and at rest, bedridden.

Treatment of heart failure—as in almost all other therapeutic situations—requires an integrated approach to achieve lifestyle modifications; nutritional adaptations, including those for alcohol, tobacco, and caffeine; and initiate drug therapy. While the aims of treating arterial hypertension contain a small symptomatic component (headache, sleep disorders, stress angina may improve by treatment, and patients may only recognize this by the absence of those symptoms), heart failure treatment has two dimensions: to improve prognosis and to ameliorate symptoms (except for NYHA I = no symptoms, but structural heart disease such as myocardial infarction in the past). The indication for drugs in the treatment of heart failure has to be profiled against both claims; as mentioned, the contribution of the prognostic claim recedes with high age, and some patients consciously negate its individual relevance, which should be respected.

Existing guidelines (e.g., by the American College of Cardiology [ACC], the American Heart Association [AHA], the Heart Failure Society of America [HFSA]) are not very explicit for the treatment of the elderly and apparently assume that recommendations for younger adults are applicable to elderly patients as well if contraindications are considered. Thus, specific chapters on the elderly are short or even absent. The recommendation of the ACC and AHA mentions elderly patients in this brief statement.

Evidence-based therapy for heart failure [should] be used in the elderly patient, with individualised consideration of the elderly patient's altered ability to metabolise or tolerate standard medications (Level of Evidence C). (Hunt et al. 2005, S. e199)

The 2009 revision did not alter this sentence and the related chapter of 34 lines (Hunt et al. 2009). The executive summary of the HFSA guideline in 2010 was more elaborate and devoted a full page to this special patient group (Lindenfeld et al. 2010).

In elderly patients with heart failure, in principle all drugs used in younger patients will be considered if they provide prognostic or symptomatic benefit to the patient:
– Diuretics
– Angiotensin-converting enzyme (ACE) inhibitors/angiotensin receptor antagonists
– Beta-blockers
– Mineralocorticoid antagonists
– Digitalis preparations

On top of these drugs, anticoagulation is needed in thromboembolic conditions (atrial fibrillation); half of heart failure patients suffer from coronary heart disease (CHD), which also needs to be treated by aspirin or other platelet inhibitors and statins to lower LDL cholesterol.

Figure 4 summarizes the therapeutic options for drug treatment depending on the stage of heart failure; it is age independent and needs to be critically checked against the individual needs of elderly patients, which are elaborated in the following chapters. In this graph, the novel U.S. classification of heart failure is used, which has been developed as an alternative to the NYHA classification. In brief, it adds stage A, identifying patients at risk without structural heart disease ("not yet"). Stage B is largely congruent to NYHA I, stage C covers NYHA II and III without differentiation, and stage D is similar to NYHA IV although subtle differences exist (refractoriness of stage 4 indicates that all normal measures were without sufficient success, while NYHA IV may be improved to lower NYHA levels). In the following discussion, the functionally more useful NYHA classification is reflected in most instances.

Diuretics

Diuretics are indicated from NYHA stage II or stage C as water and salt retention is a key feature of symptomatic heart failure. Diuretic treatment addresses the major symptoms of heart failure, which are dyspnea, nocturia, and peripheral edema. After decades of clinical use in heart failure, it is still unclear whether diuretics are only beneficial regarding symptoms or also prognosis. As they may induce electrolyte disorders and these are particularly dangerous to the vulnerable aged heart, it is fair to assume that their prognostic impact will be easily overestimated in reflection of their impressive symptomatic effect. Post hoc analyses even suggested excess mortality induced by diuretics in the elderly (Fig. 5).

Therapy escalation to loop diuretics for NYHA stages III and IV (or if mandated by impaired renal function; see the general rules for the antihypertensive treatment of elderly patients) is particularly critical with regard to hypokalemia. Absorption is less of a problem if torsemide is used instead of frusemide as it exposes a more favorable, predictable bioavailability, allowing for easier titration. It should be the preferable loop diuretic for oral long-term treatment.

These critical remarks underline the necessity to restrict the application of diuretics to symptomatic patients and to use the smallest tolerable dose and diuretic strength compatible with the patient's well-being. It is even questionable whether diuretics need to be given in NYHA

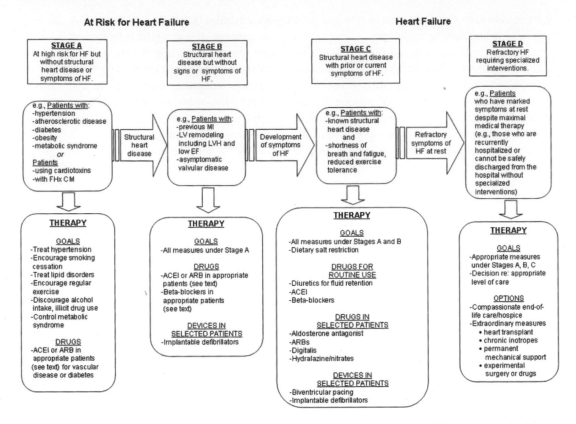

Fig. 4 Stages of heart failure and recommended therapy by stage. *ACEI* angiotensin-converting enzyme inhibitor, *ARB* angiotensin II receptor blocker, *EF* ejection fraction, *FHx CM* family history of cardiomyopathy, *HF* heart failure, *LV* left ventricular, *LVH* left ventricular hypertrophy, *MI* myocardial infarction (From Hunt et al. 2009 by permission of the American College of Cardiology Foundation and the American Heart Association, Inc.)

stage II if neurohumoral blockade (discussed in the following) is optimized and symptoms thereby minimized. As a generic rule, elderly patients are more vulnerable to diuretics than younger patients regarding electrolyte disorders, renal impairment, and dehydration precipitating orthostatic reactions; these adverse drug effects may be prognostically harmful, and the following practical advice should be considered:

– Diuretic therapy in elderly patients requires frequent monitoring of serum electrolytes, kidney function, and hydration status, with the recommendation of weekly determinations at the beginning of therapy (1–2 months) and at least monthly controls later.

– The diuretic dose needs to be checked frequently, and at the latest after 6 months of constant dosing, a dose reduction trial should be instituted under close surveillance of signs for deterioration.

The clinical control of the hydration and vascular filling status is sometimes challenging as the signs to check, such as skin folds, dry tongue, neck vein filling, and hepatojugular reflux, require advanced skills and experience in their assessment; this is not trivial like pulse taking. Unfortunately, the alternatives to measure hemodynamics, especially by right heart catherization, for the guidance of diuretic therapy are invasive and expensive and may cause strain to the patient. Adding to hemodynamic parameters, laboratory parameters may indicate overtreatment by diuretics, such as increased hematocrit (which rather tends to be at the lower limit of normal in the elderly), hyponatremia, or hyperalbuminemia.

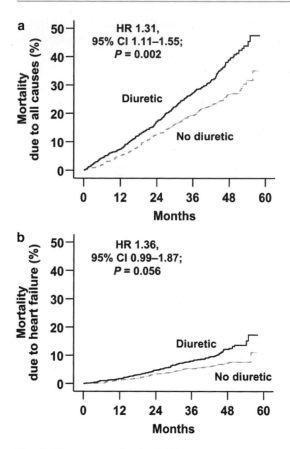

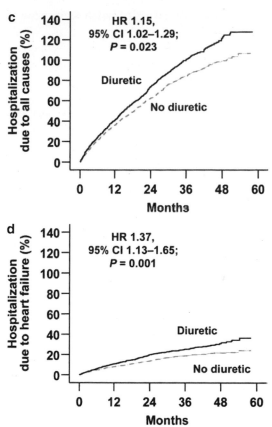

Fig. 5 Excess mortality in 8,000 patients with heart failure by diuretics. (**a**) All-cause mortality, (**b**) mortality due to heart failure, (**c**) all-cause hospitalizations, (**d**) hospitalization due to heart failure. *HR* heart rate (From Ahmed et al. 2006 by kind permission of Oxford University Press/European Society of Cardiology)

Diuretics are among the few drugs in cardiovascular medicine that are prescribed to elderly patients too often and at too high doses. The therapeutic restrictions regarding diuretics may induce more frequent decompensations in heart failure patients, but intense monitoring of patients would help to detect them early and install treatment in time.

In this context, it is important to note that the determination of potassium in serum suffers from a dangerous weakness in that it systematically tends to show falsely high values. This reflects the damage of erythrocytes during blood sampling, and serum potassium is only a weak indicator of the cellular storage of this ion. Elderly patients frequently have "no veins" as their often-extensive medical history had led to multiple punctures and thus scarring and obliteration. In this situation, blood taking may be a challenge that not rarely leads to red cell damage and related potassium release. This (in conjunction with an increased mechanical vulnerability of red cells in elderly patients) is the base for the systematic overestimation of potassium in this patient cohort.

The addition of thiazides to loop diuretics ("sequential nephron blockade") as potential escalation in refractory heart failure has been mentioned; the combination, however, seems to be more of an often unnecessary threat to elderly patients than an indispensable instrument in daily practice.

ACE Inhibitors/Angiotensin Receptor Antagonists

ACE inhibitors were the first drugs to prove the reduction of mortality of heart failure patients in large clinical trials (e.g., SOLVD, SAVE).

ACE inhibitors showed for the first time that the blockade of neurohumoral activation is beneficial in the long run; this activation is the normal response of the body to compensate for the impaired cardiac output.

In the case of ACE inhibitors, the interference with the renin-angiotensin system (RAS) is beneficial; this paradigm was followed by adrenergic inhibition later.

No studies on ACE inhibitors entirely devoted to elderly patients are available. For ethical reasons, such studies comparing ACE inhibitors to placebo cannot be performed today as the beneficial effects are convincingly shown in younger patients, and an age dependency was not detectable in larger trials. Unfortunately, only 10% of patients were 75+ years of age in the heart failure studies (Flather et al. 2000).

Criteria and rules for the safe application of ACE inhibitors have been discussed in the chapter on hypertension treatment (renal impairment, hyperkalemia). In heart failure patients, these conditions are even more critical as the impaired hemodynamics may result in more extensive fluctuations of kidney function than in healthy controls. Fosinopril may be less sensitive to such alterations of renal function than other ACE inhibitors as it is excreted both via the kidneys *and* via the liver. No large trials on heart failure have been performed with this compound, but the ACE inhibitor effects in heart failure are considered to be group effects that should be generalizable to all members of the group.

Angiotensin receptor antagonists have been studied in elderly patients with heart failure: ELITE I and II included elderly patients only (average age 71 years in ELITE II) and compared the ACE inhibitor captopril with the angiotensin receptor antagonist losartan. While the small ELITE I trial induced hope for superiority of angiotensin receptor antagonists over ACE inhibitors, the larger ELITE II trial did not show a difference. Thus, both principles are considered to be equivalent, and this conclusion is even based on studies for the aged. This equivalence is of particular relevance for elderly patients as angiotensin receptor antagonists show a better tolerability than ACE inhibitors as they do not cause coughing.

The combination of both RAS inhibitors has been studied in heart failure: In CHARM, an added benefit could be demonstrated that was absent in the older Val-HeFT. A general recommendation for this combination should not be given as the data are so heterogeneous, and side effects (hyperkalemia, hypotension) may be additive or, even worse, supra-additive. This would be especially critical in elderly patients; in addition, only a few elderly patients were included in these studies, and the finding of age-independent effects is thus only a weak argument for using the combination in the elderly.

Beta-Blockers

Chronic heart failure treatment by beta-blockers is based on the largest data pool that has been built in cardiovascular pharmacology in recent years. US-Carvedilol, MERIT, and CIBIS represented the pivotal studies to demonstrate comparably large effects of carvedilol, metoprolol, and bisoprolol on life expectancy (mortality reduction by an average of 30%). These data were instrumental to falsify the old dogma that beta-blockers are contraindicated in heart failure treatment due to their negative inotropism.

It is fortunate that a large trial on the treatment of heart failure in the elderly exists: SENIORS tested the effect of nebivolol in 2,000 elderly patients. The primary endpoint (death and hospitalizations) was significantly improved by 14%, while all-cause mortality remained unchanged (Fig. 6). Median age was 75 years, meaning that 50% of the patients were younger and 50% were older than 75 years. The overall effect was smaller than in the studies mentioned previously and was only significant in patients aged 75 years and

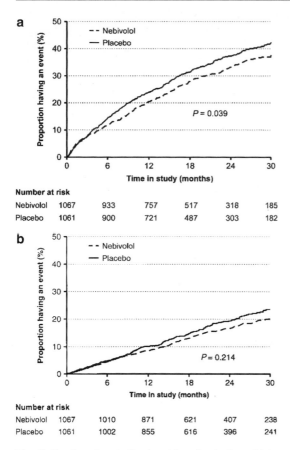

Fig. 6 Death or hospitalization (**a**) or death alone (**b**) in elderly patients with heart failure treated by placebo or nebivolol (SENIORS, from Flather et al. 2005 by kind permission of Oxford University Press/European Society of Cardiology)

younger, with an even smaller effect in patients aged 75 and older (Fig. 7).

In a post hoc analysis of MERIT, it was demonstrated that in patients aged 69 years and older the treatment effect started to dwindle; this observation could not be made at a cutoff point of 65 years (Deedwania et al. 2004). These data demonstrate that the beneficial impact of beta-blockers on the course of heart failure seems to exist even at high age, but its extent is likely to shrink. Thus, evidence to date does not support the treatment of patients aged 90 and above.

In addition to these age limitations of evidence, it should be acknowledged that beta-blockers represent a heterogeneous group of drugs: Carvedilol exerts an alpha-antagonist action on top of non-specific beta-adrenergic blockade, resulting in vasodilation, which is absent in pure beta-blockers such as metoprolol. Nebivolol has vasodilatory properties as well; however, these are based on nitroxide (NO) production in addition to beta-blockade. Carvedilol produced the largest effects on mortality, even in the head-to-head comparison with metoprolol (COMET), though the latter trial is not unanimously accepted as evidence for the superiority claim. The doses of beta-blockers compared are still a matter of debate. Nebivolol produced the smallest effects, albeit tested in elderly patients, which may explain the difference from the effect size of other beta-blockers tested in younger patients.

In this situation, the application of beta-blockers is clearly recommended also in the elderly population with heart failure and often addresses additional indications, such as hypertension, atrial fibrillation, or CHD/postmyocardial infarction.

Successful beta-blocker treatment of heart failure in the elderly absolutely mandates low starting doses, which are slowly increased.

As a rule of thumb, one tenth of the final dose in hypertension treatment is the starting dose, which should be doubled in 2- to 4-week intervals under close and meticulous clinical observation. The final dose should be close to the regular daily dose used in hypertension treatment (2×25 mg carvedilol, 100–200 mg metoprolol, 5–10 mg bisoprolol). Signs of decompensation during the uptitration require standard treatment (especially diuretics) and temporary dose reduction, which should be increased again after stabilization.

– As a note of caution, it is extremely important that beta-blocker therapy should not be started during decompensation; it is absolutely mandatory to initiate therapy only if the patient has maintained the optimal status of compensation for 4 weeks.

– The patient needs to be informed about the fact that the symptoms and well-being may initially deteriorate for 4–6 weeks; however, according to all studies, symptomatic improvement and increased quality of life will almost certainly occur after this initial phase of deterioration ("vale of tears").

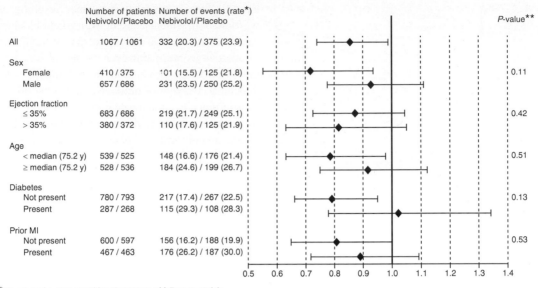

	Number of patients Nebivolol/Placebo	Number of events (rate*) Nebivolol/Placebo		P-value**
All	1067 / 1061	332 (20.3) / 375 (23.9)		
Sex				0.11
Female	410 / 375	¹01 (15.5) / 125 (21.8)		
Male	657 / 686	231 (23.5) / 250 (25.2)		
Ejection fraction				0.42
≤ 35%	683 / 686	219 (21.7) / 249 (25.1)		
> 35%	380 / 372	110 (17.6) / 125 (21.9)		
Age				0.51
< median (75.2 y)	539 / 525	148 (16.6) / 176 (21.4)		
≥ median (75.2 y)	528 / 536	184 (24.6) / 199 (26.7)		
Diabetes				0.13
Not present	780 / 793	217 (17.4) / 267 (22.5)		
Present	287 / 268	115 (29.3) / 108 (28.3)		
Prior MI				0.53
Not present	600 / 597	156 (16.2) / 188 (19.9)		
Present	467 / 463	176 (26.2) / 187 (30.0)		

0.5   0.6   0.7   0.8   0.9   1.0   1.1   1.2   1.3   1.4

* Number of events per 100 patient-years of follow-up at risk

** P-value for interaction: age and ejection fraction considered as continuous variables

Fig. 7 Subgroup analysis of SENIORS: Patients aged 75 and above did not benefit to the same extent as younger patients. *MI* myocardial infarction (From Flather et al. 2005 by kind permission of Oxford University Press/ European Society of Cardiology)

While an age-dependent attenuation of beneficial effects has not been shown for RAS inhibition (lack of data? see previous discussion), beta-blockade at high age should be indicated with greater caution and not be *forced* too vigorously in the very elderly, especially in patients aged 85 years and above. In particular, frequent side effects and contraindications in the cardiovascular (heart block) or respiratory (e.g., chronic obstructive pulmonary disease, COPD) systems must be taken into account. If beta-blocker intolerability in younger adults ranges from 10% to 15%, this figure increases to about 30% in the very elderly. This reflects two major problems:

– Decreasing efficacy
– More frequent intolerance, which also needs to be weighed against the decreasing efficacy

The typical side effects/contraindications (metabolism, cardiac side effects, asthma/ COPD) of beta-blockers are also described in chapter "Arterial Hypertension."

These limitations raise important questions in relation to elderly patients:

– Should elderly patients with heart failure who are beta-blocker intolerant be treated with a combination of ACE inhibitors and angiotensin receptor antagonists?
– Should aldosterone antagonists (see following material) be more generously applied in this situation?

Answers to these questions need to be given by future clinical trials.

Aldosterone Antagonists

RALES demonstrated a reduction of mortality of patients with NYHA class III and IV heart failure by 30% and thereby recovered aldosterone as a matter of interest for cardiovascular pharmacology. High plasma levels of aldosterone cause damage to cardiovascular structures as they induce cardiac and vascular fibrosis, hypercoagulability, and arrhythmias. The RAS stimulates the production of aldosterone in heart failure (secondary aldosteronism), and its deleterious effects can be antagonized by the "old" mineralocorticoid antagonist spironolactone. This compound is not specific for mineralocorticoid receptors but also binds to other steroid receptors, such as the androgen receptors. Binding to these receptors induces ADRs, mainly gynecomastia in about 10% of patients. This disadvantage is not shared by the modern congener eplerenone, which is specific for mineralocorticoid receptors. EPHESUS demonstrated a limited 15% reduction of mortality in patients with postmyocardial infarction heart failure. In addition, in the EMPHASIS-HF, eplerenone reduced the composite risk of death from cardiovascular causes and heart failure hospitalization by 38% in patients with NYHA class II heart failure. In a prespecified subgroup analysis, RALES showed the beneficial effects without age dependency, and significant effects were also seen in patients aged 67 years and above. In contrast, mortality effects in EPHESUS were only significant for patients younger than 65 years. It is important to note that only a few patients in RALES were on beta-blockers, leaving ample space for positive effects of spironolactone. In the later study, EPHESUS, beta-blockade was much more common, possibly explaining the lower mortality effect.

Recommendations for the treatment of elderly heart failure patients should be limited to those who are intolerant to beta-blockade.

This restrictive recommendation also reflects the relatively high threat by serious adverse effects, especially hyperkalemia. It is accentuated in the presence of ACE inhibitors (or other RAS inhibitors), which have to be given first line, and by renal failure.

Renal failure as a contraindication (estimated creatinine clearance <30 ml/min) needs to be complied with under any circumstances and is very relevant to the elderly. Even at clearances between 60 and 30 ml/min, serum potassium needs to be monitored more frequently than in the absence of this drug. Without this precaution, increased incidences of deadly hyperkalemias or at least indications for acute dialysis will be seen as they were seen soon after publication of RALES. Despite the low doses of only 25 mg/

day in this indication, spironolactone has a large potential to cause trouble in the elderly. In addition, its effects may not extrapolate to the (very) elderly, especially in the presence of betablockers. Aldosterone antagonists should not be administered in patients with a baseline serum potassium in excess of 5.0 mEq/L. When initiating these agents, close monitoring of potassium is crucial. Both serum potassium and renal function should be checked in 3 days and at 1 week after beginning therapy and at least monthly for the first 3 months.

Digitalis Preparations

Digoxin or digitoxin are the main digitalis compounds used in heart failure treatment. In the United States, a more rationalistic use of these preparations is practiced than in parts of Europe (in particular Germany). It is estimated that toxicity would not allow for a modern marketing authorization of this "old" group of drugs.

In DIG, digoxin proved to be beneficial to alleviate symptoms and reduce hospitalization related to heart failure but did not reduce mortality. There is still an ongoing debate on the reasons for this apparent discrepancy, but it is likely that positive effects (inotropy) are balanced by toxic effects (arrhythmogenicity), resulting in no net effect on mortality. Negative outcomes were associated with high plasma levels of digoxin (e.g., levels exceeding 1.2 ng/ml) (Rathore et al. 2003). As digoxin excretion critically depends on renal function and this is impaired both at high age and by hemodynamic sequelae of heart failure, this compound seems relatively unsafe in the elderly. Digitoxin is metabolized in the liver, but its long half-life causes a threat in long-term treatment as well. The remaining indication for these drugs is the comorbidity of heart failure and atrial fibrillation; heart failure will be symptomatically improved and a rapid ventricular heart rate reduced in atrial fibrillation as well. Therapy needs to be monitored closely by therapeutic drug monitoring (TDM). Goal digoxin levels should be maintained between 0.7 and 0.9 ng/ml, ideally less than 1.0 ng/ml, and checked within 1 week of beginning therapy. Many drugs can increase serum digoxin concentrations more than two-fold such as amiodarone, dronedarone, macrolide antibiotics, quinidine, and propafenone. Whether or not a therapeutic trial should be undertaken in elderly patients who are symptomatic despite adequate standard therapy remains an open question. Extreme caution should be exercised for this group of drugs in the elderly, who are vulnerable to side effects, excretory problems, and prolonged action (long half-life).

Other Interventions

Inotropic agents (e.g., milrinone or dobutamine), calcium antagonists (with the exception of long-acting dihydropyridines in hypertension) and direct vasodilators (with the exception of isosorbide dinitrate/hydralazine as an ACE inhibitor equivalent or as add-on therapy in African Americans) are not indicated for chronic treatment of heart failure. Nitrate use should be limited to acute decompensations or patients who suffer from symptoms despite optimized standard therapy. This restrictive use recommendation is highly relevant to elderly patients, who are more sensitive to hypotension and headaches induced by nitrates. In the VeHFT II trial, enalapril conferred a greater reduction in mortality compared to the combination of hydralazine-isosorbide dinitrate. However, both treatments were found to increase left ventricular ejection fraction. The combination of both hydralazine and isosorbide dinitrate mimics the lowering of pre- and afterload by ACE inhibitors separately. In the A-HeFT trial, the addition of hydralazine-isosorbide dinitrate to standard background therapy with an ACE inhibitor, diuretic, and beta-blocker significantly increased survival and reduced the rate of heart failure hospitalization in African American patients with advanced heart failure.

Electrotherapy (implantable cardioverter-defibrillator [ICD] or synchronization therapy by pacemakers) should just be mentioned here but is not in the focus of this book.

In conclusion, heart failure treatment in the elderly should preferably be based on life-prolonging principles, which in the first line are RAS blockers (ACE inhibitors *or* angiotensin receptor antagonists) and in the second line are beta-blockers. Symptomatic therapy, especially on decompensation, is the domain of diuretics, which however should be restrictively applied as they are toxic in the long run. Beta-blockers seem inferior to RAS inhibitors as their efficacy seems to be reduced in the elderly, and tolerability is decreased at higher age. Spironolactone is only safe at low doses and strict surveillance and management of potential complications; there is doubt about the efficacy at high age; thus, its use should be limited to beta-blocker-intolerant patients. Eplerenone is the alternative if gynecomastia limits therapy. Digitalis preparations are only indicated if concomitant atrial fibrillation needs treatment regarding rate control; strict TDM is recommended.

Heart Failure with Preserved Ejection Fraction

Diastolic heart failure, currently referred to as heart failure with preserved ejection fraction (HF-PEF), describes the increase of left ventricular filling pressure as a consequence of myocardial stiffening despite normal systolic function. The major symptom is dyspnea, reflecting pulmonary congestion due to this high filling pressure, and may eventually lead to pulmonary edema. In many clinical trials in patients with normal systolic function, specific therapies for this condition have been investigated. In the I-PRESERVE trial, irbesartan failed to reduce the composite outcome of all-cause mortality or hospitalization for a cardiovascular cause in patients with HF-PEF. In the CHARM-Preserved trial, candesartan failed to reduce the composite outcome of cardiovascular death or heart failure hospitalization. Digoxin has no role in the management of HF-PEF. In the DIG-Ancillary trial, digoxin had no effect on mortality and all-cause or cardiovascular hospitalization, with a trend toward an increase in hospitalizations for unstable angina. Currently, spironolactone is being studied (TOPCAT). However, it is still fair to say that the only scientifically proven, beneficial therapy of HF-PEF is the sufficient treatment of the underlying disease, which is in nearly all cases arterial hypertension. There is no reason to assume that those principles outlined in chapter "Arterial Hypertension" on the treatment of arterial hypertension in the elderly need to be modified in the presence of HF-PEF; symptomatic treatment by diuretics or nitrates may be required acutely, but this mainly reflects undertreatment of hypertension. In rare cases, restrictive cardiomyopathy without accompanying hypertension requires treatment, which would be only symptomatic and employ ACE inhibitors, diuretics, and eventually, nitrates.

Acute Heart Failure

Acute left ventricular decompensations are to be treated under strict hemodynamic control also in the elderly; treatment is primarily driven by symptoms. Like younger patients, elderly patients will receive diuretics, which need to act rapidly and strongly; thus, intravenous preparations of loop diuretics need to be applied, with frusemide preferred over torsemide as frusemide exposes a compound-specific additional action on venous tone (instant reduction of preload). Early application of ACE inhibitors is recommended; their side effects and limitations in elderly patients have been described. In addition, intravenous vasodilators (e.g., nitroprusside, nitroglycerin, or nesiritide) may be considered in patients with acute decompensated heart failure who have persistent severe heart failure despite aggressive treatment with diuretics and standard oral therapies. In the case of nitroprusside, caution is warranted in patients with hepatic or renal dysfunction due to the potential risk of cyanide toxicity. Inotropes may be given temporarily to bridge the situation until a more causal treatment may become accessible (e.g., revascularization). This includes catecholamine preparations such as dopamine or dobutamine or phosphodiesterase inhibitors such as milrinone. In patients with renal dysfunction, doses of milrinone will need to be lowered. Unfortunately, the prognosis of elderly patients with inotrope-dependent heart failure not amenable to causal therapy (revascularization too late, infarction completed) is quite desperate. This especially applies to catecholamine therapy at increasing doses and escalation to more powerful compounds such as epinephrine as these drugs are very arrhythmogenic.

Classification of Drugs for the Treatment of Chronic Heart Failure According to Their Fitness for the Aged (FORTA)

In this classification of drugs for the treatment of chronic heart failure according to their Fitness for the Aged (FORTA), the same compounds may receive alternative marks if applied in different indications (see chapter "Critical Extrapolation of Guidelines and Study Results: Risk-Benefit Assessment for Patients with Reduced Life Expectancy and a New Classification of Drugs According to Their Fitness for the Aged").

Diuretics	B
Beta-blockers (metoprolol, carvedilol, bisoprolol, nevibolol)	A (B in the very elderly)
RAS inhibitors	
ACE inhibitors	A
Angiotensin receptor antagonists	A
Spironolactone	B
Digitalis preparations	C

Note the differences in the classification of the same drug for the treatment of arterial hypertension and heart failure (e.g., beta-blockers A for heart failure, B for hypertension)

Study Acronyms

A-HeFT African American Heart Failure Trial
CHARM Study of Candesartan in Heart Failure—Assessment of Reduction in Mortality and Morbidity

CIBIS Cardiac Insufficiency Bisoprolol Study

COMET Carvedilol or Metoprolol European Trial

DIG Study of the Digitalis Investigation Group

ELITE Evaluation of Losartan in the Elderly Study

EMPHASIS-HF Eplerenone in Patients with Systolic Heart Failure and Mild Symptoms

EPHESUS Eplerenone Post-Acute Myocardial Infarction Heart Failure Efficacy and Survival Study

I-PRESERVE Irbesartan for Heart Failure with Preserved Ejection Fraction

MERIT Metoprolol Controlled Release/ Extended Release (CR/XL) Randomized Intervention Trial

PPP Pravastatin Pooling Project

RALES Randomized Aldactone Evaluation Study

SAVE Survival and Ventricular Enlargement Study

SENIORS Study of Effects of Nebivolol Intervention on Outcomes and Rehospitalisation in Seniors with Heart Failure

SOLVD Study of Left Ventricular Dysfunction

TOPCAT Treatment of Preserved Cardiac Function Heart Failure with an Aldosterone Antagonist

Val-HeFT Valsartan Heart Failure Trial

V-HeFT II Vasodilator in Heart Failure Trail II

References

Ahmed A, Husain A, Love TE et al (2006) Heart failure, chronic diuretic use, and increase in mortality and hospitalization: an observational study using propensity score methods. Eur Heart J 27: 1431–1439

Brunner-La Rocca HP, Buser PT, Schindler R, Bernheim A, Rickenbacher P, Pfisterer M, TIME-CHF investigators (2006) Management of elderly patients with congestive heart failure—design of the Trial of Intensified versus standard Medical therapy in Elderly patients with Congestive Heart Failure (TIME-CHF). Am Heart J 151:949–955

Bulpitt CJ (2005) Secondary prevention of coronary heart disease in the elderly. Heart 91:396–400

Chen J, Mormand SL, Wang Y et al (2011) National and regional trends in heart failure hospitalization and mortality rates for Medicare beneficiaries, 1998–2008. JAMA 306:1669–1678

Cowie MR, Wood DA, Coats AJ, Thompson SG, Poole-Wilson PA, Suresh V, Sutton GC (1999) Incidence and aetiology of heart failure; a population-based study. Eur Heart J 20:421–428

Deedwania PC, Gottlieb S, Ghali JK et al (2004) Efficacy, safety and tolerability of beta-adrenergic blockade with metoprolol XL in elderly patients with heart failure. Eur Heart J 25:1300–1309

Flather MD, Yusuf S, Kober L et al (2000) Long-term ACE-inhibitor therapy in patients with heart failure or left-ventricular dysfunction: a systematic overview of data from individual patients. ACE-Inhibitor Myocardial Infarction Collaborative Group. Lancet 355:1575–1581

Flather MD, Shibata MC, Coats AJ et al (2005) Randomized trial to determine the effect of nebivolol on mortality and cardiovascular hospital admission in elderly patients with heart failure (SENIORS). Eur Heart J 26:215–225

Ho KKL, Pinsky JL, Kannel WB, Levy D (1993) The epidemiology of heart failure—the Framingham study. J Am Coll Cardiol 22:A6–A13

Hunt SA, Abraham WT, Chin MH et al (2005) ACC/ AHA 2005 guideline update for the diagnosis and management of chronic heart failure in the adult: a report of the American College of Cardiology/ American Heart Association Task Force on practice guidelines (Writing Committee to update the 2001 guidelines for the evaluation and management of heart failure): developed in collaboration with the American College of Chest Physicians and the International Society for Heart and Lung Transplantation: endorsed by the Heart Rhythm Society. Circulation 112:e154–e235

Hunt SA, Abraham WT, Chin MH et al (2009) 2009 focused update incorporated into the ACC/AHA 2005 guidelines for the diagnosis and management of heart failure in adults: a report of the American College of Cardiology Foundation/American Heart Association Task Force on practice guidelines: developed in collaboration with the International Society for Heart and Lung Transplantation. Circulation 119: e391–e479

Jugdutt BI (2010) Aging and heart failure: changing demographics and implications for therapy in the elderly. Heart Fail Rev 15:401–405

Lindenfeld J, Albert NM, Boehmer JP et al (2010) Executive summary: HFSA 2010 comprehensive heart failure practice guideline. J Card Fail 16: 475–539

Rathore SS, Curtis JP, Wang Y et al (2003) Association of serum digoxin concentration and outcomes in patients with heart failure. JAMA 289:871–878

Roger VL, Go AS, Lloyd-Jones DM et al (2011) Heart disease and stroke statistics—2011 update. A report from the American Heart Association. Circulation 123:e18–e209

von Leibundgut G, Pfisterer M, Brunner-La Rocca HP (2007) Drug treatment of chronic heart failure in the elderly. Drugs Aging 24:991–1006

Wong CY, Chaudhry SI, Desai MM et al (2011) Trends in comorbidity, disability, and polypharmacy in heart failure. Am J Med 124:136–143

Zuccala G, Onder G, Marzetti E et al (2005) Use of angiotensin converting enzyme inhibitors and variations in cognitive performance among patients with heart failure. Eur Heart J 26:226–233

Coronary Heart Disease and Stroke

Martin Wehling

Relevance for Elderly Patients, Epidemiology

Although at declining incidence, cardiovascular diseases still represent the leading causes of death in the Western world, and myocardial infarction occupies the largest share within these deaths. In 2006, 26% of all 2,426,264 deaths in the United States resulted from cardiac diseases, 23% from malignant diseases; 6% were caused by cerebrovascular diseases. Cardiac deaths had a male/female ratio of 1.5. From 1999 to 2006, there was a decline of the total annual death rate from cardiac disease from 260 to 211 per 100,000 inhabitants. This rate is 207 at age 55–64 years and rises to 1,383 at age 75–84 years and even to 4,480 at age 85+ years (Heron et al. 2009). This indicates that although cardiac diseases as a major cause of death are on the decline, the immense increase at higher age is an important feature of aging societies. The life expectancy at birth in 2006 was 75 years for males, 80 years for females, with the difference mainly reflecting the underrepresentation of women in the incidence of cardiac disease.

These numbers clearly underline the paramount importance of prevention and treat- ment of cardiac disease, which is mainly myocardial infarction, in the elderly.

The epidemiology of cerebrovascular disease mainly representing stroke is analogous: From 1999 to 2006, there was a decline of the total annual death rate from cerebrovascular disease from 60 to 46 per 100,000 inhabitants; this rate was 33 at age 55–64 years and rose to 335 at age 75–84 years and even to 1,040 at age 85+ years (Heron et al. 2009). The age-related increase from 55–64 to 85+ years thus is even greater (32-fold) than for myocardial infarction (22-fold).

In the following chapters, practically relevant features of chronic treatment in the elderly should be emphasized; the special intensive care modalities for acute disease are not comprehensively discussed.

As chronic treatment of myocardial infarction includes the pharmacological protection of viable myocardium, while chronic stroke treatment mainly addresses the control of risk factors (hypertension, atrial fibrillation) and rehabilitation, stroke is only briefly mentioned here. Treatment of arterial hypertension as the most important preventive measure against stroke, and its recurrence is discussed in chapter "Arterial Hypertension", atrial fibrillation in chapter "Atrial Fibrillation". Lipid therapy and platelet inhibition for stroke prevention are not essentially different from treatment of coronary heart disease (CHD) and are thus covered here.

M. Wehling (✉)
University of Heidelberg, Maybachstr. 14, Mannheim 68169, Germany
e-mail: martin.wehling@medma.uni-heidelberg.de

M. Wehling (ed.), *Drug Therapy for the Elderly*,
DOI 10.1007/978-3-7091-0912-0_8, © Springer-Verlag Wien 2013

Therapeutically Relevant Special Features of Elderly Patients

The pathophysiology of myocardial infarction is not essentially different in elderly and younger patients. The incidences of related deaths are, however, very different (see previous discussion). This reflects the fact that in the elderly more patients suffer from multivessel disease, and diffuse myocardial damage is more likely to exist than in younger patients. This damage frequently reflects long-standing arterial hypertension, leading to myocardial hypertrophy and fibrosis, called hypertensive heart disease. Both facts may lead to more extensive changes in coronary circulation than in younger patients. Adding to this, the vulnerability of the aged myocardium to arrhythmogenic triggers is increased, and more than 50% of myocardial infarction patients die of arrhythmias, mainly ventricular fibrillation.

It is important to pay attention to the fact that the clinical presentation of acute coronary syndromes changes with age, and symptoms become less indicative and specific (dyspnea, nausea, syncopes, dizziness, disorientation may indicate various diseases in elderly patients). Even the electrocardiogram (ECG) loses specificity, and the leading clinical appearance may be that of heart failure rather than that of an acute coronary syndrome.

Therefore, atypical symptoms in elderly patients must induce a vigorous diagnostic check for CHD (Task Force for Diagnosis and Treatment of Non-ST-Segment Elevation Acute Coronary Syndromes of European Society of Cardiology et al. 2007).

Massive coronary pathologies with multiple-vessel disease, long stenotic processes including smaller vessels, and extensive calcifications are typical for elderly patients with CHD; revascularization may thus be more difficult than in younger patients, and complication rates are higher, including those at the access vessels for interventional cardiologists (femoral/iliac/brachial arteries). Despite this, there is no doubt that even

at high age revascularization for acute coronary syndromes, particularly by interventional cardiology (PTCA [percutaneous transluminal coronary angioplasty] with stents), is superior to drug-only therapy (The TIME Investigators 2001). It is commonly accepted today that there is no age limit for coronary interventions; however, limitations by high complication rates and concomitant diseases, including dementia, need to be carefully weighed against potential benefits, which is the general rule in all treatment strategies for the elderly. This and the reduced life expectancy at high age should lead to a more conservative approach, which is increasingly driven by symptoms. As an example, in a 95-year-old patient with acute coronary syndrome who has severe anginal pain despite the application of all standard drugs, coronary angioplasty is a valuable alternative that should not be withheld. Unfortunately, this book cannot extensively cover this important ethical discussion on non-medical treatment.

Chronic coronary insufficiency may induce the growth of collaterals, which protect the myocardium against regional blood flow reductions. Without collaterals, the myocardium is particularly vulnerable for regional vessel occlusions as no perfusion from neighboring areas can substitute for the blockade. Collaterals will only grow if the vascular occlusion is slowly progressive. This is the case for elderly patients, in whom calcifications of coronary arteries stabilize atherosclerotic plaques, and scarring slowly obstructs blood flow. In younger patients, hemodynamically insignificant plaques may suddenly rupture, and the rapidly growing thrombus instantly occludes the vessel. No time is left for collaterals to grow. Thus, myocardial infarctions in younger patients paradoxically may be larger and cause more dramatic cardiac damage than in elderly patients. Thus, the elderly patient with CHD is more often handicapped by chronic angina pectoris, which tends to be stable and amenable to medical treatment. In younger patients, plaques tend to be unstable, and related symptoms are also frequently unstable; if not properly diagnosed and treated, myocardial infarctions evolve frequently.

Another feature of CHD in elderly patients is of importance: The contribution of the established risk factors is increasingly investigated and has shown differences if compared with younger patients. As a general rule, these traditional risk factors lose their contributory impact in the elderly: If a 90-year-old patient has become that old despite high serum cholesterol values, the threat for CHD, although increasing sharply with age, has less and less to do with cholesterol. This has an impact on treatment recommendations under preventive aspects. An exception seems to be high blood pressure as a risk factor for stroke, which does not lose its contributory capacity even at high age (see previous discussion). An ongoing controversy circles around the question whether smoking cessation should be recommended in the very elderly. Should one ask a 90-year-old smoker without complications so far to stop smoking? There are studies pointing to a potential benefit by smoking cessation even at that high age: In very elderly patients (mean age 82 years), a 2.2-fold higher incidence of coronary events was found in smokers compared to nonsmokers (Aronow and Ahn 1996). There is no choice even in the oldest patients if smoking has led to coronary symptoms: Angina will deteriorate in the presence of smoking as smoke, especially its major active ingredient, nicotine, further reduces coronary blood flow and thus may precipitate anginal attacks and even myocardial infarctions or arrhythmias. In addition, cardiovascular risk returns to normal after 5 years of abstinence, although this has not been investigated in the very elderly. Thus, smoking cessation should almost always be recommended. Adjunctive pharmacological treatments to aid smoking cessation (nicotine replacement, bupropion, varenicline) are not well studied in the elderly.

Therapeutically relevant special features of CHD in elderly patients relate to both the importance of accepted risk factors and the pathology of often-severe forms of CHD with large myocardial infarctions associated with significant heart failure and high mortality.

Evidence-Based, Rationalistic Drug Therapy and Classification of Drugs According to Their Fitness for the Aged (FORTA)

This chapter focuses on acute therapeutic situations (acute coronary syndrome in brief) and in particular chronic therapy with preventive orientation.

Acute Coronary Syndromes

Modern therapeutic strategies for acute coronary syndromes with or without ST elevation (STEMI, ST-elevation myocardial infarction; NSTEMI, non-ST-elevation myocardial infarction) comprise multiple components:
- Early revascularization (PTCA, in most cases with stent implantation),
- Fibrinolysis (in STEMI if early PTCA is not possible),
- Anticoagulation,
- Platelet inhibition, and
- Anti-ischemic drug therapy.

TACTICS-TIMI-18 demonstrated for NSTEMI that the invasive strategy is superior to medical treatment, with a particularly clear result in the age group of 75+ years (Bach et al. 2005). The limitations of the invasive approach at high age have been described as well, which comprise life expectancy, comorbidities, and personal preferences, in particular in reflection of increased procedural complications. The last limitation especially applies to aortocoronary bypass operations.

In STEMI patients, early *fibrinolysis* (by emergency doctors) should be considered if a standby interventional catherization laboratory cannot be reached within 90 min (in some guidelines, 120 min) after the beginning of symptoms. Regarding elderly patients, data on fibrinolysis are heterogeneous: Bleeding complications are increased in elderly patients compared to younger patients, and efficacy was not detectable in the Fibrinolytic-Therapy-Trialists (FTT) study in 75+-year-old patients (FTT Collaborative Group 1994). Only in a later analysis including more patients could a net benefit be demonstrated in the elderly ($p < 0.03$), while other studies even showed damage. These data call for caution regarding thrombolysis in the very elderly (aged 85+ years); under any circumstances, early invasive intervention is preferable if the time window is met. Although bleeding complications were elevated, r-TPA (alteplase) was superior to streptokinase in patients aged less than 85 years (Kyriakides et al. 2007). The list of contraindications against lysis is long and includes all risk factors favoring bleeding complications, such as cerebral lesions, ulcers, uncontrolled hypertension, recent surgery, intramuscular injections, falls; at higher age, contraindications will be more frequent, and thus lysis become less of an option.

Acetylsalicylic acid (Aspirin®) has proven its efficacy in acute coronary syndromes at all ages, including very elderly patients (Krumholz et al. 1995). A dose of 325 (500) mg will be acutely applied orally. In some European countries, an intravenous preparation is available, which is preferable as the onset of action is more rapid, and elderly patients with dysphagia will benefit from this route of application. As this formulation is not readily available in the United States, it should be mentioned that noncapsulated aspirin needs to be employed in this situation; capsulated aspirin is thought to reduce gastric complications but will retard the effect unacceptably in the acute coronary syndrome.

The additional instant anticoagulation by *unfractionated heparin or low molecular weight heparin* in acute coronary syndromes results in increased bleeding complications in elderly patients. Low molecular weight heparins such as enoxaparin seem to be more efficacious than unfractionated heparin, but again induce a higher rate of bleeding. In addition, their activity cannot be easily monitored as a useful biomarker like thrombin time for unfractionated heparin is missing, and no antidote is available. In all patients, but especially in the elderly, low molec-

ular weight heparins require dosing in reflection of renal function, which needs to be estimated by formulas such as the Cockcroft-Gault formula. The same applies to other anticoagulants, such as bivalirudin, which is frequently used in the United States. Fondaparinux (not labeled for acute coronary syndromes in the United States) seems to be safer in patients with kidney impairment but may also not be given if clearance is below 30 ml/min. Figure 1 shows a summary of studies on the efficacy of heparins in NSTEMI patients.

Clopidogrel is the second important platelet inhibitor that is routinely given on top of aspirin; it acts through the ADP (adenosine diphosphate) receptor. In CURE, its addition to aspirin in NSTEMI resulted in increased benefits, which were also observed in elderly patients. Increased bleeding rates did not result in increased mortality; they thus were minor bleeding. This compound is standard in NSTEMI or interventionally treated STEMI and needs to be given with an initial bolus of 300 (600) mg (4–8 tablets of 75 mg each). It is not known which bolus dose (hard to swallow for elderly patients) is really indicated in the elderly, but the U.S. label for the initial bolus is 300 mg anyway. Prasugrel and ticagrelor are novel compounds that have pharmacokinetic advantages, but even fewer experiences in the treatment of elderly patients are available for those compounds than for clopidogrel.

Glycoprotein (GP) IIb/IIIa antagonists such as tirofiban, eptifibatid, or abciximab also block platelets and seem to be less efficient at high age, but lead to an increased rate of bleeding (Boersma et al. 2002). In this meta-analysis, the benefit decreased from 14% in patients less than 60 years old to only 4% in patients older than 70 years. Clear-cut recommendations for their use in the elderly population do not exist; both economical implications and lack of data mandate restrictive use, which in daily practice is mainly driven by coronary morphology and complexity of interventions. If the latter are predictive of complications, additional platelet inhibition by these drugs may be exceptionally advisable even in the elderly.

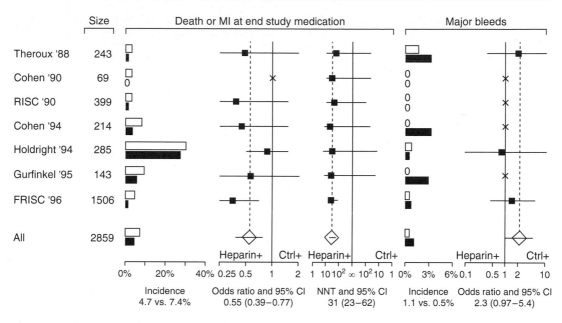

Fig. 1 Summary of studies on early anticoagulation in non-ST-elevation myocardial infarction (NSTEMI) by unfractionated or low molecular weight heparins (*dark columns*) versus placebo (*open columns*). Endpoints including bleedings are shown (From Task Force 2007 by kind permission of Oxford University Press/European Society of Cardiology)

Beta-blockers are being applied in acute coronary syndromes in the absence of contraindications orally (e.g., 50 mg metoprolol q.i.d.). The intravenous route of application should only be utilized by experienced emergency doctors as bradycardia is more frequent than after oral application. At present, treatment rules are changing in that instant application of beta-blockers at the first patient contact with the doctor is discouraged. It should be delayed for the short time necessary to reach the hospital as a safer environment and to gain more experience on the course of the individual patient.

Beta-blockers are beneficial as they reduce myocardial oxygen consumption, with heart rate lowering the major contributor. In the large COMMIT study, metoprolol was given in acute myocardial infarction and significantly reduced the risk of reinfarction and ventricular fibrillation. Effects were not different for patients under and over 70 years of age (COMMIT Collaborative Group 2005). As a note of caution, it has to be emphasized that especially in the elderly patients the exclusion of contraindications is of paramount importance (see chapter "Arterial Hypertension"). In particular, this applies to heart block at the sinus or atrioventricular levels, COPD at severe stages, and asthma, which is, however, rare at higher age.

Exclusion of left ventricular systolic dysfunction in consequence of large myocardial infarctions is elementary. The slightest suspicion of heart failure should deter less-experienced doctors from early beta-blocker application in elderly patients.

In the case of doubt, echocardiography (and the obligatory ECG) should be performed first and beta-blockade started when systolic dysfunction is minor or absent.

Angiotensin-converting enzyme (ACE) inhibitors should be initiated early in the course of STEMI as they reduce the negative impact of remodeling after myocardial infarction and lower mortality in myocardial infarction (SAVE, AIRE). The application to elderly patients has to be cautioned with similar restrictions as for beta-blockers, especially in the presence of hypotension or renal failure, which are both side effects and (relative) contraindications for ACE inhibitors. They indicate

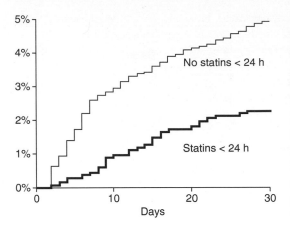

Fig. 2 Mortality of ST-elevation myocardial infarction (STEMI) patients with and without early (<24 h) statin application who survived the first 24 h (From Lenderink et al. 2006 by kind permission of University Press/European Society of Cardiology)

high risk in STEMI patients. This situation restricts the life-prolonging therapy with ACE inhibitors to patients with smaller STEMI, and elderly patients with larger STEMI or renal failure are frequently excluded from those benefits of early application. This, however, does not exclude the possibility to stabilize the patient first and, after survival of the critical initial phase, to initiate ACE inhibitor (and/or beta-blocker) therapy secondarily.

HMG-CoA (3-hydroxy-3-methylglutaryl-coenzyme A) reductase inhibitors (statins; discussed separately in the following material) are important in the instant treatment of acute coronary syndromes: MIRACL or A to Z were the studies that showed a beneficial mortality effect if high-dose statins (80 mg/day atorvastatin) were given early and independently from the lipid status (Fig. 2). More recently, this effect was confirmed for STEMI, but not for NSTEMI, although the limitations of a register study apply to this case (Lenderink et al. 2006). For this situation, no convincing data are available for elderly patients; thus, the recommendation to treat them like younger patients is empirical. However, as this treatment is short term only (long-term treatment will be instituted only after assessment of the lipid status and other risk factors about 4 weeks later), it should not be withheld from elderly patients.

Nitrates are only symptomatically beneficial; they do not prolong life. If they are chronically applied, this indicates in most cases that revascularization needs to be optimized and other medications escalated. An absolute prerequisite for their safe use is the exclusion of hypotension (<100 mmHg systolic) before applying, for example, nitroglycerin from a metered spray and subsequent hemodynamic monitoring. In the elderly, only one puff should be employed at a time, rather than the two puffs normally given to younger patients. A fatal interaction with severe hypotension occurs if nitrates and phosphodiesterase (PDE) 5 inhibitors (e.g., sildenafil) are given together; sildenafil use is not uncommon in elderly men.

Dihydropyridine calcium channel blockers such as nitrendipine or amlodipine are no valid therapeutic choice in acute coronary syndromes and should be used only to lower hypertension if other antihypertensive drugs are insufficient.

Registry data showed that recommendations for the treatment of acute coronary syndromes are less often consistently applied to elderly than to younger patients. In particular, invasive procedures are often withheld although indicated. Beta-blockers and ACE inhibitors are underutilized as well. The most deleterious deviation from common practice was reflected by a longer time needed to reach the hospital if elderly patients were compared with younger patients (Schuler et al. 2006).

In conclusion, elderly patients with STEMI or NSTEMI require a careful analysis of risk and benefit regarding antithrombotic interventions, including the assessment of kidney function. The CRUSADE data clearly showed that relative excess dosing of anticoagulatory compounds was associated with increased bleeding rates. There is no age limit for recommended therapeutic interventions, including the invasive ones. Unfortunately, higher age is associated with more frequent contraindications to some drugs, in particular beta-blockers and lysis drugs. Presentation of the disease often is atypical; acute coronary syndromes are more often missed in elderly than younger patients. Treatment of acute coronary syndromes in the elderly is more restrictive than in younger patients, and avoidable delays of invasive interventions are common, thereby clearly reducing chances of recovery and survival.

Acute coronary syndromes in elderly patients need to be diagnosed and therapeutic decisions taken as fast as in younger patients. Restrictions of the therapeutic intensity and choice of options need to reflect the overall appearance of the patient, comorbidities, expected complications, biological age and resulting remaining life expectancy, and personal preferences.

The typical 80-year-old patient would principally receive all treatments younger patients would receive, but glycoprotein IIa/IIIb antagonists, beta-blockers, and statins (lack of evidence) would not be given as frequently as in younger patients. The relatively high rate of contraindications against lysis could be balanced by invasive procedures, although in practice this does not seem to occur. Patients with symptomatic acute coronary syndromes who do not receive invasive treatment should be rare as PTCA is a powerful symptomatic procedure. However, it is conceivable that a 95-year-old patient who is symptom free in response to drug treatment alone may be left without invasive procedure. The prognostic implications of PTCA are still unclear at this age as data even for this frequent and serious condition are lacking. This is even more pressing as 95-year-old patients are not rare today.

Classification of Drugs for the Treatment of Acute Coronary Syndromes According to Their Fitness for the Aged (FORTA)

In this classification of drugs for the treatment of acute coronary syndromes according to the Fitness for the Aged (FORTA), the same compounds may receive alternative marks if applied in different indications (see Chapter "Critical Extrapolation of Guidelines and Study Results: Risk-Benefit Assessment for Patients with Reduced Life Expectancy and a New Classification of Drugs According to Their Fitness for the Aged").

Acetylsalicylic acid (aspirin)	A
Unfractionated and low molecular weight heparins	A
Clopidogrel	A
GP IIb/IIIa-antagonists	C
Thrombolytics, rTPA, if invasive procedures are delayed	B
Heart-rate-lowering beta-blockers	A
RAS inhibitors	
ACE inhibitors	A
Statins	B
Nitrates, long term	C
Nitroglycerin spray, acute, on demand	A

Chronic Drug Therapy of Postmyocardial Infarction Patients

Chronic drug therapy of postmyocardial infarction patients should be divided into directly cardioprotective interventions (by Aspirin, beta-blockers, ACE inhibitors) and modifications of risk factors (smoking cessation aids and diabetes, lipid, and hypertension control).

Directly Cardioprotective Interventions

For aspirin, beta-blockers and ACE inhibitors, life-prolonging or relapse-preventing effects have been demonstrated in large trials on postmyocardial infarction patients.

Aspirin was tested in more than 20,000 patients by the Antithrombotic Trialists' Collaboration and significantly reduced myocardial infarction recurrence and stroke by 36 events per 1,000 patients in 2 years (number needed to treat [NNT] 28). These effects were age independent. In an observational study of 1,400 patients aged 85+ years, myocardial infarction relapses were reduced by 59% within 3 years.

Aspirin at doses between 75 and 325 mg/day should be given lifelong to postmyocardial infarction patients of all ages.

Gastrointestinal (GI) side effects even at low doses are the major disadvantage of aspirin; as a rule of thumb (not exact, but easier to memorize), in

- 30% of patients any GI side effects, in
- 3% gastric or duodenal ulcers and in
- 0.3% upper GI bleeding are noted.

Exact data are difficult to obtain as many elderly patients also apply classical nonsteroidal anti-inflammatory drugs (NSAIDs) such as diclofenac, and the culprit of GI side effects is unidentifiable. In any case, elderly are clearly more vulnerable to GI side effects of aspirin than younger patients as motility is reduced (longer contact time), mucous membranes are thinner, and mucous secretion is reduced. Adding to this is the fact that NSAIDs temporarily block the receptors (cyclooxygenase) on platelets; concomitantly applied aspirin will find its receptors occupied and not bind, but receptors are freed later and platelet reactivated as NSAIDs reversibly bind to them (unlike aspirin, which is covalently bound to them). In this combination, aspirin may lose its protective effect. The optimal dose of 100 mg/day certainly induces GI side effects less frequently than higher doses of aspirin or NSAIDs as pain medication. Unfortunately, this dose is hard to obtain in the United States, with splitting a 325-mg tablet into quarters representing a suboptimal solution.

If GI side effects occur, ulcers and a *Helicobacter* infection need to be excluded endoscopically. *Helicobacter* infections are easily accessible to medical eradication. In any case, *proton pump inhibitors* (e.g., omeprazole racemate, 40 mg/day) should be given if GI side effects occur. In the United States, proton pump inhibitors are recommended prophylactically in every patient aged 65+ years on NSAIDs even without GI history or symptoms. As chronic therapy with proton pump inhibitors also carries the risk of side effects (drug-drug interactions, which are less frequent with newer compounds such as pantoprazol; osteoporosis, pneumonia for all compounds), a careful balance between risk and benefit should be sought in elderly patients. Those without GI history and without symptoms (which need to be meticulously and frequently searched for by asking for typical and atypical pain, heartburn, and by physical examination, including deep epigastric palpa-

tion) on aspirin must not necessarily be treated by proton pump inhibitors, at least according to European guidelines.

If side effects despite administration of a proton pump inhibitor or a GI ulcer occur, clopidogrel (75 mg/day) is a good alternative without GI side effects, and according to CURE in patients aged 65+ years is even an effective additive (if the patients tolerates aspirin). This dual platelet inhibition must be given to all patients after coronary stent implantation, with drug-eluting stent (DES; liberating paclitaxel or sirolimus to inhibit local tissue proliferation) for 12 months, with bare metal stent for 4 weeks. In the newer guidelines, dual platelet inhibition (aspirin plus clopidogrel or alternatives) is recommended for all patients for 12 months. It is however unclear (lack of data) if a 90-year-old patient benefits from dual platelet inhibition. As most postmyocardial infarction patients are not continued on dual inhibition past those time frames mandated by the presence of stents, it seems a bit far from reality to debate this extended combination treatment in the very elderly, although a clear tendency for this extension exists in the current scientific discussion. The extent of the additional effect on top of aspirin is small, relatively costly, associated with an elevated bleeding risk, and its size is likely to shrink at higher age. Thus, in my opinion dual platelet inhibition in the very elderly beyond the time frame mandated by stents is only justified in selected cases (absence of frailty, dementia, and other serious limitations of life expectancy) at present. Of course, this does not apply to the alternative treatment by clopidogrel if aspirin is not tolerated.

Heart-rate-lowering *beta-blockers* are a mainstay in the long-term treatment of postmyocardial infarction patients as they protect the myocardium (heart rate reduction, reduction of oxygen consumption, antiarrhythmic action, blood pressure reduction), indisputably prolong life, and lower myocardial infarction recurrences. In meta-analyses on studies on 55,000 patients after myocardial infarction in total, mortality was reduced by 23%; in smaller trials and retrospective analyses, these effects were even detected in patients aged 80+ years. In one study, this effect amounted to 43% in 2 years.

Heart-rate-lowering beta-blockers (such as metoprolol, carvedilol, bisoprolol) are devoid of a so-called intrinsic sympathomimetic activity (ISA; pindolol as an example with ISA), which abrogates the heart-rate-lowering action and thus the cardioprotective and mortality effects.

These data underline the postmyocardial infarction indication for beta-blockers as one of the most stringent ones in cardiovascular pharmacology. Contraindications have to be considered, and their prevalences increase with age, in particular because of heart block issues. Still, the number of beta-blocker-intolerant patients has receded as heart failure as a former major contraindication has been converted into a strict indication (see chapter "Heart Failure"). If heart block is present, the indication for a pacemaker needs to be discussed with priority as its implantation would render the patient beta-blocker tolerable. If a patient with atrioventricular block grade II or sinoatrial block exposes a history of vertigo or even syncope, which is not rare in elderly patients, the implantation of a simple DDD pacemaker seems justified.

The aim of medical care should be to increase beta-blocker utilization rates of only 22% (as in the study mentioned) to more than 70% in the elderly patients, a figure acknowledging the fact that intolerance may go up to 30% in the very elderly.

ACE inhibitors have proven their life-prolonging effect in large postmyocardial infarction patient trials as well, such as in HOPE for ramipril. These effects were age independent and could be observed in patients aged 65+ years, who comprised 55% of the study population (10,000 patients) as well. All caveats mentioned (hypotension, renal failure, hyperkalemia) need to be considered in this context, but the ACE inhibitor should not be missing in the postmyocardial infarction patient, even in those with good systolic function. While remodelling is a major target of ACE inhibitors in the postmyocardial infarction situation, a direct antiatherosclerotic action is thought to add to this effect and may be the only reason for its application. This indication is independent of hypertension or

heart failure. Angiotensin receptor antagonists will be the alternative if coughing is clinically relevant (only 5–10% of all patients).

As already mentioned, long-term treatment with oral *nitrates* (isosorbide dinitrate as an example) only alleviates symptoms but does not prolong life or reduce recurrences. Their application therefore should be driven by refractory symptoms occurring at low levels of exercise, which often indicate that revascularization is not complete or sufficient. Increasing doses of beta-blockers are often beneficial if an invasive strategy has failed despite optimization, but maximal doses should only be approached under close ECG surveillance.

Dihydropyridine calcium channel blockers are not indicated in postmyocardial infarction patients except for those who require additional antihypertensive treatment.

Verapamil or diltiazem may—in bail-out situations as a last option only—be added to beta-blockers if angina pectoris cannot be controlled by revascularization and maximization of beta-blocker and nitrate dosages, and ventricular function is normal. This combination is dangerous due to negative inotropism of both compounds, especially in the elderly, and should be avoided by all means in daily practice. As substitutes for beta-blockers in cases of intolerance, they have a small indication slot but are still dangerous drugs.

Antiarrhythmics, which would be discussed on several pages in an older book, are only briefly mentioned here: In postmyocardial infarction patients suffering from life-threatening ventricular arrhythmias (mainly sustained ventricular tachycardias), class I antiarrhythmics (e.g., flecainide, chinidine, procainamide) and sotatol (racemate of beta-blocker and class III antiarrhythmic drug) caused excess mortality. The only exception seems to be amiodarone, which requires deep insights and broad experiences to cope with its excessive toxicity (in particular, pulmonary fibrosis and hypertension at daily doses of 200 mg and higher, skin alterations, light sensitivity, corneal and retinal damages, liver toxicity, thyroid function alterations). Elderly patients with impaired prognosis (very high age; malignancy; severe concomitant diseases, including dementia) may benefit from this compound as a noninvasive alternative to the implantation of expensive automated implantable cardioverter/defibrillators (AICDs). In MADIT-II, the last intervention has proven its efficacy even in patients aged 75+ years with life-threatening arrhythmias and reduced left ventricular function (ejection fraction <30%): Sudden cardiac death was reduced by 68%. Although not the topic of this book, it is noted that AICD treatment is by far the safest and most efficacious intervention in this context, even for the elderly. It should, however, not be forgotten that the prevention of sudden cardiac deaths by AICD may not seem ethical in multimorbid palliative care patients, and end-of-life considerations should moderate the abundant use of AICDs in those patients.

For patients who are not amenable to this treatment (own wish, high risk of operation, end-of-life considerations), amiodarone as the only valuable alternative may be given, but with caution and at the lowest possible doses (preferably not more than 100 mg/day as a maintenance dose). The metabolism of amiodarone, which is extensively stored in tissues, is complex and for elderly patients almost unknown.

Hormone replacement (mainly estrogen) therapy (HRT) for elderly women did not prove to have any beneficial effect on the cardiovascular system, at least if started almost a decade after menopause. This has been shown in large studies (WHI and HERS), and HRT may rather produce more cardiovascular endpoints. Menopause symptoms may be treated by HRT only temporarily (1–2 years maximum).

As an important intervention that only seemingly has nothing to do with cardiovascular medicine, *influenza vaccination* needs to be mentioned here. It prolongs life in postmyocardial infarction patients and is recommended for these patients and all persons aged 65+ years. In the U.S. ACC/AHA (American College of Cardiology/American Heart Association) guidelines, the related statement is a class I, evidence level B recommendation.

Risk Factor Modification

Treatment of arterial hypertension and diabetes mellitus type 2 (obesity) is described elsewhere; smoking cessation previously in this chapter. Here, only lipid-lowering therapies are discussed; in the past 15 years, this therapeutic area has seen an unprecedented development initiated by the introduction of HMG-CoA reductase inhibitors, called statins. The inhibition of this enzyme mainly reduces the endogenous synthesis of cholesterol that exceeds the nutritional supply by far (about tenfold).

The large studies (4S, HPS, LIPIDS, CARDS) clearly demonstrated statin effects on mortality and morbidity by lowering low-density lipoprotein (LDL) cholesterol as their main action. The extent of this effect, however, critically depends on the initial LDL cholesterol level and on the overall risk factor assembly of the individual patient. Although all humans may benefit from statin therapy in principle, the net benefit shrinks with the initial risk to suffer from a cardiovascular event. In contrast, toxicity remains unchanged, and there will be a breakeven point of no net benefit when toxicity is equal to benefit.

This is the reason for a staggered recommendation depending on the initial LDL cholesterol level, which represents a treatment threshold in reflection of overall risk (for example, in the United States, the ATPIII recommendation in its modification of 2004; Grundy et al. 2004). If hypercholesterolemia is the only risk factor or only one additional risk factor is present (with age >45 years in men, >55 years in women or male sex representing one count each), a LDL cholesterol concentration of less than 190 mg/dl is acceptable without statin therapy. In the presence of two or more risk factors, the target level of LDL cholesterol is

- 160 mg/dl if the estimated 10-year risk for a cardiovascular event is below 10%, and
- 130 mg/dl if this risk is 10–20%. It is
- 100 mg/dl in high-risk patients (10-year risk >20%) who either have CHD or a so-called risk equivalent (such as diabetes). The goal is even at only
- 70 mg/dl at very high risk (e.g., CHD *and* diabetes).

The coronary risk as mentioned may be estimated from the individual risk factor assembly by using different scores, such as the Framingham score, EURO score, and many more.

In the overall treatment concept, changes of lifestyle need to be implemented: weight reduction; fat-reduced nutrition; reduction of alcohol, caffeine intake, smoking; increased physical activities, all of which are also beneficial even at low cholesterol values.

At present, large controlled clinical trials include 170,000 patients (Cholesterol Treatment Trialists' CTT Collaboration 2010); in 90,000 patients who were on statins for an average of 5 years, a decrease of serious coronary endpoints by 21% was observed for a reduction of 1 mmol LDL cholesterol (Baigent et al. 2005). This shows that the absolute extent of endpoint prevention by LDL cholesterol lowering depends on the initial cholesterol level; the more you have, the more you get, and at lower LDL cholesterol levels, the absolute gain becomes smaller. The threshold at which the absolute benefit and the risk of side effects are no longer in balance needs to be defined for each individual patient. For elderly patients, this is particularly critical as their reduced life expectancy needs to be taken into account as well.

Statin therapy is one of the few areas for which data on elderly patients from controlled trials exist. The Heart Protection Study (HPS; MRC/BHF Heart Protection Study 2002) was the first megatrial (20,563 patients included) in which the number of elderly patients (up to 80 years of age) included was large enough to allow for meaningful statistical analysis. Patients at high cardiovascular risk (history of CHD, diabetes mellitus type 2, arterial hypertension, stroke, or peripheral arterial occlusive disease) with average or even low levels of cholesterol were treated with 40 mg/day simvastatin for 5 years. At entry, 5,806 patients were 70+ years old, and of those, 1,263 patients were 75+ years. In this cohort of elderly patients, all-cause mortality was lowered by 13% ($p = 0.003$). Vascular mortality was reduced by 17% ($p < 0.0001$) and the risk of stroke by 25% ($p < 0.0001$). The risk of cardiovascular events remained unchanged during the first year, but decreased by 27% later ($p < 0.0001$). This reduction was also significant in patients aged 75+ years. To prevent one vascular event in patients aged 70+ years, only 20 patients had to be treated for 5 years (NNT). The results of HPS showed that elderly patients aged

70–80 years at high cardiovascular risk benefitted from treatment with 40 mg simvastatin.

In PROSPER, 5,804 patients aged 70–82 years (mean age 75 years) were included and treated by 40 mg pravastatin versus placebo (Shepherd et al. 2002). So far, this is the only trial on this subject that has been performed in elderly patients only, including sufficient numbers of women ($n = 3,000$). Mean observation time was 3.2 years. Inclusion criteria were cardiovascular risk factors (diabetes mellitus, arterial hypertension, smoking) or CHD. The primary endpoint consisted of death by coronary event, myocardial infarction, or stroke. This endpoint was reduced by 15% in the statin group compared to placebo ($p = 0.014$; Fig. 3). The NNT was 26 in this trial.

These data show that there is no plausible reason to withhold statins from elderly patients if they are at high cardiovascular risk. Unfortunately, there are no clear guidelines for the treatment of elderly patients in this area despite the fact that evidence is available. The modified ATPIII guideline mentioned does not explicitly state how to treat elderly patients. Should centenarians be treated the same way as younger adults would be? Which are the criteria for not treating high-risk patients? When is it not "worth it"?

The recommendation of the Mannheim Center of Gerontopharmacology has been mentioned in chapter "Critical Extrapolation of Guidelines and Study Results: Risk-Benefit Assessment for Patients with Reduced Life Expectancy and a New Classification of Drugs According to Their Fitness for the Aged" (Döser et al. 2004). It should not only guide statin treatment in the elderly but also exemplify how extrapolation into the very elderly (for whom we still do not have data on statins) might be done.

The most important basis of this extrapolation is the estimate for the remaining lifetime of a given patient as preventive measures like statin therapy always need to be gauged against life expectancy. If all statistics show that centenarians have one more year to live on average, it must be assumed that mortality reduction by 25% will prolong life by a few months only. If in a younger patient the remaining lifetime is

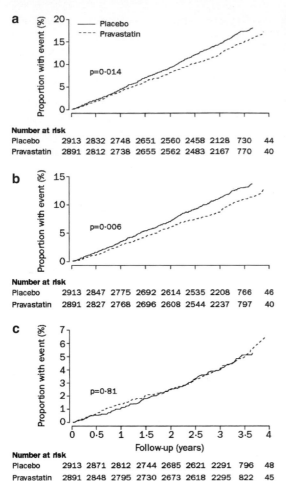

a

Proportion with event (%)

— Placebo
--- Pravastatin

p=0·014

Number at risk

Placebo	2913	2832	2748	2651	2560	2458	2128	730	44
Pravastatin	2891	2812	2738	2655	2562	2483	2167	770	40

b

Proportion with event (%)

p=0·006

Number at risk

Placebo	2913	2847	2775	2692	2614	2535	2208	766	46
Pravastatin	2891	2827	2768	2696	2608	2544	2237	797	40

c

Proportion with event (%)

p=0·81

Follow-up (years)

Number at risk

Placebo	2913	2871	2812	2744	2685	2621	2291	796	48
Pravastatin	2891	2848	2795	2730	2673	2618	2295	822	45

Fig. 3 The primary endpoint [(**a**) death by coronary event, myocardial infarction, or stroke), death by coronary event, myocardial infarction (**b**) or fatal or nonfatal stroke (**c**) in PROSPER (Prospective Study of Pravastatin in the Elderly at Risk); patients were aged 70–82 years (From Shepherd et al. 2002 by kind permission of Elsevier)

10 years, the same treatment effect would translate into a gain of several years. As shown in Table 1 of the chapter "Critical Extrapolation of Guidelines and Study Results: Risk Benefit Assessment for Patients with Reduced Life Expectancy and a New Classification of Drugs According to Their Fitness for the Aged", the average life expectancy of an 80-year-old male in the United States is 7.8 years; in a 95-year-old male, it is still 2.9 years.

The estimate of the remaining lifetime needs to be considered in all preventive therapeutic decisions in the very elderly, although the determination should be based on the biological rather than the chronological age, which carries problems of its own.

Unfortunately, patients aged 80+ years will often not be treated with statins because they are simply "too old." Even in the country that "invented" statins clinically, Norway, undertreatment of the very elderly is dramatic: Up to age 80 years, 71% of the patients who require statin treatment according to guidelines receive it. This rate drops to a mere 11% at age 80+ years, which in reflection of the data mentioned is absolutely unacceptable.

In Table 2 of chapter "Critical Extrapolation of Guidelines and Study Results: Risk-Benefit Assessment for Patients with Reduced Life Expectancy and a New Classification of Drugs According to Their Fitness for the Aged", a recommendation for the treatment of elderly patients with statins is described; it is based on the assumption derived from HPS and PROSPER that up to age 80 years, treatment rules of younger adults should be employed. The NCEP ATPIII guideline briefly states that patients over 65 years of age should be treated as younger patients would be, although an upper age limit for this guidance is missing. Prescription practice seems to support the assumption that this non-differentiating guideline results in the undertreatment issue mentioned for Norway as an example.

Even patients above 65 years should be subject to an estimate of life expectancy. If this estimate is below 10 years (malignancies, premature aging, severe dementia as examples) patients would only be treated as if they were in category 2 or, if life expectancy is only 3 years, category 3.

In all categories, starting and treatment of LDL cholesterol levels are specified. If LDL excess is small (less than 30 mg/dl), lifestyle treatment is initiated prior to statins, which may be started instantly at larger deviations.

The recommendations for categories 2 and 3 for the very elderly (80–90 and 90+ years old) represent consensus statements as no data support them. In both categories, the cutoff levels for LDL cholesterol have been raised to increase the expected treatment effect despite reduced life expectancy. The recommendation is based on the unproven assumption that the percentage decrease of mortality is the same as in younger patients; at higher initial levels, the absolute effect is bigger than at lower levels (see previous discussion). This increased effect is balanced by the overall decrease of life expectancy at high age. Considering an extreme example might be helpful: A 60-year-old male has a remaining life expectancy of about 20 years, and mortality reduction effects will be considerably larger than in a 95-year-old patient with a remaining life expectancy of 2.9 years.

Statin treatment in the so-called situation of primary prevention (no CHD known) will only be indicated in category 2 in the presence of two and more risk factors and not indicated for any patient in category 3. That means that primary prevention at very high age should be considered as ineffi-cient, although even in this category asymptom-atic CHD patients (secondary prevention) will be treated. In this situation, a starting level of LDL cholesterol of 190 mg/dl with a target level of 160 mg/dl is proposed. If life expectancy is esti-mated to be less than 3 years, chronic statin treat-ment should not be initiated. Whether this aspect of the recommendation that originally was pro-posed for elderly patients only (for instance, with malignancies) should be expanded to younger patients is debatable. In the light of the general increase of life expectancy from 2004 (when the recommendation was first published) to date, the age limits for categories 2 and 3 have been raised from 85 to 90 and from above 85 to above 90 years in this book, respectively.

The most frequent side effects of statins are elevations of transaminases (about 2% of patients), myopathies, and rhabdomyolyses. Ele-vations of transaminases are dose dependent, mostly asymptomatic, and reversible. Patients with known active liver diseases or cholestasis should not receive statins, although the progres-sion of these diseases has not been shown.

Patients with muscle pain or weakness are often highly symptomatic; in the elderly, muscle weakness may have a variety of causes, such as hypokalemia or sarcopenia. The incidence of statin-related muscle symptoms in patients is estimated to range up to 5%.

Rhabdomyolysis is a rare, but potentially lethal, complication of statin therapy as it may rapidly lead to acute renal failure. The risk for the fatal course is estimated to be less than 1 per one million treatments. To cope with this threat, regular and frequent controls of serum creatine kinase (CK) need to be performed and the patient informed about the symptoms of myopathy.

According to the general recommendations, statin medication needs to be instantly stopped in the presence of a tenfold elevation of CK (or threefold elevation of transaminases). In elderly patients without a clear statin-independent cause (such as a fall or injury), a cessation threshold of fivefold CK elevation should be accepted with the exception of the acute coronary syndrome. A threefold elevation of CK (1.5-fold elevation of transaminases) requires close monitoring, and the statin should be stopped in the case of pro-longed elevations above those levels. Patients suffering from hypothyroidism or renal failure have an increased risk of myopathy, and these risk factors are frequent in the elderly. Polyphar-macy and altered drug metabolism increase the risk for myopathies, as does alcohol. In particular in elderly women, renal function will be over-estimated as low muscle mass reduces creatinine production and thus serum creatinine elevation despite low renal function (see previous discus-sion). Prior to statin treatment, hypothyroidism needs to be excluded or treated, and the statin dose in patients with low body weight or renal failure adequately reduced. Rhabdomyolyses in the presence of cerivastatin were most frequent in dehydrated elderly patients in nursing homes who insufficiently drank and ate but regularly received the normal statin doses. Marasmus, sar-copenia, and dehydration should be taken as risk factors for side effects of statin therapy, in par-ticular in nursing homes; if those factors are not already limiting statin use by the reduced life expectancy assessment, they should be seen as additional caveats for this therapy.

Drug-drug interactions in elderly patients are another source of trouble for the treatment with statins, and interacting drugs should be avoided whenever possible. This particularly applies to fibrates, which are not rated effective in the elderly (see following discussion), but have been present in various cases with rhabdomyoly-sis under statins. If interacting drugs cannot be avoided, the statin dose should be reduced and safety monitoring as described above intensified. Rhabdomyolysis is seen as a class effect of all statins, although the cerivastatin example demonstrated that the incidence may be very different for the individual statins. In contrast to myopathies, clinically relevant rhabdomyolyses are almost only seen in response to drug-drug interactions. In this context, the CYP (cytochrome P) 450 system is most important: The variant 3A4 is responsible for the metabolism of most statins (atorvastatin, simvastatin, lovastatin), the variant 2C9 for the metabolism of fluvastatin, while pravastatin is not metabolized and rosuvastin only by 10%. Grapefruit juice and St. John's wort contain substances to be metabolized by the CYP450 system and should thus be avoided; the same applies to the drugs in Table 1 (incomplete list). The most relevant interactions with statins are compiled in this table.

To treat LDL cholesterol to target is feasible in 70–80% of patients with the optimal dose of a statin. In elderly patients, the highest marketed doses should not be employed. A stronger statin rather than the highest dose of a weaker statin should be used. The order of strength is simvastatin < atorvastatin < rosuvastatin if LDL cholesterol lowering per milligram of substance is analyzed.

Combinations of statins with fibrates or ezetimibe are not well studied in the elderly and should be avoided, also because of the potential for interactions of statins with fibrates. In ENHANCE, ezetimibe (cholesterol uptake inhibitor) has disappointed as a partner of statins; its addition did not further reduce cardiovascular endpoints. Nicotinic acid (niacin) should be used very restrictively in the elderly as it produces intolerable side effects (flush, headaches, hypotension) and thus is inacceptable to many patients. The cardiovascular strain induced by the side effects should be seen as another caveat for its use in the elderly. The combination with laropripant that suppresses side effects is not available in the United States, although approved in Europe. In addition, a National Institutes of Health (NIH) trial on cardiovascular endpoints was prematurely stopped recently as niacin failed to show additional effects on top of statins.

In the light of these data, patients aged up to 80 years should generally be treated as younger patients. Beyond that age (or in other situations of reduced life expectancy), therapeutic intensity is reduced in relation to the overall cardiovascular risk profile and life expectancy. Therapeutic nihilism, however, is no choice.

Classification of Drugs for the Chronic Treatment of Postmyocardial Infarction Patients According to Their Fitness for the Aged (FORTA)

In this classification of drugs for the chronic treatment of postmyocardial infarction patients according to their fitness for the aged (FORTA), the same compounds may receive alternative marks if applied in different indications; (see chapter "Critical Extrapolation of Guidelines and Study Results: Risk-Benefit Assessment for Patients with Reduced Life Expectancy and a New Classification of Drugs According to Their Fitness for the Aged").

Acetylsalicylic acid (aspirin) (75–325 mg/day)	A
Clopidogrel	B (A for stent patients or in Aspirin-intolerance)
Heart-rate-lowering beta-blockers	A
Renin-angiotensin system inhibitors: ACE inhibitors	A
Nitrates, chronic treatment	C
Nitrates, occasional acute treatment as spray on demand	A
Statins	A (B in very elderly patients)
Fibrates	C
Niacin (nicotinic acid)	C
Ezetimibe	C
Influenza vaccination (split vaccine)	A
Class I–III antiarrhythmics	D
Exception: amiodarone	C
Dihydropyridine calcium channel blockers (if no hypertension)	D
Verapamil or diltiazem: addition to beta-blockers	D (rare exceptions)
Verapamil or dilthiazem: alternative to beta-blockers in symptomatic patients	C

Table 1 Most important/frequent interactions of statins with other drugs (list incomplete)

Augmented effects of statins by elevated plasma levels (inhibition of CYPP450 2C9)	Cimetidine
	Metronidazole
	Omeprazole
	Ranitidine
Augmented effects of statins by elevated plasma levels (inhibition of CYPP450 2D6)	Chinidine (not FDA approved)
	Paroxetine
	Propafenone
	Thioridazine
Augmented effects of statins by elevated plasma levels (inhibition of CYP3A4)	Antimycotics (azole type, including itraconazole, increase of statin AUC by 300 %), ketoconazole
	Cyclosporine
	Fluvoxamine
	Grapefruit juice (20.4 % increase of AUC by 240 ml)
	HIV protease inhibitors
	St. John's wort
	Macrolide antibiotics, including clarithromycin (AUC, increase of statins by 80 %), erythromycin (AUC, increase of statins by 56 %)
	Nefazodone
Augmented effects of these drugs	Digoxin
	Ethinyl estradiol
	Norethisterone (not FDA approved)
	Phenytoin
	Warfarin
Displacement from plasma protein binding by these drugs	Immunosuppressants, including cyclosporine
	Gemfibrozil
	Nicotinic acid (niacin)
	Erythromycin
Increased threat of myopathy because of reduced elimination	Amiodarone
	Antimycotics, including itraconazole
	Diltiazem
	Erythromycin
	Gemfibrozil and other fibrates
	HIV protease inhibitors
	Immunosuppressants, including cyclosporine
	Macrolide antibiotics, including clarithromycin, erythromycin
	Nefazodone
	Nicotinic acid (niacin)
	Verapamil
Reduced statin effect by	Resins (ion exchangers)
	Antacids at simultaneous application
Reduced statin effect by decreased plasma levels	Rifampine (AUC of statins lowered by 50 %)

Source: From Döser et al. 2004 by permission

AUC area under the curve, *CYP* cytochrome P, *FDA* Food and Drug Administration

Stroke

The primary treatment of stroke should be reserved for specialists and requires specialized "stroke units." Its major component—as far as drug treatment is involved—is lysis treatment, which needs to be indicated with the same scrutiny (exclusion of potential bleeding complications, in particular intracerebral hemorrhage, with a computed tomographic [CT] scan mandatory before lysis) described. As a prerequisite for lysis, the arterial blood pressure should not exceed 185/110 mmHg, and proper drug treatment may be necessary to achieve this. Blood pressure reduction to values much lower than those limits is seen critical in acute ischemic strokes for about 24 h as marginal perfusion of the infarcted brain areas (penumbra) may be impaired. Lysis in the very elderly will not be possible in a progressive number of patients as bleeding complications increase with age, and contraindications prevail. Invasive procedures (stenting, bypass operations) are also critical at this age, and data for the very elderly are still sparse. Acute application of platelet inhibitors requires the exclusion of cerebral hemorrhage by a CT scan but is otherwise indicated (325 mg/day aspirin in the United States, 100 mg/day in Europe), commencing during day 1 or 2. Anticoagulation (by heparins) is not indicated according to the ASA Guidelines of 2007 (Adams et al. 2007).

In secondary prophylaxis, some of the interventions discussed in the previous chapter on postmyocardial infarction patients are recommended here as well, although their weight is different. The most important intervention is the control of arterial hypertension starting about 1 week after the acute ischemic event. In the first week, systolic pressures between 150 and 170 mmHg are seen beneficial as improved perfusion of the marginal areas (penumbra) may save and revitalize tissue in the acute phase. Only after this acute phase, treatment of arterial hypertension will be intensified to finally reach a consistent and durable control of blood pressure

as described in chapter "Arterial Hypertension". Treatment of diabetes mellitus; lifestyle modifications, including reduction of body weight, harmful nutrients (alcohol, caffeine), or habits (smoking, no exercise); are identical to those recommendations mentioned.

Platelet inhibition by aspirin, which is indicated in secondary prophylaxis of ischemic stroke, may be augmented by extended-release dipyridamol according to ESPS2. This combination is marketed as Aggrenox® (200 mg dipyridamol plus 25 mg aspirin b.i.d.). In the U.S. recommendation, both aspirin alone and this combination are recommended (Adams et al. 2008), although data are not homogeneously showing an additional effect of dipyridamol. This compound may cause orthostatic reactions in the elderly, who are not separately mentioned in this recommendation. Therefore, caution should be exercised for the use of the combination in the elderly. Aspirin side effects mandate its replacement by clopidogrel.

No doubt exists about the beneficial effect of statins for secondary (and primary) stroke prevention (PPP, SPARCL), although the extent of effects seems smaller than in myocardial infarction prevention. Fatal and nonfatal strokes were reduced by 16% in PPP and by high-dose atorvastatin (80 mg/day) in SPARCL by 16% (Fig. 4). Given that the assumptions for the indication of statins in the very elderly patients as described are correct, the use of statins in this indication should be even more restrictive than for postmyocardial infarction prevention. We do not yet know whether patients aged 80+ years benefit from statin prophylaxis against recurrent stroke. In the new modification of the AHA/ASA guideline (Adams et al. 2008), strong lowering of LDL cholesterol by 80 mg/day atorvastatin is recommended for all patients, with no age limit given. The mean age in SPARCL (63 years) was not mentioned in this recommendation. In PPP, effects were insignificant in patients aged 62+ years. I thus do not recommend statin treatment without consideration of LDL cholesterol levels (as it is the case in the AHA/ASA guideline) if the patient

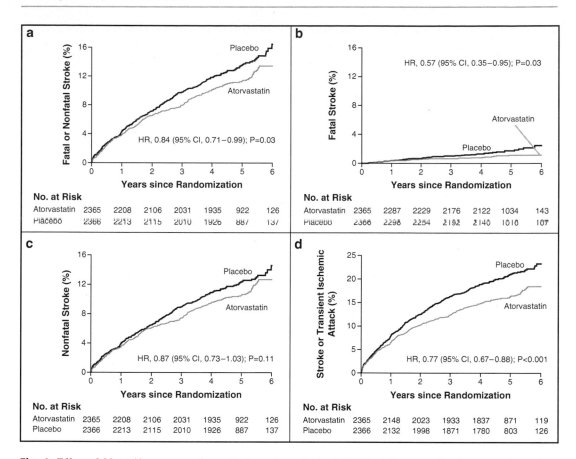

Fig. 4 Effect of 80 mg/day atorvastatin on stroke endpoints in SPARCL: (**a**) fatal and nonfatal stroke; (**b**) fatal stroke; (**c**) nonfatal stroke; (**d**) stroke or transient ischemic attack. *SPARCL* stroke prevention by aggressive reduction in cholesterol level (From Amarenco et al. 2006 by kind permission of the Massachusetts Medical Society)

is aged 75+ years. Even up to this age, statin toxicity may be considerable (polypharmacy, interactions, dehydration, renal failure) and needs to be carefully considered. At higher age, a risk-related, more restrictive approach like the one described for myocardial infarction prophylaxis should be employed. This example of missing data for very elderly patients who frequently suffer from the disease discussed and recommendations that are ignorant of age-related problems is typical for gerontopharmacology. The extrapolation that is envisioned here as in the postmyocardial infarction situation is not trivial as the effects are even smaller for stroke. As far as it is known to me, not even a consensus process has been started to address this important question.

If *cardiac thromboembolism* in atrial fibrillation is underlying the stroke, consequent anticoagulation is very effective and strictly indicated as described in chapter "Atrial Fibrillation".

In elderly/very elderly patients, long-term drug treatment of stroke, in addition to neurological drugs such as muscle relaxants, consists of the consequent treatment of arterial hypertension (combination therapy in most cases) plus aspirin with or without dipyridamol plus critically indicated and closely monitored statin therapy. This simple approach results in dramatic reductions of endpoints by 30–50 % (e.g., 42 % stroke reduction in SYST-EUR) also in elderly/very elderly patients. Unfortunately, many patients do not benefit from this

enormous opportunity as underutilization is very common in medical reality.

Study Acronyms

AIRE Acute Infarction Ramipril Efficacy Study

COMMIT Clopidogrel and Metoprolol in Myocardial Infarction Trial

CRUSADE Can Rapid Risk Stratification of Unstable Angina Patients Suppress Adverse Outcomes with Early Implementation of the ACC/AHA Guidelines National Quality Improvement Initiative Database

CURE Clopidogrel in Unstable Angina to Prevent Recurrent Events Trial

ENHANCE Ezetimibe and Simvastatin in Hypercholesterolemia Enhances Atherosclerosis Regression Study

FTT Fibrinolytic Therapy Trialists

HERS Heart and Estrogen/Progestin Replacement Study

HOPE Studie Heart Outcomes Prevention Study

HPS Heart Protection Study

MADIT-II Multicenter Automatic Defibrillator Implantation Trial II

MIRACL Myocardial Ischemia Reduction with Aggressive Cholesterol Lowering Study

PROSPER Prospective Study of Pravastatin in the Elderly at Risk

SAVE Survival and Ventricular Enlargement Study

SPARCL Stroke Prevention by Aggressive Reduction in Cholesterol Level Study

TACTICS-TIMI-18 Treat Angina with Aggrastat and Determine Cost of Therapy with an Invasive Conservative Strategy

WHI Studie Women's Health Initiative Study

References

Adams HP Jr, del Zoppo G, Alberts MJ et al (2007) Guidelines for the early management of adults with ischemic stroke: a guideline from the American Heart Association/American Stroke Association Stroke Council, Clinical Cardiology Council, Cardiovascular Radiology and Intervention Council, and the Atherosclerotic Peripheral Vascular Disease and Quality of Care Outcomes in Research Interdisciplinary Working Groups: the American Academy of Neurology affirms the value of this guideline as an educational tool for neurologists. Stroke 38:1655–1711

Adams RJ, Albers G, Alberts MJ et al (2008) Update to the AHA/ASA recommendations for the prevention of stroke in patients with stroke and transient ischemic attack. Stroke 39:1647–1652

Amarenco P, Bogousslavsky J, Callahan A 3rd et al (2006) Highdose atorvastatin after stroke or transient ischemic attack. N Engl J Med 355:549–559

Aronow WS, Ahn C (1996) Risk factors for new coronary events in a large cohort of very elderly patients with and without coronary artery disease. Am J Cardiol 77:864–866

Bach RG, Cannon CP, Weintraub WS et al (2005) The effect of routine, early invasive management on outcome for elderly patients with non-ST-segment elevation acute coronary syndromes. Ann Intern Med 141:186–195

Baigent C, Keech A, Kearney PM et al (2005) Efficacy and safety of cholesterol-lowering treatment: prospective meta-analysis of data from 90,056 participants in 14 randomised trials of statins. Lancet 366 (9493):1267–1278

Boersma E, Harrington RA, Moliterno DJ et al (2002) Platelet glycoprotein IIb/IIIa inhibitors in acute coronary syndromes: a meta-analysis of all major randomised clinical trials. Lancet 359(9302):189–198

Cholesterol Treatment Trialists' CTT Collaboration, Baigent C, Blackwell L et al (2010) Efficacy and safety of more intensive lowering of LDL cholesterol: a meta-analysis of data from 170,000 participants in 26 randomised trials. Lancet 376:1670–1681

COMMIT Collaborative Group (2005) Early intravenous then oral metoprolol in 45,852 patients with acute myocardial infarction: randomized placebo-controlled trial. Lancet 366:1622–1632

Döser S, Marz W, Reinecke MF et al (2004) Empfehlungen zur Statintherapie im Alter: Daten und Consensus. Internist (Berl) 45:1053–1062

Fibrinolytic Therapy Trialists' (FTT) Collaborative Group (1994) Indications for fibrinolytic therapy in suspected acute myocardial infarction: collaborative overview of early mortality and major morbidity results from all randomised trials of more than 1,000 patients. Lancet 343(8893):311–322

Grundy SM, Cleeman JI, Merz CNB et al (2004) Implications of recent clinical trials for the national cholesterol education program adult treatment panel III guidelines. Circulation 110:227–239

Heart Protection Study Collaborative Group (2002) MRC/BHF Heart Protection Study of cholesterol lowering with simvastatin in 20,536 high-risk individuals: a randomised placebo-controlled trial. Lancet 360:7–22

Heron MP, Hoyert DL, Murphy SL, Xu JQ, Kochanek KD, Tejada-Vera B (2009) Deaths: final data for 2006.

National vital statistics reports, vol 57, no 14. National Center for Health Statistics, Hyattsville

Krumholz HM, Radford MJ, Ellerbeck EF et al (1995) Aspirin in the treatment of acute myocardial infarction in elderly Medicare beneficiaries. Patterns of use and outcomes. Circulation 92:2841–2847

Kyriakides ZS, Kourouklis S, Kontaras K (2007) Acute coronary syndromes in the elderly. Drugs Aging 24:901–912

Lenderink T, Boersma E, Gitt AK et al (2006) Patients using statin treatment within 24 h after admission for ST-elevation acute coronary syndromes had lower mortality than nonusers: a report from the first Euro Heart Survey on acute coronary syndromes. Eur Heart J 27:1799–1804

Schuler J, Maier B, Behrens S, Thimme W (2006) Present treatment of acute myocardial infarction in patients over 75 years—data from the Berlin Myocardial Infarction Registry (BHIR). Clin Res Cardiol 95:360–367

Shepherd J, Blauw GJ, Murphy MB et al (2002) Pravastatin in elderly individuals at risk of vascular disease (PROSPER): a randomised controlled trial. Lancet 360:1623–1630

Task Force for Diagnosis and Treatment of Non-ST-Segment Elevation Acute Coronary Syndromes of European Society of Cardiology, Bassand JP, Hamm CW et al (2007) Guidelines for the diagnosis and treatment of non-ST-segment elevation acute coronary syndromes. Eur Heart J 28:1598–1660

The TIME Investigators (2001) Trial of invasive versus medical therapy in elderly patients with chronic symptomatic coronary- artery disease (TIME): a randomised trial. Lancet 358:951–957

Atrial Fibrillation

Martin Wehling

Relevance for Elderly Patients, Epidemiology

Atrial fibrillation (AF) is a very common and relevant disease of the elderly (Fig. 1). Of the general population, 1%, but 10% of the 80+-year-old age group, suffer from it. In the United States alone, 2.2 million patients have AF, with an unknown number of undiagnosed cases (which may represent another two million patients), and this figure is expected to at least double by 2050. In Europe, the number of AF patients is estimated to be around six million.

Mortality of AF patients is twice that of age-matched persons without AF. The rate of stroke is increased fivefold, and 65+-year-old patients have a rate of cardiogenic thromboembolism of 4–12% per year. These numbers demonstrate that AF is one of the most important age-related diseases. Its relevance is not only underlined by these epidemiological data, but also by the fact that treatment is very successful if properly performed. The major problem of AF is thromboembolic disease originating from the heart atria, which causes strokes and peripheral occlusions (such as mesenteric or leg artery occlusions). It is accepted that 20–30% of all strokes in the elderly originate from AF. Fortunately, all studies on the major therapeutic principle, namely anticoagulation, show positive results, and this includes a sufficient number of elderly study patients. The disease is among the very few for which several studies have a dominant participation of elderly patients (>65 years) in controlled clinical trials (mean age in AFFIRM 70 years). Relating to this book, this is the only situation for which actually more data on elderly than on younger patients are available.

Therapeutic effects have been clearly demonstrated, in particular in elderly patients. On average, the rate of embolic stroke as a major complication was lowered by 40–80% if anticoagulation was tested against placebo. Therefore, in a patient with AF, the question is not whether anticoagulation should be initiated, but only whether there are compelling, proven, and nonmodifiable reasons against it.

Anticoagulation as embolism prophylaxis is the only indisputably beneficial therapeutic option in this context.

Two additional therapeutic goals may be addressed by pharmacotherapy:

- Heart rate control (ventricular rate control if tachycardia is present)
- Restoration of sinus rhythm (Fig. 2)
  Generally, in all age groups different forms of AF are diagnosed:
- Paroxysmal (rare, short episodes)
- Persistent: for more than 7 days or requiring therapy to convert to sinus rhythm
- Long persistent: for more than 1 year

M. Wehling (✉)
University of Heidelberg, Maybachstr. 14, Mannheim 68169, Germany
e-mail: martin.wehling@medma.uni-heidelberg.de

M. Wehling (ed.), *Drug Therapy for the Elderly*,
DOI 10.1007/978-3-7091-0912-0_9, © Springer-Verlag Wien 2013

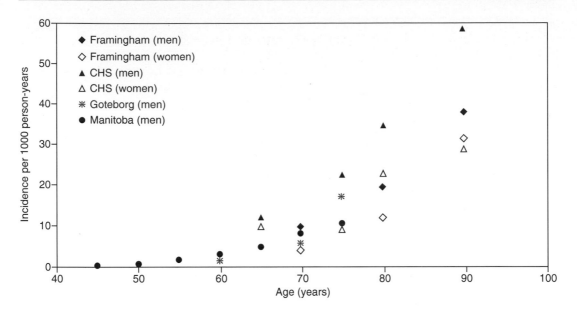

Fig. 1 Incidence of atrial fibrillation versus age, data from large epidemiological studies (From Savelieva and Camm 2001 by kind permission of Wiley-Blackwell) *CHS*: cardiovascular health study

– Permanent: accepted (not convertable by cardioversion).

The last two categories are also termed chronic AF.

Underlying diseases or conditions are as follows:

– Arterial hypertension (the disease with the largest contribution)
– Coronary heart disease
– Dilative cardiomyopathy
– Valvular heart disease

But also, endocrine and other disorders may be underlying:

– Thyrotoxicosis (including iatrogenic cases)
– Pheochromocytoma
– Fever
– In particular nutritional toxins, especially alcohol, caffeine

Excessive consumption of the last toxins, in particular alcohol, is a common and avoidable cause of paroxysmal AF. This disease is one of the many catecholamine-dependent disorders explaining the triggering of AF by stress of all causes (such as surgery, infections, excessive physical stress). Obviously, many of the triggers, including thyrotoxicosis, can be treated or avoided.

Therapeutically Relevant Special Features of Elderly Patients

As AF is a disease of the elderly, its features in this age group are the typical ones, and the younger patients would rather deserve a special discussion. In younger patients, severe cardiac diseases may be the culprits, as opposed to "lone atrial fibrillation," which is without organic correlate but is thought mainly to reflect catecholamine excess. Alcohol as a trigger (excesses on the weekend, main adrenergic stimulation on withdrawal on Monday morning, which is the main manifestation day of this form) is not rare and is a typical threat to stressed managers. Aberrant atrial tissue in the pulmonary veins may be another cause mainly manifesting the disease at younger age and is successfully treated by ablation techniques.

In elderly patients, the classic structural damages by arterial hypertension, coronary heart disease, or valvular heart disease prevail. Thyrotoxicosis in the elderly may present with AF as the only symptom.

Heart block syndromes at the level of the sinus or atrioventricular nodes may cause problems on

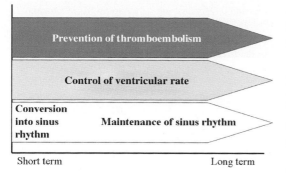

Fig. 2 Atrial fibrillation: three therapeutic goals of drug therapy

restitution of sinus rhythm and lead to syncopes. This is aggravated by the fact that during AF such heart blocks are not detectable by standard electrocardiographic (ECG) recording, and pharmacological treatment by beta-blockers and, in particular, antiarrhythmics may precipitate asystole with all life-threatening consequences.

The leading symptoms of AF in descending order of prevalence are

– Tiredness
– Palpitations
– Subjective tachycardia
– Dyspnea
– Weakness
– Sleep disorders

In the very elderly, direct symptoms of arrhythmias may remain unrecognized or are felt subjectively at low intensity. Cognitive impairment and mood instability may be the only subtle symptoms, which are hard to detect.

Syncopes are frequent in elderly patients and should always trigger the search for AF in one or more Holter ECG readings.

The rate of thromboembolic complications of AF strongly increases with age, leading to the dilemma that the elderly require strict anticoagulation even more stringently than younger patients. Unfortunately, they have more frequent contraindications (such as frequent falls) as well and, in this case, cannot be treated by current drugs (vitamin K antagonists, VKAs). The new oral anticoagulants (see the following) give hope to address the dilemma with greater success than currently achievable.

Other age-related special features are discussed in the context of the pharmacotherapy details as they are generic.

Evidence-Based, Rationalistic Drug Therapy and Classification of Drugs According to Their Fitness for the Aged (FORTA)

The "ACC/AHA/ESC Guidelines for the Management of Patients with Atrial Fibrillation" of 2006 and their 2011 amendment (Fuster et al. 2006, 2011) mentioned age-related aspects punctually but did not devote a special chapter to the very elderly. This is in contrast to the obvious fact that a 90-year-old patient may have other limitations and special issues to cover than a 60-year-old patient. In reflection of this lack of guidance, this book has to leave the relatively safe grounds of international recommendations and use the empirical and rational route in the typical way described and exemplified in many chapters of this book.

Anticoagulation

Without doubt, the most important therapeutic intervention in AF is anticoagulation, which has proven its impressive efficacy even in the geriatric population in many controlled clinical trials. The ultimate treatment goal of AF is the induction of stable sinus rhythm, which, however, is less and less often achieved at increasing age. Therefore, its relative contribution to the overall success is decreasing or even vanishing in the elderly and very elderly cohort, with anticoagulation (and rate control) becoming even more important and solitary.

In the typical therapeutic situation, an 80-year-old patient will receive anticoagulation (if no contraindications exist, such as high fall risk) and drugs for rate control. The patient will not receive antiarrhythmics (except for beta-blockers and/or verapamil or diltiazem).

To date, oral VKAs represent the main principle of long-term, oral anticoagulation, with warfarin (United States) or phenprocoumon (Europe) the main drugs from this group. These compounds reduce the production of the coagulation factors II, V, VII, IX, and X in the liver.

All interventional studies on VKAs showed extensive reductions of thromboembolic events, especially strokes; the homogeneity of data from several trials is remarkable and exemplary in medicine. The large trials AFASAK, BAATAF, CAFA, EAFT, SPAF, and SPINAF demonstrated a reduction of stroke events by oral anticoagulation of 60% versus placebo. For an average annual stroke rate of 5%, this indicates an absolute reduction by 3%. The annual number needed to treat (NNT) is only $100/3 = 33$: 100 patients need to be treated for 1 year to prevent 3 strokes or 33 patients to prevent 1 stroke. These and other trials also defined the conditions of successful oral anticoagulation. For the risk-benefit calculation, a risk for cerebral hemorrhages of 0.5–1% per patient year is assumed. This risk sharply rises with the intensity of anticoagulation (up to 3% at an international normalized ratio [INR] of 5) and with age. The recommendations derived from those studies try to optimize the risk-benefit ratio in that an optimal point is sought at which the lowering of embolism clearly produces a larger benefit than compensated for by increased bleeding risk.

If the risk of embolism is low, the bleeding risk under VKAs may exceed the benefit; thus, for low-risk patients aspirin is seen as sufficient. Oppositely, at very high risk of thromboembolism, more intense anticoagulation by VKAs may be useful, and the INR target may be 4–5 rather than 2–3 as in the average case.

According to the guideline of 2006/2011 (by kind permission of Wolters Kluwer Health), as mentioned, the following class I recommendations should be employed:

Patient under 60 years, no risk factors (heart failure, left ventricular ejection fraction <35%, arterial hypertension)	Aspirin 81–325 mg/day or nothing
Patient under 60 years, cardiac disease, but no risk factors	Aspirin 81–325 mg/day

(continued)

Patient 60–74 years, no risk factors	Aspirin 81–325 mg/day
Patient 60–74 years, CHD or diabetes mellitus	Oral anticoagulation (INR 2–3)
Patient >75 years, women	Oral anticoagulation (INR 2–3)
Patient >75 years, men, no risk factors	Oral anticoagulation (INR 2–3) or aspirin 81–325 mg/day
Patient >65 years, heart failure	Oral anticoagulation (INR 2–3)
Ejection fraction <35%, or "fractional shortening" <25%, and arterial hypertension	Oral anticoagulation (INR 2–3)
Rheumatic heart disease (mitral stenosis)	Oral anticoagulation (INR 2–3)
Prosthetic heart valves	Oral anticoagulation (INR 2–3 or higher)
Prior thromboembolism	Oral anticoagulation (INR 2–3 or higher)
Persisting atrial thrombus in transesophageal echo	Oral anticoagulation (INR 2–3 or higher)

This summary demonstrates that although the risk factor concept is differentiated, it still cannot provide unequivocal recommendations for all situations.

Why Is Anticoagulation So Critical and Needs Strict Targets?

The therapeutic index of current VKAs is narrow, and plasma concentrations are subject to multiple interactions. Thus, the INR needs to be monitored frequently; home determination by the patient may improve adjustments. INR checks need to be intensified at any instance of changing additional medications, with respect to both dose and drug cessation/initiation. This reflects the large potential of VKAs to participate in drug-drug interactions, mainly at the pharmacokinetic level. A list of potential interactions is given in Table 1.

The last line of the table needs to be emphasized as the impact of nutrition on VKA effects depends on the vitamin K supply. It is obvious that this supply may vary extensively if patients change their nutritional behavior or environment (relocation to nursing home). This point is

Table 1 Drug-drug interactions of vitamin K antagonists (VKA), warfarin or phenprocoumon

Clinically *relevant* augmentation of effect of VKA (*increased bleeding risk*) by concomitant medication	Acetylsalicylic acid (Aspirin)
	Allopurinol
	Amiodarone
	Chloramphenicol
	Cloxacillin
	Disulfiram
	Erythromycin and derivatives
	Fibrates
	Imidazole derivates
	Methyltestosterone and other anabolic steroids
	Phenylbutazone and analogues
	Piroxicam
	Thyroid hormones
	Tamoxifen
	Tetracycline
	Triazole derivatives
	Trimethoprim-sulfmethoxazole and other sulfonamides
	Tricyclic antidepressants
Clinically *possible* augmentation of effect of VKA (*increased bleeding risk*) by concomitant medication	Cefazoline
	Cefotaxime
	Cefpodoxime proxetil
	Ceftibuten
	Chinidine (not FDA approved)
	Heparinoids
	Low molecular weight heparins
	N-Methylthiotetrazole cephalosporins
	Platelet inhibitors or mucosal damage in the gastrointestinal tract by drugs, mainly NSAID
	Propafenone
	Unfractionated heparins
Reduced effect of VKA (*increased thromboembolism rates*) by concomitant medication	Barbiturates
	Carbamazepine
	Colestyramine
	Corticosteroids
	Diuretics
	Glutethimide (aminoglutethimide)
	6-Mercaptopurine
	Rifampin
	Propylthiouracil
Interaction by induction of microsomal (CYP450) enzymes, upon cessation of drug and unchanged dosing of VKA risk of excessive anticoagulation, frequent INR monitoring necessary	Barbiturates
	Carbamazepine
	Glutethimide
	Rifampin
Activation of CYP450 system. Frequent monitoring at initiation and cessation of therapy with consequent dose adaptations required	St. John's wort preparations
Complex interactions with VKA (acute effect: augmentation of VKA effect; chronic effect: attenuation, except for patients with hepatic failure: augmentation)	Ethanol

(continued)

Table 1 (continued)

Hypoglycemia possible if concomitant use of VKA and	Sulfonyl ureas
Increased clearance of VKA without obvious impact on anticoagulation	Estrogen/progesterone anticonceptives
Variable interactions of VKA with nutritional vitamin K supply; both augmentation and attenuation possible	Food

Source: Modified from Rossol-Haseroth et al. 2002 by permission
Both compounds are seen analogous in this context
CYP cytochrome P, *FDA* Food and Drug Administration, *INR* international normalization ratio, *NSAID* nonsteroidal anti-inflammatory

particularly critical for the elderly, and the nutritional instability is larger in the elderly compared to younger patients. This is one of the major contributors to therapeutic failures and complications in the elderly. The extensive list of interacting drugs (Table 1 is still incomplete) again is of major importance for elderly patients as they are at high risk to receive polypharmacy (see parts "General Aspects" and "Further Problem Areas in Gerontopharmacotherapy and Pragmatic Recommendations").

On the one hand, an improved quality of anticoagulation in the elderly is important as bleeding risk is elevated in patients 80+ years of age; on the other hand, the number of patients who cannot receive VKAs due to contraindications steeply rises in this age group.

High fall risk is one of the major issues of oral anticoagulation in the elderly, which is often caused or at least worsened by dementia impairing postural reflexes.

This and other functional deficits are largely underestimated in relation to their potential to interfere with adherence to complex drug therapies. Visual impairment (either uncorrected or permanent with no healing perspective such as in macular degeneration) as a leading example disables patients to

– Regularly apply drugs,
– Recognize missed medications, and
– Read information slips and use instructions.

A white pill in a white pill box may not be found by the visually impaired patient and will be missed. Manual dexterity may be limiting as well: If a patient is unable to write due to neurological or rheumatological disorders, it will be difficult to split tablets into parts. VKA pills tend

to be small, and typical dosing schemes often contain half or even a quarter of a tablet. Such patients urgently need help to apply the right dose at the right time and to control INR properly if applicable; this has to be provided by caregivers, such as relatives or friends if professional care is not yet available.

The functional capacity of elderly patients should be routinely tested before oral anticoagulation is initiated.

The following tests may be employed to achieve this:

– Money-counting test, which measures and quantifies the visual capacity, fine motor skills, and cognitive competence.
– "Timed-up-and-go" test, Tinetti test, and one-leg stand test help as functional tests to quantify the fall risk. They should be performed on top of routine testing for fall risk, including Holter monitoring, if a fall has been reported to have occurred in the last 3 months.
– Dementia testing is indispensable, and a decreasing speed of informational transfer and processing is a strong fall risk factor. If the patient cannot find spatial orientation rapidly enough, falls are inevitable. A simple observation may give a hint in this regard: If a patient has to stop walking to talk to someone, this proves that dual tasking is no longer possible and underlines the impairment of cognition. A related clinical test on standing and walking abilities has been described by Tinetti; it includes a stroke against the patient's chest and the observation of the reaction to prevent a fall.
– Before commencing oral anticoagulation, the fall risk should be diagnosed and classified in

each elderly patient. It is, however, unclear which fall rate represents a contraindication. One fall per month may be acceptable, one fall per day certainly not. In addition, the fall causes (sudden blackout, high risk of injury vs. slow reduction of consciousness, lower risk of injuries) are important for the assessment.

- Protective and prophylactic tools such as hip protectors or rollators (wheeled walkers) should be utilized if indicated, and side effects of central nervous system (CNS) and other drugs (so-called FRIDs [fall-risk-increasing drugs]) excluded.

In general, elderly patients should receive two thirds of the regular dose of VKA, particularly on initiation, and frequent INR checks starting on day 4–6. VKA loading should be done with one tablet/day; no rapid saturation is advisable. Bridging with low molecular weight heparins thus may be prolonged.

The problems discussed here are the main reasons for significant undertreatment in daily practice. It is commonly assumed that only 50% of patients requiring oral anticoagulation according to the recommendations mentioned receive this treatment (Nieuwlaat et al. 2006). Given the extensive benefit of oral anticoagulation, in the presence of relative contraindications VKAs should not be withheld but given at low doses, aiming at an INR at the lower limit of the therapeutic range (INR 2). This is certainly better than nothing and better than aspirin, which has a very limited effect (if any) in this indication.

Long-term treatment with low molecular weight heparins as an alternative to VKAs is expensive and often requires frequent support of elderly patients by social services. As a disadvantage, the lack of an antidote should be mentioned. The treatment effect does not require monitoring like VKA therapy; this may be seen both as an advantage (no determinations needed) and as a disadvantage (no biomarker for the treatment efficacy).

In acute AF that cannot be reverted to sinus rhythm within 48 h, rapid anticoagulation is necessary. This is normally started by low molecular weight (dose adaptation to weight and renal function) or unfractionated heparins (5,000 IU b.i.d. or t.i.d.). Particularly the latter heparins may cause heparin-induced thrombocytopenia (HIT); platelet counts need to be controlled twice per week. HIT I is frequent, rapidly reversible on cessation, and clinically generally benign; HIT II is rare and reflects an immune reaction and may progress even after cessation of the drug and cause severe, life-threatening bleeding. The latter form may start within hours of application if immunization has already occurred in the past. Lepirudine (United States) and danaparoid (Europe) are alternatives in these cases.

Long-term treatment with VKAs is difficult and seen as dangerous. Great hope is therefore raised by the novel oral anticoagulants (such as dabigatran, rivaroxaban, apixaban), which are orally available inhibitors of thrombin (dabigatran) or factor Xa (rivaroxaban, apixaban). They are thought to be easier to handle ("one dose fits all," no monitoring required). They have proven their efficacy and safety in chronic treatment of AF (RE-LY, ROCKET-AF, ARISTOTLE) and are in the process of marketing approval; at the time of writing, dabigatran and rivaroxaban have been approved in the European Union and the United States for anticoagulation in AF. All had been approved for short-term treatment for perioperative prophylaxis of venous thromboembolism in knee and hip surgery. These new drugs will help to improve the underutilization issue mentioned for VKAs, although it still has to be seen whether all promises hold in reality. There are doubts about the singular dose approach and safety issues in the very elderly. Labeling will contain notes of caution and dose adjustment recommendations for the very elderly and patients with renal impairment. Although primarily tested in elderly patients, further experiences are required to determine their position in the treatment options. Soon after marketing approval of dabigatran, "Dear Doctor letters" (remedial communication required by the FDA if drug safety/efficacy issues have to be dealt with) had to be issued as lethal bleeding complications associated with renal failure became obvious.

Comparative assessments of these compounds are necessary to further define the conditions of safe use in the "real world." The predominant renal excretion route of dabigatran (as opposed to the predominant hepatic route of apixaban) would have mandated a closer monitoring of renal function and dose adaption beforehand. These measures of precaution are now being installed.

The innovation by these drugs is real; only their expected high costs are likely to prevent their widespread use.

Excursion: Prophylaxis of Venous Thromboembolism in Elderly Patients

Venous thromboses are frequent in the elderly population, and a short excursion on this topic is inserted here (also see chapter "Immobility and Pharmacotherapy"). Above age 60, the incidence doubles with every decade, and 12% of all patients admitted to an acute geriatric hospital show an asymptomatic pulmonary embolism scintigraphically. Pulmonary emboli originate from deep venous thromboses in 90% of cases, for which serious diseases, especially malignancies, heart failure, immobilization, infections, and surgery are the risk factors.

In this context, prophylaxis and acute/chronic treatment of thrombosis need to be separated. Prophylaxis of thrombosis in the perioperative setting or in bedridden patients should be performed by unfractionated heparin, 5,000 IU s.c. q.d. or b.i.d., or preferably with low molecular weight heparins ("low dose") once daily. Especially in elderly patients, renal function and body weight need to be considered for correct dosing as effect determinations or therapeutic drug monitoring (plasma levels of low molecular weight heparins) are not easily accessible in clinical practice. It should be noted that not all low molecular weight heparins are alike; tinzaparin does not accumulate in renal failure to the same extent as enoxaparin and thus appears to be safer in elderly patients.

Clinical studies showed that this prophylaxis is effective in patients aged 75+ years, such as in the MEDENOX Studie (Alikhan et al. 2003;

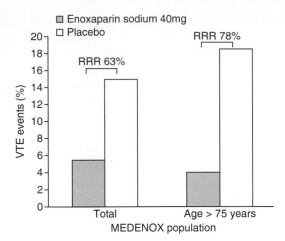

Fig. 3 Reduction of venous thromboembolism events by enoxaparin: no effect difference between the total population and the subgroup of 75+-year-old patients. *MEDENOX* Prophylaxis in Medical Patients with Enoxaparin Study, *RRR* relative risk ratio, *VTE* venous thromboembolism (From Spyropoulos and Merli 2006 by kind permission of Wolters Kluwer)

Fig. 3). Aspirin is no adequate replacement for heparins in this indication.

Generally, this prophylaxis is underutilized, and many thromboembolic events could be prevented, particularly in the elderly. As mentioned, bleeding risk also increases with age, and the estimation of the risk-benefit ratio is important in situations of long-term or even lifelong immobilization. In reflection of this, recommendations concerning thromboembolic prophylaxis need to be rather complex. In our institution, structured and detailed recommendations have been consensually developed (Rossol-Haseroth et al. 2002, Harenberg et al. 2010) that are more sophisticated than the eighth recommendation by the ACCP (American College of Chest Physicians; Geerts et al. 2008). Mobility and other important risk factors for venous thromboembolism are important contributors to the therapeutic approach, and a consensual scoring attempt is shown in Fig. 4. The differentiated recommendations for different clinical situations in which prophylaxis is indicated are compiled in Table 2 in reflection of this risk stratification. This complex recommendation is an example for the therapeutic situation of elderly patients that requires a rationalistic, multidimensional approach for optimal treatment.

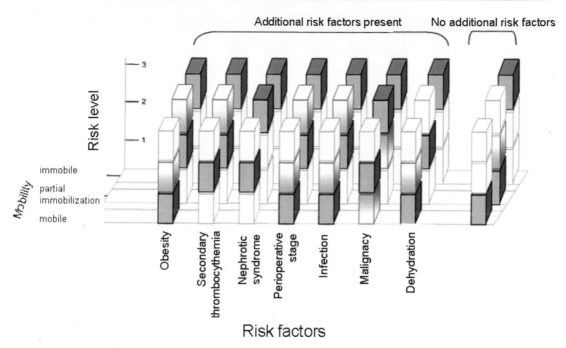

Fig. 4 Stratification of risk for venous thromboembolic disease in elderly patients: The risk level ranges from low (*1*) through intermediate (*2*) to high (*3*) and implies the intensity of the therapeutic intervention. It depends on the mobility status and major risk factors. *Dark segments* of the columns reflect the consensus assessment of risk for the particular mobility/risk factor situation, *shaded segments* indicate the assessment for severe forms of the respective risk factor. If more than one risk factor are present, risk is increased by one step per additional risk factor (Modified from Rossol-Haseroth et al. 2002)

Unfortunately, there are only very few structured analyses and consensus results comparable to this one. Obviously, important aspects of these recommendations are extrapolated, deducted, and not based on solid data. As all consensus recommendations, they represent opinion averaging, and deviations are all but prohibited.

The treatment of thromboembolic diseases as opposed to the prophylaxis described is initiated by unfractionated or low molecular weight heparins at high ("therapeutic") doses; typically, this means two injections of low molecular weight heparins in doses adapted to weight and renal function or 15,000 IU unfractionated heparin per day. Oral anticoagulation will then be started. The duration of anticoagulation ranges from 3 months for distal leg deep vein thrombosis up to a year for proximal thrombosis, including iliac disease. After recurrences, particularly those with pulmonary embolism, the duration of treatment should be increased to 2 years or even

to lifelong therapy in patients with hereditary thrombophilic diathesis or frequent recurrences of thromboembolic events.

Heart Rate Control

Symptoms of AF relate to excessive ventricular heart rates in many patients. If left ventricular systolic function is normal, patients are able to compensate for the lack of atrial filling of the left ventricle, although this contributes to cardiac output by about 10%. At high ventricular rates, this compensation potential is rapidly exhausted, and signs of heart failure, such as dyspnea or angina pectoris, may occur. A well-known model of heart failure is the rapidly stimulated dog heart, which will fail within a few hours of rapid pacing. This situation will occur even in healthy humans at heart rates continuously elevated above 180 beats/min,

Table 2 Age-specific consensus recommendations for the prophylaxis of venous thromboembolic diseases in reflection of risk factors (see Fig. 3)

	Age <65 years		Age 65–75 years		Age >75 years	
Risk sum (Fig. 3)	1 + 2	3	1 + 2	3	1 + 2	3
Primary prophylaxis, in hospital, acute care	—	F	—	F	—	F
Primary prophylaxis, outpatient	—	G	—	G	—	G
Secondary prophylaxis, distal DVT[a]	A	B	A	B	A	B
Secondary prophylaxis, proximal DVT[a]	B	B	B	B	B	B
Secondary prophylaxis after clinically apparent PE[a]	B	C	B	C	B	C
Secondary prophylaxis after recurrence of DVT or PE *without* *anticoagulation*	D	D	D	D	D	D
Secondary prophylaxis after recurrence of DVT or PE *with* *anticoagulation*	E	E	E	E	D	D
Thrombophilic diathesis and other permanent risk factors	E	E	E	E	D	D

Source: Modified from Rossol-Haseroth et al. 2002
A OAC 6 weeks; in addition: rapid mobilization, compression stockings
B OAC 3–6 months; in addition: compression stockings
C OAC up to 12 months
D long-term OAC (INR 2–3); alternative: LMWH (adapted dose)
E long-term OAC (INR3–4); alternative: LMWH (adapted dose)
F LMWH
G at high risk: LMWH (adapted dose)
DVT deep vein thrombosis, *PE* pulmonary embolism, *OAC* oral anticoagulation, *LMWH* low molecular weight heparins, *ASA* acetylsalicylic acid
[a]Except for patients with thrombophilic diathesis

but at much lower heart rates in elderly patients and those with cardiac damage. The threshold may be as low as 100 beats/min. To prevent the heart from failure by this mechanism in AF, almost all patients require ventricular rate control. In AF, the atria produce 500–600 electrical stimuli per minute, which need to be filtered by the atrioventricular node to protect the ventricles against overstimulation. In many patients, this mechanism is not effective enough, at least not in most situations, including those with physical activities. Exercise and adrenergic stimulation (e. g., exerted by emotional stress) lead to a significant reduction in the filtering function of the node, and high ventricular rates are the consequence. The patient will try to avoid all situations that trigger these compromising and unpleasant sensations.

In addition to anticoagulation, heart rate control is the second-most-important measure in the treatment of AF as the restoration of sinus rhythm, which would be a valuable alternative, is only rarely successful.

Rate control in AF typically requires the application of beta-blockers, digoxin/digitoxin, or—exceptionally—verapamil/diltiazem. Acute application of amiodarone also lowers the heart rate (see discussion in the following paragraphs), but this treatment should be carefully indicated as even short-term amiodarone treatment may cause thyroid abnormalities.

Digitalis treatment should be initiated in elderly patients by the normal maintenance dose of 0.25 mg/day without a preceding loading dose for safety reasons. If treatment is urgent (e.g., in the presence of rate-dependent heart failure), intravenous application may be necessary. A cumulative first-day dose of 1.5 mg should not be exceeded as a latency of effects by up to 2 h may seduce the doctor to reinject too shortly after former injections.

As digoxin is predominantly excreted through the kidneys, the oral maintenance dose of 0.125–0.375 mg/day needs to be adapted to the renal function. This treatment is one of the few for which therapeutic drug monitoring is mandatory in the elderly as the therapeutic range is narrow.

Plasma concentrations should not exceed 1.5 ng/ml, although the normal therapeutic range is considered to be between 1 and 2 ng/ml.

Elderly patients are threatened by digoxin intoxication, mainly resulting from the impairment of renal function triggered by gastrointestinal infections, dehydration, or renin-angiotensin system (RAS) inhibition. This intoxication may result in nausea, vomiting, weight loss, depression, or cognitive impairment; viewing of colors as a "famous" sign of intoxication is rare in elderly patients. Weight loss, inappetence, and other nonspecific disturbances of well-being in an elderly patient on digitalis must be taken seriously and an intoxication excluded. Even "normal" plasma concentrations do not exclude intoxication, and a dose reduction or cessation trial should be ordered at the slightest suspicion.

Drug-drug interactions are another problem of digitalis preparations: Digoxin concentrations may critically rise in the presence of antiarrhythmics, especially verapamil, but also chinidine or amiodarone, and statins (this is only a small, incomplete list).

Digitoxin is mainly hepatically cleared, which is a more stable way of excretion in the elderly than renal elimination. However, a half-life time of up to 3 weeks (1 week in younger adults) in the elderly appears to be unsafe, and accumulation may occur. As renal function can be measured, estimated, and—within limits—controlled, digoxin *at adapted doses* appears to be safer in the elderly.

Digitalis preparations represent the second-most-dangerous drug treatment in AF (the most dangerous therapy is anticoagulation), and this is almost their last resort.

Given these limitations, other drugs to control the ventricular rate are even more important: First-line treatment should be done by heart-rate-lowering *beta-blockers*, which are important in this indication as well. The contraindications and dosing restrictions in heart failure are detailed in chapters "Arterial Hypertension" and "Heart Failure." A problem may be the yet unrecognized sinuatrial (SA) block, which cannot be detected in the presence of AF. On restitution of sinus rhythm, it may become apparent by bradycardic symptoms with

dizziness and syncope, and a beta-blocker may aggravate this situation. History taking thus should focus on former episodes of bradycardia and vertigo, although patients' descriptions are often inconclusive. Without an emergency situation, oral rather than intravenous application of beta-blockers should be preferred as the latter route is associated with a higher rate of complications, such as heart block or heart failure.

In many patients, beta-blockers have more than one indication as hypertension, postmyocardial infarction, heart failure, and AF often exist concomitantly.

In many patients, beta-blockers help to reduce or even withdraw digitalis preparations. An attempt to get rid of digitalis should be undertaken after dose optimization of beta-blockers in elderly patients as they are particularly sensitive toward digitalis toxicity (especially cardiac arrhythmias). In addition, digitalis is not very efficient to suppress stress-induced tachycardias, which is the domain of beta-blockers and a major, if not the main problem in many patients.

Nondihydropyridine calcium channel blockers (*verapamil or diltiazem*) are very effective for rate control in AF. As a major drawback, both compounds, in particular verapamil, are negative inotropes and thus should only be given to patients with normal systolic left ventricular function. This prerequisite will remain unmet by an increasing number of elderly, especially very elderly patients. In the case of doubt and with no means of assessment at hand (echocardiography), this contraindication should be assumed to exist in an elderly patient until disproven. Therefore, the use of verapamil or diltiazem should be very restrictive in this age group, and application without prior assessment of left ventricular function is prohibited. Verapamil at 40 mg b.i.d. or t.i.d. should be preferred to any intravenous application, which is relatively unsafe for all reasons mentioned, but at an even higher risk. Intravenous verapamil should only be given in intensive care units.

Verapamil and diltiazem have produced much trouble in elderly patients with AF and unclear left ventricular function in daily practice.

Conversion to Sinus Rhythm, Maintenance of Sinus Rhythm

In principle, restoration of sinus rhythm is the ultimate goal in the treatment of AF as any further treatment could theoretically be stopped. This, however, is only rarely achieved unless a treatable cause of the disorder is found, such as thyrotoxicosis or valvular disease. In all other cases, the long-standing culprit diseases, in particular arterial hypertension and coronary heart disease, maintain the electrical instability of the atria, and recurrences are the rule rather than the exception.

The large clinical trials supported this critical view of the feasibility of rhythm restoration treatment. They compared the clinical outcomes for patients on rate control drugs (see previous discussion) versus those with additional treatments for the restoration and maintenance of sinus rhythm (rhythm control). AFFIRM, RACE, and recently AF-CHF did not show a consistent advantage of rhythm control over rate control. In AF-CHF, including 1,300 patients (mean age 67 years) with heart failure and AF, endpoint curves were identical for all major events (death, stroke; Fig. 5), and no benefit of rhythm control was detectable (Roy et al. 2008).

Thus, there are no strong arguments to force a patient into sinus rhythm. In AF-CHF, one or two cardioversions followed by amiodarone were employed. Cardioversion is the least-aggressive method for the restoration; class I antiarrhythmics such as flecainide or propafenon are proarrhythmogenic (up to 10% of patients) and negative inotropes. Thus, they are not a good choice for the elderly population.

Amiodarone (class III antiarrhythmic) is much safer in relation to these side effects and thus more suitable for the restoration and maintenance of sinus rhythm in the elderly. Given the sobering results of AF-CHF in elderly patients, it should still be very critically indicated as its long-term application is limited by serious side effects. Their listing is long:

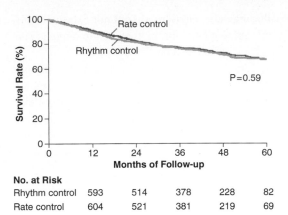

Fig. 5 Cardiovascular death; rhythm versus rate control (From Roy et al. 2008 by kind permission of Massachusetts Medical Society)

- Hyper-/hypothyreosis
- Skin coloring, photodermatosis (light sensitivity, strong sun shield required)
- Cornea/retina damage
- Pulmonary fibrosis, pulmonary hypertension
- Hepatic failure

There are many more. Pulmonary hypertension, which may be fatal, is only common at doses of 200 mg/day and higher. Thus, the maintenance dose should not exceed 100–150 mg/day.

Restoration treatment only seems promising if
- AF does not exist for more than a year.
- Left atrial diameter is less than 5 cm.
- Major valvular disease is absent.

So far, these data did not support vigorous restoration attempts in many elderly patients, especially those with long-standing AF. In this context, data from ATHENA on dronedarone are interesting as this amiodarone analogue (not containing iodine) was the first antiarrhythmic ever to lower mortality and cardiovascular endpoints in elderly patients with AF (Hohnloser et al. 2009). In PALLAS, patients with permanent AF did not benefit from dronedarone, and the study had to be terminated prematurely due to excess mortality. Unfortunately, dronedarone has entered the European Society of Cardiology (ESC) guidelines in a prominent position before its potential is fully understood. In addition, there have been reports of fatal liver damage. The more restrictive listing by the mentioned U.S. guideline as an experimental drug is more adequate, and its use for the very elderly is not backed by experience anyway.

Those data, in particular the side effects of drug treatment, do not support a wide use of restoration/maintenance approaches in elderly patients with long-standing AF. If the inclusion criteria mentioned are met and the patients suffer from major symptoms, electrical cardioversion is preferable. Maintenance therapy should start with a beta-blocker (if not already previously tested), which, however, is not very successful in this indication. Amiodarone then is still the drug of choice but should only be started by a cardiologist and only in selected cases.

Causal treatment of underlying disease is often possible and should be started or optimized even if AF is not reverted to sinus rhythm. This applies particularly to arterial hypertension.

The elderly patient with AF must receive proper treatment of all cardiovascular risk factors, with arterial hypertension the most important one.

Classification of Drugs for the Chronic Treatment of AF According to Their Fitness for the Aged (FORTA)

In this classification of drugs for the chronic treatment of AF according to their Fitness for the Aged (FORTA), the same compounds may receive alternative marks if applied in different indications (see chapter "Critical Extrapolation of Guidelines and Study Results: Risk-Benefit Assessment for Patients with Reduced Life Expectancy and a New Classification of Drugs According to Their Fitness for the Aged").

Acetylsalicylic acid (aspirin, 81–325 mg/day)	C (rarely sufficient, minimal efficacy)
Oral anticoagulation	
Warfarin, phenprocoumon	A, likely to turn to B
Dabigatran, rivaroxaban, apixaban	B, likely to turn to A
As an alternative: low molecular weight heparins	B

(continued)

Heart rate lowering beta-blockers	A
Digoxin	B
Digitoxin	C
Diltiazem, verapamil	C
Class I–III antiarrhythmics	D
Except for amiodarone	C
Dronedarone	D

Study Acronyms

AFASAK Copenhagen Atrial Fibrillation, Aspirin, Anticoagulation Study

AF-CHF Atrial Fibrillation and Congestive Heart Failure

AFFIRM Atrial Fibrillation Follow-up Investigation of Rhythm Management

ARISTOTLE Apixaban for the Prevention of Stroke in Subjects with Atrial Fibrillation

ATHENA A Placebo-Controlled, Double-Blind, Parallel Arm Trial to Assess the Efficacy of Dronedarone 400 mg bid for the Prevention of Cardiovascular Hospitalization or Death from Any Cause in Patients with Atrial Fibrillation/Atrial Flutter

BAATAF Boston Area Anticoagulation Trial for Atrial Fibrillation

CAFA Canadian Atrial Fibrillation Anticoagulation Study

EAFT European Atrial Fibrillation Trial

MEDENOX Prophylaxis in Medical Patients with Enoxaparin Study

PALLAS Permanent Atrial Fibrillation Outcome Study Using Dronedarone on Top of Standard Therapy

RACE Studie Rate Control Versus Electrical Cardioversion of Persistent Atrial Fibrillation Study

RE-LY Randomized Evaluation of Long Term Anticoagulant Therapy

ROCKET AF Rivaroxaban Once Daily Oral Direct Factor Xa Inhibition Compared with Vitamin K Antagonism for Prevention of Stroke and Embolism Trial in Atrial Fibrillation

SPAF Studie Stroke Prevention in Atrial Fibrillation Study

SPINAF Studie Stroke Prevention in Nonrheumatic Atrial Fibrillation Study

References

Alikhan R, Cohen AT, Combe S et al (2003) Prevention of venous thromboembolism in medical patients with enoxaparin: a subgroup analysis of the MEDENOX study. Blood Coagul Fibrinolysis 14:341–346

Fuster V, Ryden LE, Cannom DS et al (2006) ACC/AHA/ESC 2006 guidelines for the management of patients with atrial fibrillation: a report of the American College of Cardiology/American Heart Association Task Force on Practice Guidelines and the European Society of Cardiology Committee for Practice Guidelines (Writing Committee to revise the 2001 guidelines for the management of patients with atrial fibrillation): developed in collaboration with the European Heart Rhythm Association and the Heart Rhythm Society. Circulation 114:e257–e354

Fuster V, Rydén LE, Cannom DS et al (2011) 2011 ACCF/AHA/HRS focused updates incorporated into the ACC/AHA/ESC 2006 guidelines for the management of patients with atrial fibrillation: a report of the American College of Cardiology Foundation/American Heart Association Task Force on practice guidelines. Circulation 123:e269–e367

Geerts WH, Bergqvist D, Pineo GF et al (2008) Prevention of venous thromboembolism: American College of Chest Physicians evidence-based clinical practice guidelines (8th edition). Chest 133(6 suppl):381S–453S

Harenberg J, Bauersachs R, Diehm, C et al (2010) Antikoagulation im Alter [Anticoagulation in the elderly] Internist (Berl) 51:1446–1455, in German

Hohnloser SH, Crijns HJ, van Eickels M et al (2009) Effect of dronedarone on cardiovascular events in atrial fibrillation. N Engl J Med 360:668–678

Nieuwlaat R, Capucci A, Lip GY, Euro Heart Survey Investigators et al (2006) Antithrombotic treatment in real-life atrial fibrillation patients: a report from the Euro Heart Survey on atrial fibrillation. Eur Heart J 27:3018–3026

Rossol-Haseroth K, Vogel CU, Reinecke F et al (2002) Empfehlungen zur Thromboembolieprophylaxe bei internistischen Patienten im Alter. Internist (Berl) 43:1134–1147

Roy D, Talajic M, Nattel S et al (2008) Atrial fibrillation and congestive heart failure investigators. Rhythm control versus rate control for atrial fibrillation and heart failure. N Engl J Med 358:2667–2677

Savelieva I, Camm AJ (2001) Clinical trends in atrial fibrillation at the turn of the millennium. J Intern Med 250:369–372

Spyropoulos AC, Merli G (2006) Management of venous thromboembolism in the elderly. Drugs Aging 23:651–671

Diabetes Mellitus

Heinrich Burkhardt

Relevance for Elderly Patients, Epidemiology

The prevalence of diabetes is increasing across the world, not only in more economically developed countries, and diabetes is one of the most significant chronic diseases. More than 90% of all patients with diabetes disclose type 2 diabetes or non-insulin-dependent diabetes, which is associated with the metabolic syndrome and a sedentary lifestyle. Epidemiologic studies and surveys consistently show an increase of the prevalence with advancing age (Fig. 1). Diabetes is a major cause for reduced life expectancy and aggravated morbidity. This is due to both vascular complications and loss of metabolic control, leading to hyper- or hypoglycemia. As far as morbidity is concerned, this includes reduced functional capacities in daily activities, loss of independence in everyday life, and reduced quality of life. Last but not least, this poses enormous costs on society. Estimations from economic surveys in Western countries found up to 17% of global health insurance budget spent for the treatment of diabetes and its complications.

H. Burkhardt (✉)
IVth Department of Medicine, Geriatrics, University Medical Centre Mannheim, Theodor-Kutzer-Ufer 1-3, Mannheim 68167, Germany
e-mail: heinrich.burkhardt@umm.de

Therapeutically Relevant Special Features of Elderly Patients

Patients with diabetes represent a heterogeneous population not only according to the subtype of disease, with insulin resistance or β-cytotropic deficiency as dominant causes. There are further issues triggering therapeutic decisions, with duration of disease and presence of vascular complications the leading ones. In case of type II diabetes, a longer duration of disease is usually accompanied by advancing insulin resistance and decline of β-cytotropic activity, which in turn trigger therapeutic decisions. For instance, the ADA (American Diabetes Association) clearly states that in case of advanced vascular complications, strict metabolic control has to be questioned as a primary therapeutic goal (American Diabetes Association 2009). This is particularly true for the elderly as further limiting characteristics influencing therapeutic decisions may frequently exist. These are remaining life expectancy, comorbidity, geriatric syndromes, and self-care competence. However, those characteristics are often overlooked in textbooks or general treatment recommendations, despite the fact that in real life they are the most significant patient characteristics. All together, these factors form a complex and dynamic interplay and determine individual treatment decisions (Fig. 2).

The especially heterogeneous population of elderly patients with diabetes has to be treated by a highly individualized approach.

M. Wehling (ed.), *Drug Therapy for the Elderly*,
DOI 10.1007/978-3-7091-0912-0_10, © Springer-Verlag Wien 2013

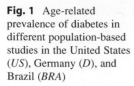

Fig. 1 Age-related prevalence of diabetes in different population-based studies in the United States (*US*), Germany (*D*), and Brazil (*BRA*)

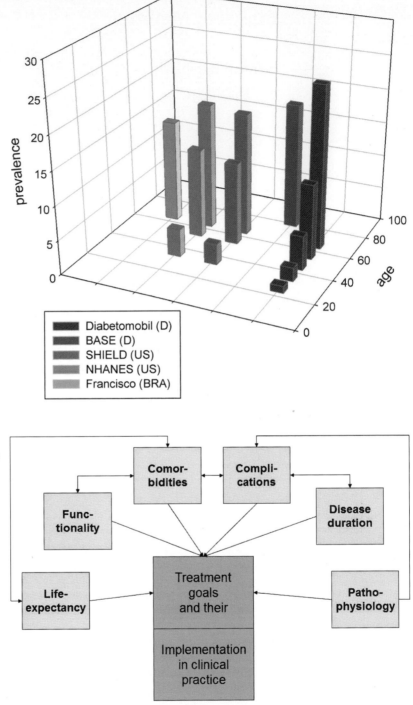

Fig. 2 Interference of different aspects influencing treatment decisions and implementation in clinical practice

In general, three treatment goals exist in diabetes:

1. Prevention of severe acute complications like hypoglycemia or ketoazidosis.

2. Improvement of direct sequelae of hyperglycemia, such as polyuria, polydipsia, exhaustion, pruritus, and increased susceptibility to infectious diseases.

3. Decreased incidence of long-term vascular complications (both micro- and macrovascular diseases).

Therapeutic strategies in diabetes are multimodal and cannot be reduced to pharmacotherapeutic measures, although they are often indispensable for the control and prevention of hyperglycemia and acute complications of the disease.

A significant and successful diabetes treatment includes lifestyle interventions and optimizing physical activities and nutritional behavior.

Without lifestyle interventions, optimal benefit from a pharmacotherapeutic approach cannot be achieved. Although these issues—physical activity and nutrition—are also of significance in the elderly, special considerations in this population may mandate the deviation from recommendations given for younger adult patients with diabetes. For instance, in the elderly malnutrition is an increasing problem, and restrictive diets are discouraged in general (discussed in more detail in the following). Another example is endurance training, which will not be as feasible and useful as in the younger adults. Although these issues are important as well, this chapter focuses on pharmacotherapy as the major topic of this book.

In diabetes, two major pharmacotherapeutic principles are employed:
1. Achieving control of metabolism by antihyperglycemic medication(s); the goal is normoglycemia.
2. Reducing vascular risk by additional medication(s) (RAS inhibition, lowering lipid levels, platelet inhibition, optimizing blood pressure control).

The results from the Danish STENO study (Gaede et al. 2003) made clear that an optimal benefit in the pharmacotherapeutic approach for patients with type 2 diabetes—significant reduction of mortality and morbidity risk—can only be achieved by a combined approach, including both principles.

In the elderly, the risk-benefit ratio of pharmacotherapy may be influenced by several factors. First, general factors have to be mentioned (see part "General Aspects"):
– Functional limitations hampering the implementation of certain pharmacotherapeutic strategies (e.g., insulin therapy and loss of visual acuity)
– Reduced life expectancy, rendering a preventive approach less significant if the prevented event is to be expected in a rather long time range (e.g., strict metabolic control in patients with estimated life expectancy of less than 1 year)

Besides these general issues in the elderly, more special problems exist in elderly patients with diabetes:
1. With advancing age, perception of thirst decreases. Therefore, in the elderly patient with diabetes, polydipsia is often less pronounced than in younger adults, posing a significant risk of dehydration in the case of poor metabolic control (e.g., serum glucose above 200 mg/dl and osmotic diuresis) (Phillips et al. 1984).
2. With advancing age, the risk of hypoglycemia increases (Shorr et al. 1997). Besides this, the subjective perception of hypoglycemia decreases (Thomson et al. 1991).

The significance of hypoglycemia was recently highlighted by the results of three large studies in patients with type 2 diabetes (ACCORD 2008; ADVANCE 2008, and VADT). In these studies, hypoglycemic episodes did not necessitate a softer metabolic control; the strict control yielded no additional beneficial effect on the incidence of vascular complications. On the contrary, this strategy was associated with a higher risk of cardiovascular events (Skyler et al. 2009).

Although several studies consistently demonstrated a higher incidence of hypoglycemia with advancing age as an independent risk factor in multifactorial analyses (Abram et al. 2006), it is still not clear whether this is due to an increasing rate of functional limitations, such as cognitive decline, or depends on age-related changes in glucose metabolism. From a geriatric point of view, it seems fair to assume that those functional limitations are predictors of higher

Table 1 Self-management requirements in different antidiabetic treatment strategies

Strategy		Requirement	Comment
Oral antidiabetics	Metformin	Suspend treatment before surgery or anesthesia	—
	Sulfonylureas	Hypoglycemia	[a]
	Metiglinides	Hypoglycemia (self-management of carbohydrate intake)	[b]
	Thiazolinediones	Hypoglycemia	[b]
	Acarbose	—	—
Insulin	Basal supported oral treatment (BOT)	Hypoglycemia, application of insulin, self-measurement of glucose	[a]
	Conventional therapy (CT)	Hypoglycemia, application of insulin, self-measurement of glucose (self-management carbohydrate intake)	[c]
	Prandial adjusted therapy; supplementary therapy (SIT), intensified therapy (ICT)	Hypoglycemia, application of insulin, self-measurement of glucose, complete nutritional self-management, including quantifying carbohydrate intake	[d]

No additional requirements compared to counseling and education usually demanded at beginning of any long-time pharmacotherapy (indication, dosage, effects, adverse drug reaction [ADR])

[a]Need for an additional education concerning two special issues

[b]Need for an additional education concerning one special issue

[c]Need for an additional education concerning more than two special issues

[d]Need for detailed education concerning including individual diet management, insulin dosing, and glucose monitoring

vulnerability and more frequent failure in the self-management of drug therapy; these aspects should be added to the list of identified general risk factors of hypoglycemia originally provided by Cryer et al. (2003):

– Prescription of sulfonylureas
– Prescription of insulin
– Alcohol
– Erratic eating habits
– Erratic physical activity
– Advancing age
– Advancing diabetes duration
– Functional limitations (cognitive decline, reduced visual acuity, etc.)

An individualized therapeutic approach should cover all strategies to reach these treatment goals. This approach has to take the patients' individual resources and barriers into account. This is especially true for patients with diabetes because in this case self-care and disease control require a high level of patient competence. Patients with diabetes often have to take responsibilities for significant treatment decisions; therefore, patient education and counseling are very important issues. This is in particular the case if more complex treatment strategies such as meal-oriented insulin therapy have to be established. In the elderly, even simple strategies can result in confusion and excessive strain (e.g., when treatment monitoring and self-measurement of blood glucose have to be performed by the elderly patient). Table 1 provides an overview concerning different common treatment strategies in diabetes and related self-management requirements.

Evidence-Based, Rationalistic Drug Therapy and Classification of Drugs According to Their Fitness for the Aged (FORTA)

In general, data from large, randomized control trials concerning elderly patients with diabetes are sparse. These patients are clearly underrepresented in most studies or primarily excluded as in the UKPDS (1998) cohort. This is particularly remarkable as a large and significant portion of type 2 diabetes patients is older than 70 years. As for many conditions in the elderly, evidence has to be translated and adapted from study results in younger cohorts bearing the risk of a misleading risk-benefit ratio estimate.

Strategies to Normalize Blood Glucose Levels

It is generally accepted that normalization of blood glucose levels should prevent an early occurrence of vascular complications and therefore may improve morbidity and mortality in diabetes. This has been demonstrated for both insulin-dependent diabetes in the DCT cohort and non-insulin-dependent diabetes in the UKPDS cohort. Especially in type 2 diabetes patients, this preventive effect is more pronounced for microvascular complications such as diabetic nephropathy and retinopathy than for macrovascular complications such as coronary heart disease. The metabolic control aiming at normoglycemia in patients with diabetes is traditionally considered as the cornerstone and primary treatment goal in these subjects.

Since the publication of the STENO study in 2003 (Gaede et al. 2003), there has been an ongoing debate about the dogma of metabolic control mentioned here, in particular for patients with type 2 diabetes and additional vascular disease or hypertension. Today, diabetes therapy mainly follows a multifactorial approach, including control of these additional risk factors or comorbidities. The STENO cohort comprised patients with type 2 diabetes and albuminuria. The STENO investigators clearly demonstrated in this cohort that only the simultaneous control of glucose and lipid levels and hypertension and a mandatory prescription of renin-angiotensine-aldosterone-system inhibitors (RAAS) inhibitors and aspirin prevents vascular complications as opposed to metabolic control alone. As a remarkable result of this study, tight control and monitoring of this study cohort achieved the metabolic goal in less than 20% of participants, whereas 70% succeeded in blood pressure control. Although the STENO cohort did not represent the elderly, it may be assumed that success rates of achieving therapeutic goals may be similar at age 70 years and older.

The quality of metabolic control is usually assessed by the determination of HbA1c. This measure integrally covers a time period of about approximately 4 weeks, depending on erythrocyte turnover. A tight or strict metabolic control aiming at HbA1c levels below 6.5% was the primary goal in DCCT and UKPDS. However, a very important condition for achieving this goal has to be kept in mind: All strategies for metabolic control have to avoid increasing rates of hypoglycemia, or no additional benefit from strict metabolic control will be seen. This has been clearly demonstrated in the ACCORD cohort and initiated an ongoing debate about reasonable treatment goals for HbA1c. Currently, the ADA recommends HbA1c levels below 7.0% as the treatment goal for adults with diabetes and only if achievable on the grounds of an individual risk-benefit ratio assessment (American Diabetes Association 2011). A more moderate metabolic control allows HbA1c levels above 6.5%, accepts a lower preventive effect on vascular complications, but still limits blood glucose levels to avoid acute symptomatic hyperglycemia. Exact HbA1c limits for this moderate metabolic control are still under discussion. This is mainly due to a remarkable lack of scientific studies on this issue. Many investigators recommend HbA1c values below 8.0% to prevent acute hyperglycemic symptoms like polyuria.

Symptoms of hyperglycemia such as polyuria, polydipsia, pruritus, and exhaustion should be absent or rare at HbA1c levels below 8.0%. In addition, the risk of an aggravated course of acute diseases such as pneumonia is reduced.

Moderate metabolic control is a comprehensive treatment goal for every patient with diabetes and—unlike tight metabolic control—certainly achievable in most of them.

An example for the benefit of even only moderate metabolic control relates to the occurrence and course of pressure ulcers. This issue is particularly important in bedridden elderly patients and often represents a challenge for their caregivers. With moderate metabolic control, healing of pressure ulcers was more favorable than without any control (Moty et al. 2003). However, there is a remarkable lack of data concerning the achievement of moderate metabolic control in geriatric patients, its conditions, and the clinical outcome effects. For example, from a theoretical point of view one would expect lower rates of dehydration, dizziness, skin problems, and infectious diseases such as urinary tract infection. After 30 years of comprehensive research in diabetes and 20 years of research in geriatrics, such basic data are still unavailable. How may these shortcomings be explained? A major reason might be methodological problems in the elderly regarding the control for covariates or the definition of clear outcome parameters as outlined in part "General Aspects." Nevertheless, without these data at hand, the assumption seems fair that moderate metabolic control is potentially beneficial to control acute symptoms. Besides this, support comes from intensive care studies demonstrating that metabolic control improves the clinical outcome in acute diseases (Van den Berghe et al. 2001). These results were predominantly obtained in trauma patients and may not even apply to other disease categories in intensive care (e.g., septicemia), not to speak of the situation of elderly outpatients. Yet, with all uncertainties of extrapolation and deduction, at least a moderate metabolic control devoid of recurrent episodes of hypoglycemia is recommended for elderly patients with diabetes both during intermittent acute diseases and long-term treatment of diabetes as the minimum standard.

Tight metabolic control defined by HbA1c level below 7.0% is only reasonable when achievable without an increased rate of hypoglycemia and if the remaining life expectancy is compatible with the delayed time course of the vascular prevention.

Keeping this in mind, in many elderly patients strict metabolic control no longer represents a reasonable treatment goal. The decision to stop strict control and switch to moderate control has to be based on a repeated and individualized assessment of the risk-benefit ratio. This is in line with the ADA recommendation, which discourages strict metabolic control, for example, if advanced vascular complications and significant comorbidities exist (American Diabetes Association 2011). Although not explicitly stated there, this recommendation of moderate metabolic control should also be applied to patients with geriatric syndromes like cognitive impairment or severe limitations of activities of daily living. In an individual patient, however, a precise definition of such reasons for restriction often remains elusive. A more distinct definition providing cut-point levels is lacking due to the very limited scientific data on this issue and inherent methodological difficulties (e.g., definition of typical geriatric multimorbidity patterns).

Strict metabolic control (HbA1c <7.0%) is not recommended under the following circumstances:
- Multiple, clinically apparent vascular complications
  - Repeated severe hypoglycemia
  - Pronounced comorbidity (e.g., advanced malignancies), geriatric multimorbidity (> three major diseases)
  - Reduced life expectancy (e.g., advanced dementia or cancer)
  - Long disease duration and failure of metabolic control by common antihyperglycemic strategies
- Low level of functionality (e.g., loss of visual acuity, loss of activities of daily living, chronically bedridden patients, frailty)

Strategies to Reduce Vascular Risk

Like metabolic control, additional strategies to reduce the burden of vascular risk have to be based on an individual risk-benefit ratio assessment. Although lifestyle interventions are most essential to control for obesity and ameliorate the risk burden of a sedentary lifestyle, there is also a significant benefit from pharmacotherapeutic strategies. They aim at preventing vascular complications or reducing the progression of existing vascular disease.

In case of a concomitant hypertension, the principles described in chapter "Special Aspects with Respect to Organ Systems Based on Geriatric Clinical Importance" should be thoroughly utilized with RAS inhibitors such as angiotensin-converting enzyme (ACE) inhibitors as first-line drugs. Control of hypertension in patients with diabetes is essential to reduce the excess morbidity and mortality due to stroke and heart failure; according to UKPDS, hypertension control is far more effective in the prevention of macrovascular endpoints than glucose lowering interventions.

Prescription of statins is recommended to lower low-density lipoprotein (LDL) cholesterol levels to less than 100 mg/dl or even 70 mg/dl in case of concomitant coronary vascular disease. Beneficial effects are well documented in the elderly (Shepherd et al. 2002), but there are few data in patients above 75 years. The details of cholesterol-lowering strategies are described in chapter "Coronary Heart Disease and Stroke" under the section "Evidence-Based, Rationalistic Drug Therapy and Classification of Drugs According to Their Fitness for the Aged (FORTA)."

The ADA and the American Heart Association (AHA) jointly recommend platelet inhibitors in elderly diabetic patients with one or more additional risk factors of cardiovascular heart disease (hypertension, tobacco smoking, family history of cerebrovascular disease [CVD], dyslipidemia, or albuminuria). Although there might be an increased risk of bleeding in the elderly, this seems to be outweighed by the increased risk of CVD in the elderly (see chapter "Coronary Heart Disease and Stroke"). However, again, data addressing this special issue are rare. Only in the case of a severe reduction of life expectancy (e.g., lower than 1 year), a negative shift of benefit-risk ratio may render aspirin treatment inefficient or even dangerous as platelet inhibitor therapy aims at long-term effects. This effect is normally assumed to be accrued over 10 years; thus, 1 year is arbitrarily seen as too short to allow for clinically relevant positive treatment effects.

Comprehensive Evaluation of Different Drugs Prescribed for Metabolic Control

Oral Antidiabetics

Diabetes control by oral antidiabetics is obviously easier than management of parenteral insulin therapy; oral treatment therefore requires smaller self-management capacities and educational efforts (see Table 1). Functional limitations or insufficient patient education thus render this strategy preferable. In addition, a considerable fraction of type 2 diabetics exposes a significant remaining insulin secretion. Thus, without strict demand for exogenous insulin application, this treatment may become a second-line option. Nevertheless, it has to be kept in mind that hypoglycemia is the most frequent and serious adverse drug reaction (ADR) for many oral antidiabetics. Thus, it is mandatory without exception to educate patients or caregivers how to recognize and treat hypoglycemia. This is particularly true for the elderly as hypoglycemia is more frequent and often more serious in this age group (see previous discussion).

Sulfonylureas

Sulfonylurea drugs have been prescribed to patients with type 2 diabetes for decades; therefore, empirical data on ADRs are abundant. However, it needs to be kept in mind that prospective placebo-controlled clinical trials have never been performed for these drugs as they were introduced before regulatory requirements for such trials had been established.

The major representative of this group is glyburide (glibenclamide). Because of their β-cytotropic activities, sulfonylureas are the drugs of choice in patients with type 2 diabetes and preserved insulin secretion. However, they also carry a considerable risk of ADRs, in particular hypoglycemia, but also cardiac arrhythmias. This risk is increasing with decreasing renal function and longer duration of action. Therefore, most sulfonylureas are contraindicated in renal failure (estimated glomerular filtration rate <30 ml/min). Gliquidone is predominantly metabolized by the

Table 2 Risk profiles of sulfonylurea drugs

	Duration of action	Elimination	ADR	Comment
Glibenclamide	15 h	50% renal	Total prevalence 1.5–2.5%; hypoglycemia 1.46%	Best data among all sulfonylureas; multiple daily dosing not recommended (risk of nocturnal hypoglycemia)
Gliburide	24 h	60–72% renal	Total prevalence 4.7–7.6%; hypoglycemia: 0.3%	
Glipizide	8–10 h	60–80% renal	Total prevalence 3–12%; hypoglycemia 0.35%	
Gliclazide	6–12 h	60–70% renal	Total prevalence: 7.6%	
Gliquidone (not FDA approved)	5–7 h	5% renal	Hypoglycemia 7.6% (few data)	The only sulfonylurea that can be prescribed in reduced renal function (GFR <30 ml/min)
Glimepiride	12–24 h	50% renal	Lower risk of hypoglycemia discussed (<0.5%)	

ADR adverse drug reactions, *FDA* Food and Drug Administration, *GFR* glomerular filtration rate

liver and thus allows for application in renal failure patients; it is, however, not available in the United States.

Close monitoring for hypoglycemia and proarrhythmicity (Holter electrocardiogram [ECG], QT interval) is strongly recommended, and insulin therapy should be considered as an alternative.

With regard to its long duration of action, glibenclamid is the least favorable in this group (Holstein et al. 2001), although it has been extensively prescribed and analyzed (e.g., in UKPDS). As the risk of hypoglycemia is increasing with advancing age, third-generation drugs of this class should be used at higher age. ADR data are pointing to lower rates of hypoglycemia for glimepiride and glipizide. First-generation sulfonylureas (tolbutamide, chlorpropamide) should not be used in the elderly due to a high prevalence of ADRs. Although a higher rate of hypoglycemia is expected for a longer duration of action, glimepiride may be dosed once a day. This helps to simplify medication schedules and to improve drug adherence. Table 2 provides an overview of the risk profiles of sulfonylurea drugs.

Some drug-drug interactions with sulfonylureas may enhance the risk of hypoglycemia. On top of this list are ACE inhibitors, drugs very often prescribed to patients with diabetes due to common cardiovascular comorbidities. During the initial phase of ACE inhibitor therapy, there should be close monitoring of blood glucose. Other important drugs on the interaction list are nonsteroidal anti-inflammatory drugs (NSAIDs), warfarin, fibrates, and fluconazole, which interact with sulfonylureas by inhibiting drug elimination.

At comparably low adjusted doses, third-generation sulfonylurea drugs seem to be first-line treatments for elderly diabetics if endpoint effects are unlikely to become clinically relevant within the estimated life expectancy. Without this limitation (younger patients with longer life expectancy), there seems to be no "first-line" treatment in non-insulin-dependent diabetics as all present oral therapies are suboptimal (see the following chapters).

Meglitinides

Repaglinide and nateglinide are meglitinides that act through the same receptor as sulfonylureas and thus also stimulate β-cell function. As they have been introduced into diabetes therapy "only" 10 years ago, clinical experiences with meglitinides are not as abundant as those for sulfonylureas. They were also not used in UKPDS, which so far is still the only long-term study of type 2 diabetes. Smaller cohorts, however, showed acceptable drug safety and efficacy in older diabetes patients (>65 years) treated with nateglinide (Schwarz et al. 2008). The main difference compared to sulfonylureas is a pharmacokinetic one. The duration of action is rather short, and the onset of action is faster than that of sulfonylureas. Therefore, meglitinides allow for a prandial dosing schedule or even dosing on demand. Basically, they carry a risk of hypoglycemia, especially when a meal is skipped in a prandial dosing schedule and the medication has been taken. In the cohort studied by Schwarz et al. (2008), however, there was no significant risk of hypoglycemia associated with nateglinide when applying a prandial dosing schedule in elderly patients. Although this was seen in a rather small data sample, this risk appears rather low. In patients with significantly reduced renal function (estimated glomerular filtration rate [GFR] below 30 ml/min), the risk of hypoglycemia increases; therefore, in these patients meglitinides are contraindicated like sulfonylureas.

Metformin

Metformin has been prescribed for decades and was one of the standard drugs in the UKPDS cohort. Therefore, clinical experiences with this drug are abundant. Metformin is also recommended in the early stages of diabetes and for the treatment of the metabolic syndrome under preventive auspices. Its antidiabetic properties have been established for the elderly as well. Compared to other antidiabetic drugs, a major advantage of metformin is its favorable effect on body weight and insulin resistance. In addition, glucose uptake by skeletal muscles is improved and hepatic gluconeogenesis inhibited. It remains uncertain if the potentially beneficial effect on body weight shown for younger adults is also significant in the elderly population. In addition, it is questionable whether metformin's unique preventive effect and metabolic properties are identical in younger and elderly populations.

Data from the Diabetes Prevention Program point to a much smaller preventive effect of metformin in the elderly than in younger adults, although some benefit seems to remain. In a primary prevention approach, the Diabetes Prevention Program included a large cohort of elderly without significant chronic diseases (Diabetes Prevention Research Group 2006). The extrapolation of these data from primary prevention to diabetes treatment remains uncertain, and data comparing antidiabetic properties of metformin in different age groups in a longitudinal manner are still lacking. Nevertheless, obesity aggravates metabolic control also in the elderly and is therefore associated with higher drug dosages and polypharmacy. Metformin is preferable in obese patients with diabetes, and this also applies to the elderly. Moreover, the risk of hypoglycemia is very low as there is no direct effect on β-cell function. Both arguments seem to support the nomination of metformin as first-line therapy.

However, there is a serious concern about the most relevant contraindication for metformin: renal failure. In this context, renal failure is defined as reduced glomerular filtration rate below 60 ml/min (see K/DOQI (National Kidney Foundation Disease Outcomes Quality Initiative) criteria Table 3). Renal failure largely increases the risk of lactic acidosis. Although its incidence is very low and estimated to be below 1/10,000 patient years (Josephkutty and Potter 1990), this complication is potentially lethal. Furthermore, this risk increases with other comorbidities, such as impaired hepatic function, cardiac failure, and respiratory insufficiency with hypoxia. Metformin has to be discontinued in every clinical situation carrying the risk of hypoxemia or hypotension (e.g., surgery and general anesthesia) and prior to the application of x-ray contrast media (temporary renal impairment). Also dehydration—a condition that is very common in the elderly—increases the risk of lactic acidosis. Dehydration may be even more frequent in the subpopulation of frail elderly with impaired daily activities (see the section "Important Aspects of Differential Pharmacotherapy in the Elderly" in chapter "Heterogeneity and Vulnerability of Older Patients" on the activities of daily living/

Table 3 Stages of chronic kidney disease National Kidney Foundation Disease Outcomes Quality Initiative (K/DOQI)

Stage	Term	GFR (ml/min/1.73 m^2)
1	Kidney damage with normal GFR	>90
2	Kidney damage with mild reduction of GFR	60–89
3	Moderately reduced renal function	30–59
4	Severely reduced renal function	15–29
5	Kidney failure	<15

Source: Modified from National Kidney Foundation 2002
Chronic kidney disease is defined as either kidney damage or GFR reduced less than 60 ml/min/1.73 m^2 for more than 3 months; kidney damage is defined as pathological abnormality either in imaging studies or by laboratory markers (blood or urine)
GFR glomerular filtration rate

instrumental activities of daily living [ADL/IADL] concept). Antidiabetic drug therapy with metformin in the elderly therefore requires monitoring of renal function (estimation of glomerular function) and careful managing of fluid balance. In any case of suspected impaired renal function, impaired liver function, heart or respiratory failure, or increased risk of dehydration (e.g., frailty syndrome or dementia), metformin should not be applied.

Metformin should not be prescribed if the estimated GFR is below 60 ml/min.

These limitations reduce the value of metformin in the elderly despite the important fact that the risk of hypoglycemia is low for this compound.

Thiazolidinediones

Thiazolidinediones are selective agonists for the peroxisome proliferator-activated receptor-y (PPAR-y) receptor and were used for diabetes treatment as they increase insulin sensitivity in liver, fat, and muscle. Hereby, they lower insulin resistance and were recommended especially for obese patients with diabetes. Moreover, the risk of hypoglycemia is lower than that associated with sulfonylureas. They were enthusiastically introduced into diabetes treatment in the early years of this century.

However, serious safety concerns have been triggered by medium- and long-time experiences in clinical trials and practice (Lehman et al. 2010). First, thiazolidinediones are contraindicated in heart failure as they may aggravate edema and fluid retention. Although this ADR is amenable to control by close monitoring of

fluid intake and has been found fully reversible after drug removal (Dargie et al. 2007), it may lead to unnecessary hospitalizations. It remains unclear whether there is an increased risk in the elderly as fluid and sodium balances are more unstable in the elderly than in younger adults. Recommendations restricted the prescription of thiazolidinediones to elderly diabetics without heart failure. Furthermore, promotion of osteoporosis and an increased risk of bone fractures have been reported in association with thiazolidinediones (Meier et al. 2008).

Recently, a consistently higher risk for cardiovascular events was found for thiazolidinediones in study cohorts of patients with diabetes, especially in those aged 66 and over (Lipscombe et al. 2007). Rosiglitazone has already been withdrawn from the market. Pioglitazone is still available in some countries, but additional reports described an increased cancer risk associated with this drug. Drug surveillance data consistently pointed to an increased risk of bladder cancer (Piccini et al. 2011). Today, prescription of thiazolidinediones cannot be recommended, especially in the elderly, as substantial evidence of a negative risk-benefit ratio exists.

Thiazolidinediones are associated with a negative risk-benefit ratio and should not be prescribed to the elderly.

Acarbose

The action of the α-glucosidase inhibitor acarbose is restricted to the bowel; the compound therefore is largely devoid of systemic effects. In addition, there is no risk of hypoglycemia associated with this drug. Unfortunately, the antihyperglycemic effect of acarbose is limited and smaller than that of other oral antidiabetics such as sulfonylureas. Furthermore, acarbose may lead to an accumulation of oligosaccharides in the small intestine, resulting in gastrointestinal ADRs such as bloating and diarrhea. These ADRs are the main causes for poor adherence. Careful initial dosing and patient education are demanding. In elderly with limited locomotion and incontinence, bloating and diarrhea are even more significant, but special data concerning this topic are lacking. Nevertheless, Mooradian et al. (2000) found prandial doses of 25 mg acarbose sufficient to reach the maximal antihyperglycemic effect; higher doses are not recommended in the elderly.

Dipeptidyl peptidase-4 Inhibitors and Glucagon-like-peptide-1 Analogues

Sitagliptin, saxagliptin, and vildagliptin (not approved by the Food and Drug Administration [FDA]) as inhibitors of the dipeptidyl peptidase-4 (DPP-4) and exenatide and liraglutide as Glucagon-like-peptide-1 (GLP-1) analogues are the most recently developed antidiabetics. The DPP-4 inhibitors are administered as oral antidiabetics, whereas exenatide and liraglutide have to be applied parenterally. Both principles augment GLP-1 agonism, either by external GLP-1 agonist supply or by inhibition of the degradation of endogenous GLP-1. For pathophysiologic reasons, they carry a very low risk of hypoglycemia as the compounds sensitize β-cell stimulation by glucose in a near physiologic way. The mechanism becomes inert at low glucose concentrations, explaining the absence of prohypoglycemic effects. In addition, these drugs do not cause an increase in body weight typical for insulinotropic treatments, for example, by sulfonylureas or parenteral insulins. In this respect, the antihyperglycemic effect of these drugs resembles that of metformin (Drucker and Nauck 2006).

DPP-4 inhibitors and GLP-1 analogues are promising new drugs; unfortunately, experiences with long-term administration, especially in the elderly, and endpoint data are missing to date. In addition, no data on the risk-benefit ratio in the elderly as opposed to younger patients are available.

As a desirable goal for diabetes therapy in the elderly, a new formulation of exenatide that allows a once-weekly dosage would improve acceptance and adherence (Deyoung et al. 2011). Exenatide has to be given subcutaneously and is mainly manufactured as a formulation for twice-daily injection. The once-weekly dosage would be helpful for ambulatory elderly patients unable to perform self-administration of a subcutaneous drug due to cognitive impairment or other functional limitations as it allows for passing the management of drug therapy to caregivers. A slow-release preparation of exenatide for weekly injection has been recently approved by European Medicines Agency (EMA), but not by the FDA.

However, results from recent animal studies (Matveyenko et al. 2009) point to a possible risk of pancreatitis and pancreatic neoplasms associated with sitagliptin treatment. Before a clearer picture of the clinical risk-benefit ratio in the long-term treatment exists, the prescription of these drugs should be exercised with particular caution in the elderly. Conversely, these new principles are yet most promising to carry the potential of becoming first-line drugs in the near future when endpoint studies that include sufficient numbers of elderly patients will become available. A reevaluation of their position in the treatment of elderly diabetics has to be performed in close connection with expected pivotal trial outcomes.

Insulin

There are several age-associated changes in the regulation of glucose metabolism in humans (Meneilly 1999), but they did not yet support a differential approach concerning insulin therapy in the elderly. As in younger adults, prescription of insulin is indicated if metabolic control cannot be sufficiently achieved by one or two oral antidiabetics and lifestyle interventions.

Initiating insulin therapy always requires a thorough education of the patient or the caregivers.

Insulin therapy requires safe self-management concerning not only the administration of the drug but also the glucose monitoring and dosage planning; thus, insulin therapy should always be preceded by a thorough assessment of the

Fig. 3 Interaction between
patients, social networks,
and health care providers

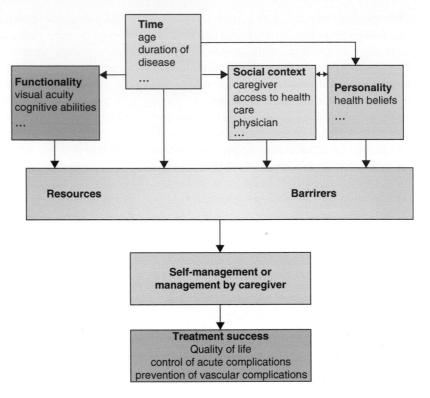

patients' ability to meet these self-management requirements. In the elderly, barriers are often missed without an appropriate assessment of the patients' abilities. The majority of nurses involved in diabetes education report difficulties in training elderly patients in appropriate insulin injection techniques, and in their opinion a significant portion of the elderly is unable ever to achieve these skills. Encouragingly, Braun et al. (2004) found that in elderly with mild functional limitations a successful training for self-management of diabetes therapy is possible if an adjusted training program to meet the needs of these elderly is instituted.

Functional limitations of self-management capacities may impair complex pharmacotherapeutic strategies such as insulin therapy; these limitations are mainly cognitive decline, impaired vision, and reduced dexterity. To assess these domains of functionality, comprehensive geriatric assessment tools need to be employed. A short and easy-to-perform screening tool is the "test of money counting," which can predict successful management of insulin self-administration

(Burkhardt et al. 2006). The assessment of functional abilities should not be performed only at the initiation of insulin therapy as the functional decline in the elderly is very heterogeneous, and regular reassessments are indispensable for the early detection of self-management problems. This is even more important as we know that elderly patients with diabetes carry a higher risk of cognitive decline and visual impairment than elderly without diabetes (Allen et al. 2004).

Further aspects need to be taken into consideration before starting insulin therapy. Social network and available caregiver resources are keystones of successful insulin therapy in many ambulatory elderly patients with diabetes. In this context, Fig. 3 provides an overview of the complex interplay between different factors determining successful therapy.

Insulin therapy carries a much higher risk of treatment errors than therapy with oral antidiabetics. Treatment errors may result from

– Dosage errors
– Errors concerning the site and mode (subcutaneous, intramuscular) of injection

– Errors in calculating insulin dosages according to energy intake and physical exercise

Insulin therapy carries a high risk of hypoglycemia if a treatment error occurs.

To avoid potentially harmful hypoglycemias, the dose of insulin has to be adapted to the amount of physical exercise and carbohydrate intake, at least if short-acting insulin or insulin analogues are used.

In elderly patients, malnutrition or irregular intake of protein or carbohydrates is an increasing issue and represents significant clinical problems; thus, this is called a geriatric syndrome (Thorslund et al. 1990). Different age-associated factors may promote this syndrome: decrease of gustatorial sensation, loss of appetite due to polypharmacy, or decreased cognitive abilities or mobility. The last may result in increased difficulties in obtaining adequate food supplies, a factor often overlooked. Also, pharmacotherapy is often not regularly checked in the case of malnutrition or nutritional problems but may be the cause for these problems (Pickering 2004). They are more frequent in elderly with diabetes than in those without (Turnbull and Sinclair 2002). As mentioned for insulin therapy in general, the management of nutritional aspects also requires functional abilities such as cognition, manual dexterity, and visual acuity (see previous discussion and Table 1). Therefore, monitoring of these aspects in elderly patients is strongly recommended. As said, the assessment of these factors should take place not only at the beginning of insulin therapy but also during follow-up. We recommend 6-month intervals.

Most complex therapy strategies with regard to insulin are prandial treatment schedules with short-acting insulin. Unfortunately, these schemes may carry the highest risk of hypoglycemia, which, however, is not absent in more popular conventional schedules with combined administration of short- and long-acting insulin. In elderly patients, treatment decisions always have to consider carefully the risk balance and self-management demands.

Among all insulin treatment schedules, the solitary administration of long-acting insulin or insulin analogues given once or twice daily carries the lowest hypoglycemic risk.

This treatment scheme is by far easier to establish than conventional insulin treatment schemes with either prandial dosing or fixed combinations. This scheme has been recommended for treatment of elderly patients with diabetes (Yki-Järvinen et al. 1992) since the 1990s. Today, very long-acting insulin analogues are available that allow for more flexible dosing, with once-daily administration reflecting individual patient's and caregivers' preferences. Table 1 summarizes common treatment schedules of insulin therapy and highlights requirements and application modes.

Algorithm for Treatment Decisions of Glycemic Control in the Elderly

The arguments mentioned concerning different drugs and pharmacotherapeutic strategies can be summarized and described as a comprehensive algorithm. This algorithm covers several steps:

1. Decision whether strict metabolic control is a comprehensive treatment goal
2. Assessment of renal function
3. Assessment of risk for hypoglycemia and of the potential amelioration by educational and other means of customizing patients' individual treatment situation (Fig. 4)

This algorithm leads to four different treatment categories, including options for treatment escalation. Acarbose is not mentioned explicitly as this drug may be used in each category, but only if well tolerated. On the other hand, thiazolidinediones and GLP-1 analogues/DDP-4 inhibitors are not mentioned due to limited experiences or severe ADR risk in the elderly. Finally, the algorithm is restricted to drugs given for metabolic control and does not cover important additional vasoprotective treatments by ACE inhibitors, statins, or aspirin.

Table 4 gives an overview and summarizes arguments that build the recommendation along Fit for the Aged (FORTA) classification

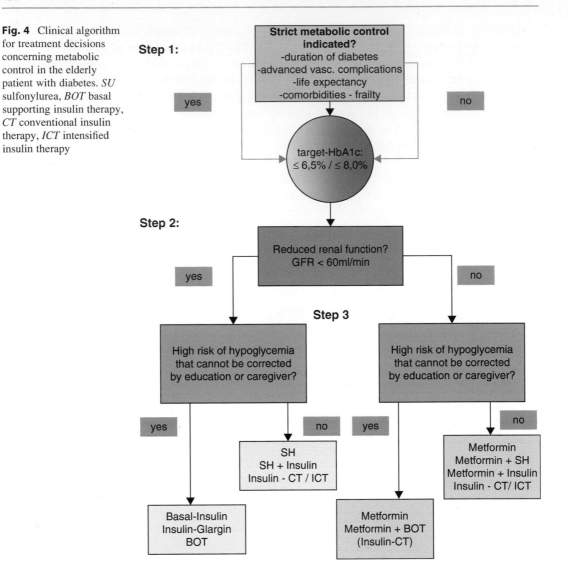

Fig. 4 Clinical algorithm for treatment decisions concerning metabolic control in the elderly patient with diabetes. *SU* sulfonylurea, *BOT* basal supporting insulin therapy, *CT* conventional insulin therapy, *ICT* intensified insulin therapy

Table 4 Antidiabetic drugs: overview and comments

	Drug	Comment
Oral antidiabetics	Sulfonylureas	Restrictive use in elderly because of increasing hypoglycemia risk
	Metformin	Only under close monitoring of renal function recommended; has to be abandoned in case of GFR <60 ml/min
	Acarbose	Limited effect
	Meglitinides	Restricted experience, restrictive use recommended because of hypoglycemia risk
	Thiazolidinediones	Severe ADR, critical risk-benefit ratio
	DPP-4 inhibitors	Limited experience, ADR under discussion
	GLP-1 analogues	Limited experience, once-weekly dosage may provide additional benefit for adherence in certain subgroups
Insulin	Insulin and insulin analogues	Risk-benefit ratio not altered in the elderly but strongly dependent on patient self-management abilities resp. caregiver management abilities

ADR adverse drug reaction, *DPP-4* dipeptidyl peptidase-4 inhibitors, *GFR* glomerular filtration rate, *GLP-1* glucagon-like-peptide-1

categories (Wehling 2009). This classification may help to optimize the overall benefit-risk ratio associated with pharmacotherapeutic strategies in the individual patient. Can all drugs for metabolic control in patients with diabetes be omitted to reduce polypharmacy in the elderly? In the vast majority of diabetic patients, this will certainly not be possible. The remaining principle can be summarized as follows:

Find the simplest and least-risky way for metabolic control. The fewer drugs you need for metabolic control, the better your therapeutic schedule will work.

Classification of Drugs for the Chronic Treatment of Diabetes Mellitus Type 2 According to Their Fitness for the Aged (FORTA)

(see chapter "Critical Extrapolation of Guidelines and Study Results: Risk-Benefit Assessment for Patients with Reduced Life Expectancy and a New Classification of Drugs According to Their Fitness for the Aged"):

Sulfonylureas (third generation)	B
Metformin	B
Acarbose	B
Meglitinides	C
Thiazolidinediones	D
DPP-4 inhibitors	C (B expected)
GLP-1 analogues	C (B expected)
Insulin, if oral antidiabetics insufficient for metabolic control	A

Study Acronyms

ACCORD The Action to Control Cardiovascular Risk in Diabetes Study

ADVANCE Action in Diabetes and Vascular Disease: Preterax and Diamicron MR Controlled Evaluation Study

DPP Diabetes Prevention Program

STENO Study by the Steno Diabetes Centers in Denmark

UKPDS UK Prospective Diabetes Study

VADT Veterans Affairs Diabetes Trial

References

Abram K, Pedersen-Bjergaard U, Borch-Johnsen K, Thorsteinsson B (2006) Frequency and risk factors of severe hypoglycemia in insulin-treated type 2 diabetes: a literature survey. J Diabetes Complications 20:402–408

ACCORD (The Action to Control Cardiovascular Risk in Diabetes Study Group) (2008) Effects of intensive glucose lowering in type 2 diabetes. N Engl J Med 358:2545–2559

ADVANCE (The ADVANCE Collaborative Group) (2008) Intensive blood glucose control and vascular outcomes in patients with type 2 diabetes. N Engl J Med 358:2560–2572

Allen KV, Frier BM, Strachan MWJ (2004) The relationship between type 2 diabetes and cognitive dysfunction: longitudinal studies and their methodological limitations. Eur J Pharmacol 490:169–175

American Diabetes Association (2009) Standards of medical care in diabetes. Diabetes Care 32:S13–S61

American Diabetes Association (2011) Executive summary: standards of medical care in diabetes—2011. Diabetes Care 34(Suppl 1):S4–S10

Braun A, Muller UA, Leppert K, Schiel R (2004) Structured treatment and teaching of patients with type 2 diabetes mellitus and impaired cognitive function—the DICOF trial. Diabet Med 21:999–1006

Burkhardt H, Karaminejad E, Gladisch R (2006) A short performance-test can help to predict adherence to self-administration of insulin in elderly patients with diabetes. Age Ageing 35:449–452

Cryer PE, Davis SN, Shamon H (2003) Hypoglycemia in diabetes. Diabetes Care 26:1902–1912

Dargie HJ, Hildebrandt PR, Riegger GA et al (2007) A randomized, placebo-controlled trial assessing the effects of rosiglitazone on echocardiographic function and cardiac status in type 2 diabetic patients with New York Heart Association functional class I or II heart failure. J Am Coll Cardiol 49:1696–1704

DCCT (The Diabetes Control and Complications Trial Research Group) (1993) The effect of intensive treatment of diabetes on the development and progression of long-term complications in insulin-dependent diabetes mellitus. N Engl J Med 329:977–986

Deyoung MB, Macconell L, Sarin V, Trautmann M, Herbert P (2011) Encapsulation of exenatide in poly-(D,L-lactide-co-glycolide) microspheres produced an investigational long-acting once-weekly formulation for type 2 diabetes. Diabetes Technol Ther (13 July epub) 2011 Nov; 13(11):1145–54

Drucker DJ, Nauck MA (2006) The incretin system: glucagon-like peptide-1 receptor agonists and dipeptidyl peptidase-4 inhibitors in type 2 diabetes. Lancet 368:1696–1705

Duckworth W, Abraira C, Moritz T, Reda D, Emanuele N, Reaven PD, Zieve FJ, Marks J, Davis SN, Hayward R, Warren SR, Goldman S, McCarren M, Vitek ME,

Henderson WG, Huang GD; VADT Investigators. Glucose control and vascular complications in veterans with type 2 diabetes. N Engl J Med. 2009 Jan 8;360(2):129–39

Gaede P, Vedel P, Larsen N, Jensen GV, Parving HH, Pedersen O (2003) Multifactorial intervention and cardiovascular disease in patients with type 2 diabetes. N Engl J Med 348:383–393

Holstein A, Plaschke A, Egberts EH (2001) Lower incidence of severe hypoglycemia in patients with type 2 diabetes treated with glimepiride versus glibenclamide. Diabetes Metab Res Rev 17:467–473

Josephkutty S, Potter JM (1990) Comparison of tolbutamide and metformin in elderly diabetic patients. Diabet Med 7:510–514

Lehman R, Yudkin JS, Krumholz HM (2010) Licensing drugs for diabetes. BMJ 341:c4805

Lipscombe LL, Gomes T, Lèvesque LE, Hux JE, Juurlink DN, Alter DA (2007) Thiazolidinediones and cardiovascular outcomes in older patients with diabetes. JAMA 298:2634–2653

Matveyenko AV, Dry S, Cox HI et al (2009) Beneficial endocrine but adverse exocrine effects of sitagliptin in the human islet amyloid polypeptide transgenic rat model of type 2 diabetes: interactions with metformin. Diabetes 58:1604–1615

Meier C, Kraenzlin ME, Bodmer M, Jick SS, Jick H, Meier CR (2008) Use of thiazolidinediones and fracture risk. Arch Intern Med 168:820–825

Meneilly GS (1999) Pathophysiology of type 2 diabetes in the elderly. Clin Geriatr Med 15:239–253

Mooradian AD, Albert SG, Wittry S, Chehade J, Kim J, Bellrichard B (2000) Dose response profile of acrabose in older subjects with type 2 diabetes. Am J Med Sci 319:334–337

Moty C, Barberger-Gateau P, De Sarasqueta AM, Teare GF, Henrad JC (2003) Risk adjustment of quality indicators in French long term care facilities for elderly people. A preliminary study. Rev Epidemiol Sante Publique 51:327–338

National Kidney Foundation (2002) K/DOQI clinical practice guidelines for chronic kidney disease: evaluation, classification, and stratification. Am J Kidney Dis 39(Suppl 1):S1–S246

Phillips P, Phil D, Rolls B et al (1984) Reduced thirst after water dehydration in healthy elderly men. N Engl J Med 311:753–759

Piccini C, Motola D, Marchesini G, Poluzzi E (2011) Assessing the association of pioglitazone use and bladder cancer through drug adverse event reporting. Diabetes Care 34:1369–1371

Pickering G (2004) Frail elderly, nutritional status and drugs. Arch Gerontol Geriatr 38:174–180

Schwarz SL, Gerich JE, Marcellari A, Jean-Louis L, Purkayastha D, Baron MA (2008) Nateglinide, alone or in combination with metformin, is effective and well tolerated in treatment-naive elderly patients with type 2 diabetes. Diabetes Obes Metab 10:652–660

Shepherd J, Blauw GJ, Murphy MB et al (2002) Pravastatin in elderly individuals at risk of vascular disease (PROSPER): a randomised controlled trial. Lancet 360:1623–1630

Shorr RI, Ray WA, Daugherty JR, Griffin MR (1997) Incidence and risk factors for serious hypoglycemia in older persons using insulin or sulfonylureas. Arch Intern Med 157:1681–1686

Skyler JS, Bergenstal R, Bonow RO et al (2009) Intensive glycemic control and the prevention of cardiovascular events: implications of the ACCORD, ADVANCE, and VA Diabetes Trials: a position statement of the American Diabetes Association and a scientific statement of the American College of Cardiology Foundation and the American Heart Association. J Am Coll Cardiol 53:298–304

The Diabetes Prevention Program Research Group, Crandall J, Schade D, Ma Y et al (2006) The influence of age on the effects of lifestyle modification and metformin in prevention of diabetes. J Gerontol A Biol Sci Med Sci 61A:1075–1081

Thomson FJ, Masson EA, Leeming JT, Boulton AJ (1991) Lack of knowledge of symptoms of hypoglycaemia by elderly diabetic patients. Age Ageing 20:404–406

Thorslund S, Toss G, Nilsson I, von Schenk H, Symbwerg T, Zetterqvist H (1990) Prevalence of protein-energy malnutrition in a large population of elderly people at home. Scand J Prim Health Care 8:243–248

Turnbull PJ, Sinclair AJ (2002) Evaluation of nutritional status and its relationship with functional status in older citizens with diabetes mellitus using the Mini Nutritional Assessment (MNA) tool. A preliminary investigation. J Nutr Health Aging 6:116–120

UKPDS (UK Prospective Diabetes Study) Group (1998) Effect of intensive blood-glucose control with metformin on complications in overweight patients with type 2 diabetes. Lancet 352:854–865

Van Den Berghe G, Wouters P, Weekers F et al (2001) Intensive insulin therapy in critically ill patients. N Engl J Med 345:1359–1367

Wehling M (2009) Multimorbidity and polypharmacy: how to reduce the harmful drug load and yet add needed drugs in the elderly? Proposal of a new drug classification: fit for the aged. J Am Geriatr Soc 57:560–561

Yki-Järvinen H, Kauppila M, Kujansuu E et al (1992) Comparison of insulin regimens in patients with non-insulin-dependent diabetes mellitus. N Engl J Med 327:1426–1433

Obstructive Lung Diseases

Martin Wehling

Relevance for Elderly Patients, Epidemiology

The major forms of obstructive lung disease are bronchial asthma and chronic obstructive pulmonary disease (COPD). Asthma is characterized by a predominantly functional bronchial obstruction that is almost entirely reversible, at least at early stages; COPD exposes structural changes and deficits of the respiratory tract, including the lung tissue, that are mostly irreversible. COPD is the typical and most prevalent chronic lung disease of the elderly, while new asthma will rarely occur, and existing asthma usually becomes milder at higher age. Therefore, the focus of this chapter is drug treatment of COPD in the elderly. Unfortunately, the epidemiological significance of COPD is not adequately recognized even today. Yet, the incidence will sharply rise in the future, and it is assumed that in 2030 COPD will be the third-most-important cause of death globally, only secondary to cardiovascular diseases and AIDS (Table 1). This epidemic reflects the aging of Western societies as COPD is an age-related disease and the lack of success against the main avoidable culprit, which is smoking, causing about 80–90% of all COPD-related deaths. Although in the United States smoking is on the decline, the increasing prevalence of smoking in women partly compensates for the success of smoking cessation. It is assumed that in 2008 there will be 12 million U.S. citizens who suffer from COPD (American Lung Association 2010), with an estimated equal number of undiagnosed cases. The prevalence of COPD in elderly U.S. citizens aged 65+ years was around 10 % in 2000 (Mannino et al. 2002) and should have risen in between. In patients aged 70+ years in Salzburg, Austria, the prevalence was at 50 % (Schirnhofer et al. 2007).

Unfortunately, medical care, academic representation, and scientific efforts are not nearly adequate to properly address this tremendous challenge of industrial, wealthy societies, not to speak of developing or underdeveloped countries. This fact is even more relevant for COPD in the elderly, whose specific problems of multimorbidity, frailty, and polypharmacy add another dimension to the challenge.

The indisputable successes of drug support for smoking cessation have been described in chapter "Coronary Heart Disease and Stroke" under the section "Therapeutically Relevant Special Features of Elderly Patients," and nonpharmacological treatment combined with drugs represents a valuable opportunity for many patients, including the elderly. Smoking cessation is never too late; symptoms of COPD may improve at any stage of the disease, although the structural changes are irreversible. Reducing progression of COPD by smoking cessation is proven and should be utilized at any stage. Inborn diseases

M. Wehling (✉)
University of Heidelberg, Maybachstr. 14, Mannheim 68169, Germany
e-mail: martin.wehling@medma.uni-heidelberg.de

Table 1 Changes in rankings for global causes of death 2002/2030

Category	Disease or injury	2002 rank	2030 ranks	Change in rank
Within top 15	Ischemic heart disease	1	1	0
	Cerebrovascular disease	2	2	0
	Lower respiratory infections	3	5	−2
	HIV/AIDS	4	3	−1
	COPD	5	4	+1
	Perinatal conditions	6	9	−3
	Diarrheal diseases	7	16	−9
	Tuberculosis	8	23	−15
	Trachea, bronchus, lung cancers	9	6	+3
	Road traffic accidents	10	8	+2
	Diabetes mellitus	11	7	+4
	Malaria	12	22	−10
	Hypertensive heart disease	13	11	+2
	Self-inflicted injuries	14	12	+2
	Stomach cancer	15	10	+5
Outside top 15	Nephritis and nephrosis	17	13	+4
	Colon and rectum cancers	18	15	+3
	Liver cancers	19	14	+5

Source: From Mathers and Loncar 2006
COPD in 2030 is on the third rank if all cardiovascular diseases, including stroke, are taken together
COPD chronic obstructive pulmonary disease

such as alpha1-antitrypsin deficiency are rare and do not significantly contribute to the problem. This disease may even be treated by substitution of alpha1-antitrypsin.

Therapeutically Relevant Special Features of Elderly Patients

An important aspect of COPD in the elderly is the fact that smoking as its common culprit causes many other diseases. Arteriosclerotic diseases, especially coronary heart disease, are most relevant in this context as this comorbidity has serious implications for the choice of the therapeutic options. It is obvious that obstructive lung disease will be treated by drugs that dilate the airways but at the same time stress the heart (such as betamimetics and theophylline). If both diseases are present, relative contraindications against those drugs may evolve, thus narrowing the array of therapeutic choices. Individualization of drug therapy, which is always mandatory, may be particularly challenging in this situation of elderly patients, and the outcome may be disappointing. Dutch data show that COPD patients aged

65+ years have two relevant additional diagnoses in 25% of cases and three in 17% of cases (van Weel 1996). A frequent cardiac comorbidity is heart failure in about 20% of elderly COPD patients. Both diseases lead to dyspnea as a key symptom, but treatment modalities are absolutely divergent; thus, an exact differential diagnosis must be established to avoid sometimes deleterious consequences (such as beta-blockers, which are indicated for heart failure but may be contraindicated in pulmonary obstructive disease).

As these age-dependent comorbidities represent the main modifiers of COPD treatment in the elderly, they are the major issue of the following chapter.

Evidence-Based, Rationalistic Drug Therapy and Classification of Drugs According to Their Fitness for the Aged (FORTA)

Figure 1 shows the treatment escalation for the different stages of COPD according to the Global Initiative for Chronic Obstructive Lung Disease (GOLD) (Rabe et al. 2007). The core

GOLD stages of COPD Escalation of treatment

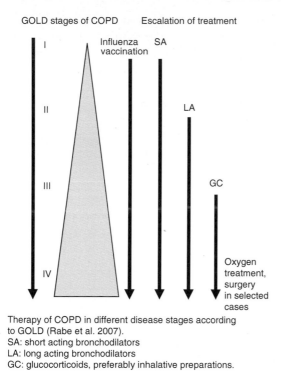

Therapy of COPD in different disease stages according
to GOLD (Rabe et al. 2007).
SA: short acting bronchodilators
LA: long acting bronchodilators
GC: glucocorticoids, preferably inhalative preparations.

Fig. 1 Therapy of chronic obstructive pulmonary disease
(*COPD*) in different disease stages according to the
Global Initiative for Chronic Obstructive Lung Disease
(GOLD; Rabe et al. 2007). *SA* short-acting bronchodila-
tors, *LA* long-acting bronchodilators, *GC* glucocorticoids,
preferably inhaled preparations

interventions remain unchanged in the revised
recommendation of 2010 (Global Initiative for
Chronic Obstructive Lung Disease (GOLD)
2010). A classification of COPD severity into
four stages is proposed, with the stages defined
by FEV_1 (forced expiratory volume in the first
second of expiration) and forced vital capacity
(FVC) values and by blood gas analysis results as
a measure of respiratory failure (stage IV). In
addition, the frequency of exacerbations by
infections is important. Even in the 2010 version
of the recommendation, no separate chapters or
even paragraphs are devoted to elderly patients.
The most important entry is the statement that
age-adapted normal values should be considered
for the interpretation of respiratory testing results
to avoid overdiagnosing of COPD in the elderly.
This reflects the fact that FEV_1 and FVC values
are declining with age even in the absence of
COPD, thus being in line with the course of

many (if not almost all) organ functions in the
aging organism. Therapeutically, elderly patients
are not even explicitly mentioned.

Beta-2 Mimetics

Short- and long-acting beta-2-mimetics are separate and only differ in regard to their half-life.
Stimulation of beta-2 receptors in the airways
(bronchi and bronchioles) results in dilation and
reduces obstruction. The prerequisite for this
beneficial action is the reversibility of obstruction, which is limited in COPD (see previous
discussion) compared to asthma. These compounds are used not only for treatment, but also
as diagnostic test agents for the separation of
both diseases: Reversibility of obstruction is
indicated if the FEV_1 improves by more than
20–30%. This is clearly a feature of asthma as
opposed to COPD and constitutes an absolute
contraindication against beta-blockers.

The effects of beta-2 mimetics in COPD are
limited and certainly smaller than in asthma;
unfortunately, they elicit the same side effects
as in asthma treatment. Given the age dependency of COPD, these toxic actions mainly hit
elderly patients and thus impaired organs in
COPD; thus, they are seemingly more toxic in
COPD than asthma treatment, but this just
reflects the increased vulnerability of elderly
patients. Despite beta-2 selectivity and slow
absorption after inhalation, drug concentrations
reaching the heart are capable of inducing all
known side effects of adrenergic compounds:

– Tachycardia,

– Inotropy,

– Bathmotropy, and

– Especially arrhythmogenicity.

The last side effect is potentially lethal, particularly in elderly patients with cardiac disease or
age-related changes. High-quality pharmacoepidemiological studies of this problem are missing
for the elderly, but large meta-analyses pointed to
this issue in the all-age patient cohort (Salpeter
2007). Thus, it is only fair to assume that in
elderly patients with a greater cardiac vulnerability and high prevalence of cardiovascular diseases

catecholamine toxicity is even worse than in younger adults. As a consequence, alternative strategies for bronchodilation and anti-inflammatory measures as described in the following need to be utilized early.

In particular, COPD treatment in elderly patients is only successful if drugs with a significant potential to cause cardiovascular harm are reduced or avoided. This note of caution applies to catecholamines and especially to theophylline, which has to be given systemically.

Treatment of GOLD stage I COPD is based on the powder inhalation of short-acting beta-2-mimetics such as fenoterol (European Union), pirbuterol, or albuterol (= salbutamol in the European Union) as on-demand drugs; in stage II, long-acting beta-2 mimetics such as formoterol or salmeterol are added.

Inhalation of drugs is a general problem in the elderly as it requires active participation of the patient. The patient's contribution is more demanding for powder than spray inhalation as the powder has to be actively and vigorously inspired in a coordinated and timed manner. Sprays result in a lower fraction of drug deposition in the airways than powder preparations (20% vs. up to 80%). Thus, local side effects (e.g., in the pharynx or larynx) are more common for sprays than powder inhalations. The latter preparations are thus preferable. Present spray preparations are generally free of fluorochlorinated hydrocarbons, which are under suspicion as causing arrhythmias as well. If patient fitness to use inhalative preparations is at borderline, sprays are easier to use and preferable under these conditions. Sprays should be combined with spacers to reduce large-droplet deposition.

A simple drawing test (copying overlapping pentagons) has been proven to be helpful in identifying patients with impaired cognition who thus are unable to apply drug by inhalation successfully (Board and Allen 2006). Hand grip strength correlates with successful inhalation and thus may be measured as an indicator as well. Nebulization of the respective compound (either as ready-to-use preparation or by dilution in physiological saline) may be used as an alternative for patients with severe dementia; this, however, requires sufficient room ventilation to avoid drug application to caregivers and relatives.

Parasympatholytics

Ipratropium is the prototype of a parasympatholytic that is poorly absorbed from the airway epithelia. Its bronchodilatory action is limited to 6–8 h; thus, the drug has to be applied three or four times a day. A limited amount of substance may be absorbed both from the airways and—after deposition in the upper airways, larynx, and pharynx—the gastrointestinal tract. This explains systemic parasympatholytic side effects such as dry mouth, blurred vision (impaired lens accommodation), or tachycardia. Still, this compound is much safer than catecholamine derivatives, but also less effective.

A newer compound, tiotropium, has striking advantages: It is long acting (24 h, q.d. application), is more efficacious than ipratropium in preventing exacerbations of COPD, and is safer than beta mimetics regarding cardiovascular side effects (Jara et al. 2007). Although not stated in the GOLD guideline of 2010, this compound seems to be preferable in elderly patients on continuous treatment (stage II and higher). The once-daily application is advantageous particularly for elderly patients, as is the lower rate of cardiovascular side effects. In the recent Prevention of Exacerbations with Tiotropium in COPD study (POET-COPD) (Vogelmeier et al. 2011), tiotropium proved to be superior to salmeterol in the prevention of COPD exacerbations, and this effect seemed to be even larger in patients aged 65+ years.

Tiotropium is an important contributor to the catecholamine-reducing strategy of elderly COPD patients. If not efficient as a single treatment, a combination with long-term beta mimetics adds to the effects. These recommendations of tiotropium as a first-line chronic treatment of COPD in the elderly are not backed by the GOLD recommendations; however, latter do not seem to reflect the special aspects of elderly patients adequately.

Table 2 Low, intermediate, and high doses of inhaled glucocorticoids

Daily doses of inhaled glucocorticoids			
Compound	Low dose (µg)	Intermediate dose	High dose
Beclomethasone	$\leq$500	$\leq$1.000	$\leq$2.000
Budesonide	$\leq$400	$\leq$800	$\leq$1.600
Ciclesonide	80–160	160	>160
Fluticasone	$\leq$250	$\leq$500	$\leq$1.000
Mometasone	200	400	800

Source: From Buhl et al. 2006, p. 165, Table 15, by kind permission of Thieme; translation by the author

Inhaled Glucocorticoids

From stage III, inhaled glucocorticoids such as budesonide or fluticasone should be added to the treatment as they are strong anti-inflammatory drugs. Systemic side effects are not to be feared at low-to-intermediate doses (Table 2); at high doses, typical signs of hypercortisolism may occur: suppression of the adrenocortical axis and increased risk of osteoporosis with fractures. While the systemic side effects are much less important than for systemic glucocorticoid application, local side effects such as hoarseness or candidiasis in the mouth, pharynx, larynx, or upper esophagus are common and at times embarrassing. They are much rarer if powder inhalation rather than spray applications are properly used. Age-related immunodeficiency is a risk factor for secondary generalization of yeast infections, such as systemic candidiasis, which has a high fatality rate in the elderly, although exact epidemiological figures are lacking.

Concerning efficacy, it should be mentioned that a synergism exists between glucocorticoids and beta mimetics in that glucocorticoids sensitize airway muscle cells for beta mimetic action. For compliance support, fixed combination preparations are preferable in elderly patients after treatment initiation with individual components and achievement of clinical stability. Most available combinations contain a long-acting beta-2 mimetic and an inhaled glucocorticoid, such as formoterol and budesonide or salmeterol and fluticasone.

Systemic Therapy

The efficacy of bronchodilation and anti-inflammatory effects in COPD is quite limited

(with the exception of infectious exacerbations, bronchitis) as this disease is characterized by structural, irreversible deficits, and constriction/ inflammation are of minor importance. In the frequent case of therapeutic failure under the regimen described, subjective improvement may be experienced by dose escalation of beta mimetics. The mechanism is unclear and does not mainly involve airway parameters; it rather seems to reflect central nervous system (CNS) effects (stimulation, well-being, "cocaine-like effects"). At increasing doses, cardiovascular side effects, especially tachycardia and arrhythmia, aggravate as well. If the therapeutic escalation is felt to be insufficient, systemic drugs will be utilized, such as theophylline (for which systemic application is the only route), oral systemic glucocorticoids, or oral systemic beta-2- mimetics.

This escalation needs to be avoided in elderly patients by all means as systemic treatment always carries a much higher risk of side effects than inhalation strategies and hits a vulnerable organism in this case. The side effects of chronic systemic glucocorticoid therapy are well known (Cushing syndrome with hypertension, heart failure, osteoporosis, skin damage, and many more symptoms); those of theophylline and systemic beta mimetics are dramatic as well (tachycardia, arrhythmias, sleeplessness, delirium).

Theophylline is a relatively unsafe drug as its pharmacokinetics are complicated, and it has a great potential of drug-drug-interactions and a small therapeutic range. Particularly in the elderly, even at high-normal plasma levels delirium syndromes may be induced. The clearance is reduced in elderly patients; thus, therapeutic drug monitoring is mandatory (treatment range

5–20 mg/l; I recommend not exceeding 15 mg/l in the elderly).

To avoid such systemic treatments, all means of nonpharmacological interventions need to be utilized, such as physical therapy, including pulmonary percussion; breathing exercises; suction of mucus. Mucolytics have no proven value (see following discussion). Only on failure of those care-intense measures should systemic therapies be instituted, knowing that they may shorten life. Risk-benefit assessment must reflect quality-of-life aspects; in geriatric cases, this may be difficult and has to comprise biological age, comorbidities, and thus life expectancy. As a result, even morphine may be considered in end-stage cases of COPD to alleviate symptoms of asphyxia, although it will definitely shorten life.

Oxygen

At GOLD stage IV with respiratory failure, long-term treatment with oxygen is indicated. The initial dose should not exceed 1.5 l/min as hypercapnic respiratory arrest may be induced at higher doses. In severe COPD, respiratory stimulation is driven by oxygen rather than carbon dioxide, which is the normal stimulant. The carbon dioxide intoxication leads to a lack of respiratory stimulation and breathing arrest if blood oxygen is elevated. The appropriate oxygen dose is adjusted to finally keep blood oxygen saturation above 90%.

Long-term oxygen therapy is the only measure that is proven to prolong life in severe COPD.

Oxygen lowers pulmonary artery pressure and improves cognition and quality of life. It should not be withheld even from the very elderly, but supportive care must be provided if dementia or impaired cognition may interfere with its proper use. A combination with lung surgery (such as the removal of bullae) may be indicated.

Newer drugs for the treatment of pulmonary arterial hypertension such as endothelin antagonists

(bosentan) or sildenafil have not be tested in elderly COPD patients with success and need to be further profiled for this indication as opposed to cases of primary, hereditary forms of pulmonary hypertension. The ultimate intervention in end-stage COPD, lung transplantation, is normally restricted to younger patients and thus is no viable option for the elderly.

Vaccinations

At any age and for all stages of COPD, yearly vaccinations against influenza are recommended (split vaccine, usually against strains A/H1N1, A/H3N2, and B, will be modified each year reflecting viral epidemiology). From age 65, pneumococcal vaccination should be performed as well. Although highly effective, vaccinations are underutilized in elderly persons: Only 63% of persons aged 65+ years in the United States received influenza vaccinations in 2005 (Centers for Disease Control and Prevention 2006) and only 50% in Germany (Muller and Szucs 2007). By increasing the utilization, a greater impact on mortality and morbidity could be achieved than by all those drugs (expect oxygen) described.

Exacerbations

Elderly patients are particularly threatened by exacerbations of COPD, which are normally caused by infections. These patients have a limited bandwidth of reactions and mechanisms to cope with infections.

As a rule, antibiotic therapy needs to be calculated and to cover a broad spectrum of pathogens; it should be started on suspicion of infection without delay, and hospitalization is mandatory for the elderly patients with COPD, who are vulnerable and do not tolerate time loss.

The choice of antibiotics against the infection has to reflect the circumstances of acquisition (nosocomial during hospitalization: very dangerous;

acquired in the "normal" community: relatively benign) and the local situation of resistance. Data on the use of antibiotics in elderly patients with COPD are rare. The choice is mandated by the diagnosed or expected pathogens; however, dosing needs to be strictly adapted to altered pharmacokinetics in the elderly, mainly relating to kidney or liver function, as described elsewhere. Fluoroquinolones are particularly toxic for the elderly brain and may induce atypical psychiatric and cognitive disturbances, including severe delirium. Betalactam antibiotics such as aminopenicillins (amoxicillin), often in combination with beta-lactamase inhibitors, or macrolides (e.g., clarithromycin) are much safer in the elderly if dosed correctly. This means reduced doses in many instances (e.g., patients with renal impairment) but not generally. Oral cephalosporins typically expose a low absorption fraction. They thus mainly remain in the gut, where they cause trouble by destroying the intestinal flora, with subsequent diarrhea or even *Clostridium difficile* infection/pseudomembranous colitis. In elderly patients, antibiotic-associated diarrhea may rapidly induce dehydration, electrolyte disorders (hypo- or hyperkalemia), and venous thromboses. In this situation, sufficient and balanced rehydration and electrolyte substitution is mandatory, which may require intravenous therapy and strict balancing/weight control.

An important and successful therapeutic supplement in COPD exacerbation is the oral application of high-dose glucocorticoids (30–40 mg/day prednisolone) for 7–10 days.

Despite numerous studies, mucolytics such as acetylcysteine or guaifenesin do not have a proven effect, but may cause side effects. Physical therapy (see previous discussion) during hospitalization and adequate hydration for the liquification of the mucus are certainly more effective. Unfortunately, physical therapy is care intense and thus restricted in many settings. This urges doctors to do "something," which may mean to recommend mucolytics. Antitussives (cough suppressants) also are not efficacious. Elderly patients should even be discouraged from buying them over the counter as coughing is important to prevent pneumonia and thus should definitely not be suppressed in the elderly.

Classification of Drugs for the Chronic Treatment of COPD According to Their Fitness for the Aged (FORTA)

In this classification of drugs for the chronic treatment of COPD according to their Fitness for the Aged (FORTA), the same compounds may receive alternative marks if applied indifferent indications (see chapter "Critical Extrapolation of Guidelines and Study Results: Risk-Benefit Assessment for Patients with Reduced Life Expectancy and a New Classification of Drugs According to Their Fitness for the Aged").

Influenza vaccination	A
Pneumococcal vaccination, age 65+ years	A
Beta-2 mimetics, inhalation	B
Parasympatholytics, long acting, inhalation	A
Glucocorticoids, inhalation	A
Oxygen, long-term therapy	A
Theophylline	C
Glucocorticoids, systemic treatment, chronic	D
Glucocorticoids, systemic treatment, acute with exacerbation	A
Antibiotics, acute with exacerbation, "calculated" or in reflection of antibiogram	A
Mucolytics	C
Antitussives	D

References

American Lung Association (2010) Trends in COPD (chronic bronchitis and emphysema): morbidity and mortality. American Lung Association Epidemiology and Statistics Unit, Research and Program Services Division. http://www.lungusa.org/finding-cures/our-research/trend-reports/copd-trend-report.pdf. Accessed 20 Jul 2011

Board M, Allen SC (2006) A simple drawing test to identify patients who are unlikely to be able to learn to use an inhaler. Int J Clin Pract 60:510–513

Buhl R, Berdel D, Criee CP et al (2006) Leitlinie zur Diagnostik und Therapie von Patienten mit Asthma. Pneumologie 60:139–177

Centers for Disease Control and Prevention (CDC) (2006) Influenza and pneumococcal vaccination coverage among persons aged > or = 65 years—United States, 2004–2005. MMWR Morb Mortal Wkly Rep 55:1065–1068

Global Initiative for Chronic Obstructive Lung Disease (GOLD) (2010). Global Strategy for the Diagnosis, Management and Prevention of COPD, http://www.goldcopd.org/uploads/users/files/GOLD-Report_April112011.pdf. Accessed 27 Jun 2012

Jara M, Lanes SF, Wentworth C 3rd, May C, Kesten S (2007) Comparative safety of long-acting inhaled bronchodilators: a cohort study using the UK THIN primary care database. Drug Saf 30:1151–1160

Mannino DM, Homa DM, Akinbami LJ et al (2002) Chronic obstructive pulmonary disease surveillance: United States, 1971–2000. MMWR Surveill Summ 51:1–16

Mathers CD, Loncar D (2006) Projections of global mortality and burden of disease from 2002 to 2030. PLoS Med 3:e442

Muller D, Szucs TD (2007) Influenza vaccination coverage rates in 5 European countries: a population-based cross-sectional analysis of the seasons 02/03, 03/04 and 04/05. Infection 35:308–319

Rabe KF, Hurd S, Anzueto A et al (2007) Global initiative for chronic obstructive lung disease. Global strategy for the diagnosis, management, and prevention of chronic obstructive pulmonary disease: GOLD executive summary. Am J Respir Crit Care Med 176:532–555

Salpeter SR (2007) Bronchodilators in COPD: impact of betaagonists and anticholinergics on severe exacerbations and mortality. Int J Chron Obstruct Pulmon Dis 2:11–18

Schirnhofer L, Lamprecht B, Vollmer WM, Allison MJ, Studnicka M, Jensen RL, Buist AS (2007) COPD prevalence in Salzburg, Austria: results from the Burden of Obstructive Lung Disease (BOLD) study. Chest 131:29–36

van Weel C (1996) Chronic diseases in general practice: the longitudinal dimension. Eur J Gen Pract 2:17–21

Vogelmeier C, Hederer B, Glaab T et al (2011) Tiotropium versus salmeterol for the prevention of exacerbations of COPD. N Engl J Med 364:1093–1103

Osteoporosis

Martin Wehling

Relevance for Elderly Patients, Epidemiology

Osteoporosis is an important age-related disease; its largest incidence occurs in postmenopausal women. Social and economical consequences are considerable as it is frequent and leads to fractures, particularly of the hip and vertebrae. In the elderly, and particularly the very elderly, fracture morbidity leads to mortality as they may be complicated by pneumonia or venous thromboembolism due to immobilization. The disease is characterized by a progressive reduction of bone density, which not only includes demineralization but also structural rarification. Typical risk factors apart from female sex are

- Low body weight,
- Malnutrition,
- Age,
- Physical inactivity,
- Smoking, and
- Systemic glucocorticoid therapy for more than 3 months.

Men acquire a greater bone density than women as their body weight and physical activity are higher, and higher androgen concentrations increase bone density to higher levels than estrogens do. Still, they may develop osteoporosis,

which on average is delayed by 10 years compared to the progress of the disease in women. Prior to menopause, endogenous estrogens protect women against a more rapid development of osteoporosis. As osteoporosis is often first diagnosed at the event of a fracture, treatment modalities have to cover both therapeutic (meaning the treatment of complications arising from existing osteoporosis) and preventive (before osteoporosis or its complications occur) aspects.

In the United States, it is estimated that 10 million citizens have osteoporosis, and 33.6 million show decreased bone mineral density of the hip (National Osteoporosis Foundation 2002). The socioeconomic impact is demonstrated by the fact that 432,000 hospital admissions and 180,000 nursing home admissions are caused by this disease per year (U.S. Department of Health and Human Services 2004). The prevalence increases from 6% in 50-year-old women to over 50% in 80-year-old women (Looker et al. 1997). At age 50, a woman has a 40% chance to suffer from an osteoporotic fracture (hip, wrist/radius, vertebrae) at least once during her remaining lifetime. Vertebral fractures are often overlooked; only one third will be properly diagnosed (measurement of body height). These fractures have a serious impact on mortality: Within 1 year after hip fracture, 20% of women and 40% of men will die (Chrischilles et al. 1991), not to mention personal dependence in nursing homes and depression as negative outcomes.

In the 2010 recommendations by the National Osteoporosis Foundation, only little attention is

M. Wehling (✉)
University of Heidelberg, Maybachstr. 14, Mannheim 68169, Germany
e-mail: martin.wehling@medma.uni-heidelberg.de

M. Wehling (ed.), *Drug Therapy for the Elderly*,
DOI 10.1007/978-3-7091-0912-0_12, © Springer-Verlag Wien 2013

paid to the special aspects of drug treatment in the elderly (with the exception of the vitamin D status and supplementation), although age is one of the strongest risk factors for this disease. Thus, its prevalence sharply rises with age.

Therapeutically Relevant Special Features of Elderly Patients

Several peculiarities of elderly, especially very elderly, patients with osteoporosis and its treatment have to be considered. An important association is that of osteoporosis and nutritional supply of vitamin D and calcium. As elderly persons often suffer from insufficient nutrition, particularly those in nursing homes, vitamin D and calcium deficiency is frequent, and substitution by nutritional supplements is indicated in most cases (see the following discussion).

Low body weight as a leading risk factor is common in elderly patients with sarcopenia ("nothing but skin and bone"). Nutrition therefore should be adequate regarding total calorie and protein intake, although excessive obesity needs to be avoided as it may induce diabetes mellitus and other cardiovascular risk factors. Conversely, elderly patients are the only ones for whom strict weight reduction recommendations are discouraged for these obvious reasons. Physical exercise is the best method to gain muscular weight and change the body composition in a bone-protective way. Its prerequisite again is adequate nutrition. Osteoporosis and related fractures are a major complication of sarcopenia, which has not yet been studied and understood properly.

Osteoporotic fractures are almost exclusively provoked by falls. This age-dependent syndrome is extensively discussed in part "Pharmacotherapy and Geriatric Syndromes." It is obvious that osteoporosis treatment per se cannot be effective if frequent falls continue to occur. Protective measures such as the hip protector or antifall training, but particularly the withdrawal of fall-risk-increasing drugs (FRIDs), are essential in the prevention of falls. Thyroid hormone and vitamin D deficiencies are associated with an increased fall risk.

Benzodiazepines, antidepressants, antiepileptics, and drugs inducing orthostasis (mainly antihypertensive drugs) are the most common FRIDs in this context.

Systemic glucocorticoid therapy exceeding 3 months and chronic use of heparins (unfractionated worse than low molecular weight heparins) or proton pump inhibitors may induce osteoporosis. This risk needs to be carefully weighed against benefits in the elderly, and the threat to the patient by osteoporosis induction or aggravation should not be estimated to be small. This side effect is one of the major reasons for the serious restrictions or contraindications that should be put forth regarding chronic glucocorticoid therapies above the Cushing threshold (7.5 mg prednisolone equivalent/day). In the elderly, the osteoporosis threshold seems to be lower, and no dose above 2.5 mg/day should be considered bone safe. Smoking and alcohol abuse are seen as risk factors, but their prevalences—unlike those of the drugs mentioned—are not increasing with age.

The majority of drugs used in the treatment and prophylaxis of osteoporosis (mainly bisphosphonates) are renally excreted and thus need to be carefully dosed in the elderly. Oral intake may be complicated by age-dependent alterations of motility in the upper gastrointestinal tract and impairment of the ability to swallow. Frequent episodes of aspiration are the consequence and may render the application of oral bisphosphonates dangerous. Parenteral preparations are to be preferred in such cases.

Evidence-Based, Rationalistic Drug (and Nutritional Supplement) Therapy and Classification of Drugs According to Their Fitness for the Aged (FORTA)

In addition to lifestyle modifications (balanced, calorically sufficient nutrition to guarantee a minimum body mass index of 20 kg/m^2, physical exercise, fall risk assessment, and treatment), the adequate supply of oral calcium and vitamin D is essential for all elderly individuals, including those without manifest osteoporosis. Total daily

Table 1 Criteria for recommending pharmacologic treatment from the U.S. National Osteoporosis Foundation guidelines

In women and men aged 50 years and older, pharmacologic therapy should be recommended for those with any one of the following
A history of hip fracture or clinical or radiographic spine fracture
T score of −2.5 or less at femoral neck or spine[a]
Low bone mass (osteopenia), T scores of −1.0 to −2.5 at the femoral neck or lumbar spine and any of the following
3% 10-year probability of hip fracture or
20% 10-year probability of a major osteoporotic fracture based on the WHO model for the United States

Source: From Donaldson et al. 2010 by permission of John Wiley and Sons
WHO World Health Organization
[a]After excluding secondary causes

calcium intake (including supplements) should not exceed 1,200 mg (National Osteoporosis Foundation 2010). After estimation of nutritional calcium content, 500–1,000 mg calcium may be needed as an oral supplement. Regarding vitamin D, the National Osteoporosis Foundation recommends a daily intake of 800–1,000 international units (IU) to achieve plasma levels of vitamin D_3 of at least 30 ng/ml. The upper limit of daily supplements was set at 2,000 IU, and in reflection of their plasma levels, some elderly patients may require that dose. Sun exposition is the natural trigger of vitamin D_3 generation and should be considered for the dose estimate. For elderly people, in particular in nursing homes, sun exposition is very limited and should be extended whenever possible (stay on a balcony or porch, excursions). As this is often insufficient given the light conditions of the Northern Hemisphere, vitamin D_3 substitution is the rule rather than the exception. Our ancestors came from Africa, and the equatorial sun produced enough vitamin D despite the dark skin; moving North required a less-pigmented skin to provide enough vitamin D for survival. As even the pale skin of elderly patients does not produce enough vitamin D under the conditions of our way of life, substitution is highly recommended in almost all patients. Intoxications at those dosages mentioned are very unlikely to occur. Inuits settle their vitamin D demand by lipid-rich fish, which contain vitamin D in its active form as the intensity of sunshine is too low in Arctic regions. Interestingly, vitamin D has now been shown to exert cardioprotective and antidementia

effects; it also reduces the risk of falls. However, if there were only the bone-protective effect of vitamin D, which is absolutely clear and evidence based, it should be seen as a sufficient reason for its substitution. This area of research is very active at present, and new insights are likely to be generated in the near future. Anyway, there is also no doubt about the deficiency in the industrial countries of the Northern Hemisphere, and the proven antiosteoporotic effect should mandate the substitution in many more patients than presently treated. This measure is very cost effective as it prevents costly complications of osteoporosis; thus, it should be reimbursed by health insurance, which is not the case everywhere (e.g., Germany).

In addition to these basic measures, which are applicable to almost all elderly patients (independent of bone status), and unspecific pain treatment in the case of symptomatic osteoporosis, specific and effective antiosteoporotic drugs are available.

In Table 1, the indications for specific pharmacotherapy of osteoporosis treatment are summarized as derived from the National Osteoporosis Foundation Guideline 2010. In this recommendation, low bone mass means a DXA (dual-energy x-ray absorptiometry) T-score between −1.0 and −2.5 at the femoral neck or spine. The T-score describes the number of standard deviations from normal values of the respective age cohort. Specific drug therapy is indicated for this range if the World Health Organization (WHO) risk prediction score criteria are met. This score may be computed on the following Web page: http://www.shef.ac.uk/FRAX. By the computation of the FRAX score, to which age contributes as a major factor, the U.S. recommendation of specific drug therapy indication is very specific for elderly and even very elderly patients, which is exceptional. Still, particular aspects of drug treatment (safety) in the elderly are not well covered (see previous discussion). It is also estimated that 49% of white men aged 75+ years in the United States would qualify for drug therapy, which seems excessive (Donaldson et al. 2010).

In summary, these guidelines recommend specific treatment in the case of fractures independently of risk factors, while in the prophylactic approach (no fractures so far), DXA T-scores, age, sex, weight, height, smoker status, glucocorticoid medication, rate of falls, and other risk factors are included in the overall risk assessment. It is obvious that this risk factor concept resembles similar concepts in the cardiovascular system or that described for venous thromboembolism. As a major shortcoming in the treatment of very elderly patients, reduced life expectancy and the delay of treatment effects are not considered in this recommendation. It is hard to conceive that in a 95-year-old male treatment effects will become significant and—more important—clinically relevant during the remaining lifetime of 2.9 years. Thus, for the very elderly these recommendations need to be individualized. However, the risk-benefit assessment remains a dilemma in such patients: No one wants a very old lady to suffer from a vertebral fracture after a minor fall, but all specific drugs also cause side effects, which at times will occur much faster than the beneficial effects. In studies of osteoporosis, treatment effects become just visible after 6 months at minimum, but are small in the beginning. To achieve significant effects, about 3 years are required. Thus, the time horizon of treatment should be 3–5 years, meaning that indications in the very elderly should be restrictive, particularly as again data are not available for them.

Drugs approved by the Food and Drug Administration (FDA) for specific osteoporosis therapy are bisphosphonates (alendronate, alendronate plus D, ibandronate, risedronate, risedronate with 500 mg of calcium carbonate, and zoledronic acid); estrogens; SERM (selective estrogen receptor modulator, raloxifen); teriparatide (parathyroid hormone analogue); and calcitonin; strontium ranelate is only available in Europe.

Bisphosphonates

Bisphosphonates inhibit osteoclasts and thereby delay bone absorption. They bind to bone matrix as a reservoir and thus may exert their effects for months or even years. There is no reasonable doubt about their efficacy in the prevention of osteoporotic fractures, in both primary (osteoporosis, no fracture so far) and secondary (postosteoporotic fractures) settings. Reductions of fracture incidences for both hip and vertebral fractures range from 20% to 60% versus placebo. It should be noted that profound experiences for bisphosphonate therapies over more than 5 years are not available. Given those long-lasting bone deposits mentioned, prolonged effects after cessation of application cannot be excluded, but the time range for this is unclear. For the first time, even a reduction of mortality could be shown for zoledronic acid in elderly patients (mean age 74.5 years) with hip fracture (Fig. 1); this also underlines the vital threat by hip fractures in the elderly population.

FDA-approved bisphosphonates are alendronate, ibandronate, risedronate, and zoledronic acid. Daily dosing (e.g., alendronate) may be replaced by applications at longer intervals, such as weekly (alendronate 70 mg/week), monthly (ibandronate 150 mg/month), or even yearly applications (zoledronate 5 mg; see Fig. 1). Compliance can be improved by these less-frequent applications, although even then they may be forgotten. The monthly and especially the yearly parenteral application must be controlled and performed by the practitioner, which is an advantage as the patient has to see the doctor at least at this occasion.

As the inhibition of bone absorption supports remineralization (which is the only parameter determined by DXA), the supply of calcium and vitamin D (see previous discussion) must be sufficient in patients receiving bisphosphonates. Without substitution, even hypocalcemia (and hypophosphatemia) may occur.

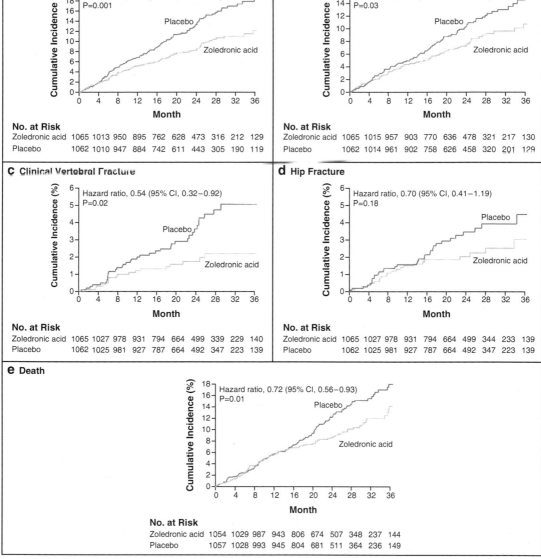

Fig. 1 Effect of 5 mg zoledronic acid per year (!) on risk of fractures and mortality in patients with hip fracture. (**a**) Any clinical fracture, (**b**) clinical nonvertebral fracture, (**c**) clinical vertebral fracture, (**d**) hip fracture, (**e**) death (From Lyles et al. 2007 by kind permission of Massachusetts Medical Society)

Unfortunately, tolerability of bisphosphonates is limited. Oral application is only allowed in the upright position, maintained for at least 30 min after swallowing, and at least 200 ml of water need to be drunk to flush the tablet into the stomach. If retained in the esophagus (mostly in front of the lower gastroesophageal sphincter), the local release of drug may cause esophageal ulcers, which do not heal and have to be surgically treated in most instances. Apart from this, gastrointestinal side effects are common after oral application, but recede with time. More serious is the so-called flu-like syndrome of fever, malaise, joint and muscle pain, and general discomfort. Again, this side effect is temporary, mostly seen after parenteral application, and will eventually disappear with longer treatment; the patient needs to be instructed about it beforehand. Acetaminophen is effective as symptomatic treatment.

Almost only at the very high doses of bisphosphonates employed in cancer metastasis treatment, osteonecrosis of the jaw (ONJ) may occur, which is fortunately very rare at osteoporosis doses. ONJ is a therapeutic disaster as the necrotic, avascular bone of the jaw does not heal and has to be surgically removed, and catastrophic results, including mutilation and functional deficits, are common. Patients at risk (cancer, radiation of the jaws or neck, glucocorticoid therapy) should be seen by the dentist to especially exclude periapical granulomas as one of the suspected starting points of ONJ.

All bisphosphonates are renally excreted; this applies to the fraction not bound to the bone or liberated from it. Kidney function thus is essential for correct dosing. Nephrotoxicity at low osteoporosis doses is not frequent. Rare side effects such as flares or phototoxicity should be recognized.

Teriparatid

Teriparatid is a parathyroid hormone analogue (n-terminal amino acids 1–34 of the human hormone) that supports bone replacement and regulates calcium transport in the gut. It may cause hypercalcemia. Daily, 20 µg need to be applied subcutaneously; this limits its use in the elderly as they are often handicapped, and nursing capacities may not be sufficient for this daily parenteral application. It is approved (like alendronat) for the treatment of males with osteoporosis. This compound is expensive and should only be applied by osteologic specialists; its use in the elderly seems problematic.

Estrogens and SERM

The antiosteoporotic effect of estrogens is indisputable; this is the reason for the rare occurrence of osteoporosis in premenopausal women and for the rapidly increasing incidence thereafter. Post-

menopausal hormone replacement therapy (HRT) has been investigated in megatrials (WHI, Women's Health Initiative; Million Women Study) studying its impact on survival and morbidity. Initiated with a delay of several years past menopause as in these studies, HRT increases the risk of thromboembolic events and hormone-dependent tumors (breast, uterus) and decreases the risk of colonic cancer and osteoporosis. In these studies, women were included who had menopause 10 and more years before inclusion, and vasomotor-related symptoms (such as flushing) were no longer significant. A rationalistic approach for HRT is thus only to use it for few years starting when menopause and related vasomotor symptoms begin. It should be limited to 1–2 years of use, which should be strictly symptom oriented (sweating, flushing). Elderly women thus would not qualify for HRT.

Raloxifen is a SERM; this compound—unlike estrogens—only partially deflects the conformation of the intracellular estrogen receptor. This ligand-receptor complex acts partially agonistically in some effector systems but partially antagonistically in others. Raloxifen thus has no potential to promote breast cancer like estrogens and is even applied as an antagonist in the treatment of this disease. The opposite is true regarding osteoporosis: Here, it is an agonist and acts like estrogen as an antiosteoporotic compound. The cardiovascular risk seems to decrease, although thromboembolic events may slightly increase. This treatment is only advisable in postmenopausal women; as a differential indication, familial risk for breast cancer should be considered, although its preventive effect against breast cancer has not been proven yet.

Denosumab

Denosumab is a human monoclonal antibody against the RANKL (receptor activator of nuclear factor kappa-B ligand) and needs to be given subcutaneously every 6 months. It was recently (2010) FDA approved for the treatment of postmenopausal women at risk or with proven osteoporosis. It may produce hypocalcemia, rashes, serious infections, and rarely ONJ. Its advantage is the dose independence from renal function. In the clinical studies, almost 10,000 women aged 65+ and 3,600 aged 75+ years were included. No age dependency of efficacy and safety was detectable. The assessment in the treatment of the elderly is still somewhat uncertain as too few data in the elderly, particularly in the very elderly, cohorts are available. The wider use in vulnerable elderly patients should be backed by greater experiences, especially under "real-life" conditions.

Calcitonin has to be parenterally applied or by nasal spray. Local and generalized allergic reactions and the mode of application requiring patient participation limit its utility in the elderly.

Strontium ranelate (not available in the United States) inhibits bone absorption and stimulates osteoblast activity. In a few studies, its efficacy has been proven, but it also induced deep vein thromboses as a side effect. Data on patients with impaired renal function are sparse, and the assessment of the fitness for the aged should be postponed until data are available. Recently, cases of toxic epidermiolysis have been reported, which support the reluctance.

Other compounds such as *fluoride, nandrolone acetate, and alfacalcidol* are less effective or more toxic. Those compounds, described previously, should suffice to prevent and treat osteoporosis in the elderly and very elderly. They have been successfully tested not only in clinical trials, but also in real life, which is equally important. Their critical use in the very elderly has been mentioned; a bedridden patient fully dependent on round-the-clock care may still benefit from specific antiosteoporotic therapy if vertebral collapse fractures are symptomatic. However, sufficient pain medications, including opioids, are by far more important in this situation. A complete and unlimited (as opposed to temporary) immobilization of frail or even moribund patients without the clearly defined, fracture-related pain should be the reason for critical reevaluation of the indication for osteoporosis drugs. Under the conditions of complete immobilization, osteoporotic symptoms will rarely occur de novo; they are almost always precipitated by the upright position.

The basic treatment with vitamin D and calcium, physical therapy, and physical activation should be provided to all patients in nursing homes. Patients who are only partially immobilized should receive specific drug therapy according to the general recommendations detailed previously. In a Canadian consensus conference (Duque et al. 2007), long-term nursing institutions were recommended to provide specific pharmacotherapy on top of basic treatment to all high-risk patients and those with fractures; the underutilization of osteoporosis treatment and prophylaxis was acknowledged by the conference as a pressing problem.

Classification of Drugs Against Osteoporosis According to Their Fitness for the Aged (FORTA)

In this classification of drugs against osteoporosis according to their Fitness for the Aged (FORTA), the same compounds may receive alternative marks if applied in different indications (see chapter "Critical Extrapolation of Guidelines and Study Results: Risk-Benefit Assessment for Patients with Reduced Life Expectancy and a New Classification of Drugs According to Their Fitness for the Aged").

Basic supplementation of calcium and vitamin D	A
Bisphosphonates (alendronate, ibandronate, risedronate, zoledronate)	A
Raloxifen	A
Teriparatide	B
Denosumab (needs revision if more data in elderly are at hand)	C
Calcitonin	C
HRT (estrogen, except past menopause for 1–2 years, symptom driven)	D
Strontium ranelate	C
Alfacalcidol	C
Nandrolone decanoate	D
Fluoride	D

References

Chrischilles EA, Butler CD, Davis CS, Wallace RB (1991) A model of lifetime osteoporosis impact. Arch Intern Med 151:2026–2032

Donaldson MG, Cawthon PM, Lui LY et al (2010) Estimates of the proportion of older white men who would be recommended for pharmacologic treatment by the new U.S. National Osteoporosis Foundation guidelines. J Bone Miner Res 25:1506–1511

Duque G, Mallet L, Roberts A, Gingrass S, Kremer R, Sainte-Marie LG, Kiel DP (2007) To treat or not to treat, that is the question: proceedings of the Quebec symposium for the treatment of osteoporosis in long-term care institutions, Saint- Hyacinthe, Quebec, November 5, 2004. J Am Med Dir Assoc 8 (3 Suppl 2):e67–e73

Looker AC, Orwoll ES, Johnston CC Jr et al (1997) Prevalence of low femoral bone density in older U.S. adults from NHANES III. J Bone Miner Res 12:1761–1768

Lyles KW, Colon-Emeric CS, Magaziner JS et al (2007) HORIZON Recurrent Fracture Trial. Zoledronic acid and clinical fractures and mortality after hip fracture. N Engl J Med 357:1799–1809

National Osteoporosis Foundation (2002) America's bone health: the state of osteoporosis and low bone mass in our nation. National Osteoporosis Foundation, Washington, DC

National Osteoporosis Foundation (2010) Clinician's guide to prevention and treatment of osteoporosis. National Osteoporosis Foundation, Washington, DC

U.S. Department of Health and Human Services (2004) Bone health and osteoporosis: a report of the surgeon general. U.S. Department of Health and Human Services, Office of the Surgeon General, Rockville

Parkinson's Disease

Heinrich Burkhardt

Relevance for Elderly Patients, Epidemiology

Parkinson's disease occurs mainly in elderly patients. Among those aged over 80 years, up to 2.6% are diagnosed with Parkinson's disease (de Rijk et al. 2000). At onset of the disease, approximately 70% of individuals were 50 years or older. As for dementia, a significant increase in its incidence is expected, with the consequence that in 2030 twice the number of patients will have to be treated for Parkinson's disease if compared with current rates. Besides these data concerning primary Parkinson's disease, there will also be an even more increasing prevalence of nonprimary parkinsonian syndromes. To date, nonprimary parkinsonian syndromes or partial symptoms thereof are reaching prevalence rates up to 51% in some subgroups of the elderly population (Bennett et al. 1996). Among nonprimary forms, drug-induced syndromes are most common, and other causes such as postinfectious, metabolic, and toxic ones are rare. The prevalence of drug-induced parkinsonian syndromes remains less clear, but reports found it to be up to 50% in nursing home residents

(Stephen and Williamson 1984). As this figure seems alarmingly high, ruling out drug-induced parkinsonian syndromes is very important as otherwise correct treatment opportunities will be missed, causing serious disadvantages for the patient. Needless to say, in drug-induced parkinsonian syndromes, the responsible drug has to be identified and discontinued instead of adding levodopa treatment.

If symptoms like akinesia, hypomimia, and rigor are found as potential indicators of Parkinson's disease, drug-induced nonprimary forms always have to be ruled out first before starting special drug treatment.

The most common triggers for drug-induced parkinsonian syndromes are antipsychotics. This adverse drug reaction (ADR) can occur in up to 60% of all patients receiving antipsychotics (Janno et al. 2004) and is often overlooked in mild forms. Those drugs are strictly contraindicated in primary Parkinson's disease and other patients if parkinsonian syndromes occur. For acute short-term treatment, anticholinergics like biperiden may be used.

Common triggers of drug-induced parkinsonian syndromes that are strictly contraindicated in primary Parkinson's disease are

- Central nervous system (CNS) active dopamine antagonists
- Metoclopramide
- Classical antipsychotics (e.g., haloperidol)
- Olanzapine
- Risperidone
- Flunarizine

H. Burkhardt (✉)
IVth Department of Medicine, Geriatrics, University Medical Centre Mannheim, Theodor-Kutzer-Ufer 1-3, Mannheim 68167, Germany
e-mail: heinrich.burkhardt@umm.de

M. Wehling (ed.), *Drug Therapy for the Elderly*,
DOI 10.1007/978-3-7091-0912-0_13, © Springer-Verlag Wien 2013

Table 1 Special therapeutic features in parkinsonian syndromes accompanying other neurodegenerative disorders

	Diagnostic characteristics	Comment to treatment of Parkinson-like motor symptoms
Multisystem atrophy (MSA)	Early autonomic disorder, additional cerebellar signs	No dopamine agonists
Lewy body dementia	Primary progressive cognitive dysfunction	No dopamine agonists
Progressive supranuclear palsy	Supranuclear vertical opthalmoparesis, early postural instability	Very little response to drug treatment
Corticobasal degeneration (CBD)	Apraxia, dysphasia, focal reflex myoclonus	Very little response to drug treatment
Frontotemporal dementia	Early behavior disorder with lethargy or disinhibition	Very little response to drug treatment
Huntington's disease	Typical hyperkinetic syndrome	If akinesia and rigidity are present try L-dopa

- Cinnarizine
- Netilmicine
- Moxonidine
- Indometacine
- Reserpine (strongly discouraged in the elderly for many other reasons).

Therapeutically Relevant Special Features of Elderly Patients

In the elderly, parkinsonian syndromes may occur also in some other neurodegenerative diseases. This may result in different treatment recommendations. Therefore, a careful diagnosis is essential and sometimes challenging. Neurodegenerative diseases associated with Parkinson-like symptoms are

- Multisystem atrophy (MSA)
- Lewy body dementia
- Progressive supranuclear paralysis
- Corticobasal degeneration (CBD)
- Frontotemporal dementia
- Huntington's disease
- Subcortical arteriosclerotic encephalopathy (SAE).

Furthermore, normal-pressure hydrocephalus—a disease that may be amenable to a curative treatment—may mimic Parkinson's disease, and there are essential tremor syndromes that have to be distinguished from Parkinson's disease and will not respond to common Parkinson's drug treatment. Table 1 gives an overview about different treatment options and highlights the need for an exact diagnosis before treatment. In the following, we focus on treatment of primary Parkinson's disease.

Although the pathophysiological cause of Parkinson's disease—depletion of dopaminergic neurons in the striatum and the substantia nigra—is well known, the underlying mechanism for the degeneration remains unclear. Under discussion are oxidative stress, intracellular accumulation of toxic products due to altered transport mechanisms, and changes in intracellular enzymes. From a clinical point of view, it is significant that these processes lead to a progressive loss of dopaminergic neurons. In fact, at the time of diagnosis, usually 50% of these neurons have already been lost.

Evidence-Based, Rationalistic Drug Therapy and Classification of Drugs According to Their Fitness for the Aged (FORTA)

General Treatment Strategies

The primary treatment goal for Parkinson's disease is to preserve the self-management capacity of patients for as long as possible. In general, a multidimensional approach has to be used, covering not only drug treatment but also non-pharmacologic interventions such as physical therapy. Drug therapy is often complex and has to be tailored to the individual needs of the patient. As for almost all therapeutic areas, data on differential treatment strategies are scarce for elderly patients with Parkinson's disease. Treatment modalities may be categorized into

1. Drug therapy to control major symptoms (akinesia, rigor, tremor)
2. Nonpharmacological treatments of gait disorders, speech disorders, dysphagia, and postural instability (physiotherapy, occupational therapy, speech therapy, and physical training),
3. Treatment of associated problems (depression, loss of cognitive function, delusions, sleeping disorders, etc.), and
4. (Neuroprotection).

Neuroprotection is listed in parentheses as to date no treatment approach has been proven to retard or stop the progressive loss of dopaminergic neurons in Parkinson's disease. Some approaches (antioxidative agents, monoamine oxidase [MAO] B inhibitors) showed beneficial effects in animal studies, but these results unfortunately did not translate into clinical settings (Parkinson Study Group 1993).

Drug treatment in Parkinson's disease should be started when motor disorders or other symptoms impair functionality and self-competence.

The optimal onset for drug treatment of Parkinson's disease has to be determined on an individual basis. If a patient is handicapped in everyday activities, treatment should begin; positive diagnostic surrogate markers such as threshold values in performance tests of motor function do not suffice by themselves. To date, the ongoing loss of dopaminergic neurons cannot be influenced, and all therapeutic approaches are symptomatic ones.

With advancing disease duration, treatment of parkinsonism gets more and more complex and has to be adjusted individually.

These ultimately almost-inevitable treatment escalations are mainly driven by the occurrence of fluctuations in motor symptoms:

– End-of-dose akinesia
– On-off phenomenon
– Freezing.

Moreover, dyskinesias associated with "peak dose" and "off dose" may occur. These problems often force very demanding treatment schedules into place. After 5 years on levodopa treatment, up to 50% of patients show motor symptom fluctuation, up to 30% dyskinesia, and 25% freezing (Poewe and Wenning 1998). Surprisingly and for unknown reasons, these problems are more prominent in younger patients compared to the elderly.

In general, the efficacy of antiparkinsonism drugs for symptomatic control is sufficiently proven by both clinical studies and daily clinical experience. However, as in other therapeutic areas, elderly are underrepresented in those studies despite the fact that the prevalence of this disease is increasing with advancing age. In typical clinical studies, mean age is about 60 years, and concerns about the extrapolation of related results to elderly patients, namely those older than 75 years, are very reasonable (Mitchell et al. 1997). Moreover, even if a few elderly patients aged above 75 years were included in some studies, no subgroup analyses are available or feasible due to the insufficient patient numbers. From a clinical and geriatric point of view, one may assume that treatment effects are not different in the elderly compared to younger patients, but this may not equally apply to ADRs. Therefore, ADRs are a major topic in the comprehensive evaluation of antiparkinsonism drugs.

Another issue that requires differential treatment decisions in the elderly is associated with levodopa. Levodopa therapy is discussed to increase the risk of motor fluctuations and dyskinesia in later stages of Parkinson's disease, although this debate is ongoing and not based on large cohort studies. However, as many elderly patients (especially those with high comorbidities and functional limitations) are expected to have a reduced life expectancy, this problem may be inferior in these subjects. It seems as if the elderly may have a reduced risk of dyskinesia, although the reasons are still unclear and poorly examined. In a small series of young-onset patients with Parkinson's disease (disease onset before age 40 years), all of them developed dyskinesias within 6 years (Quinn et al. 1987).

The risk of early progression to motor fluctuation and dyskinesia in Parkinson's disease is assumed to be lower in patients with a late onset of the disease.

Accordingly, a German guideline (German Society for Neurology 2009) differentiated between elderly and younger patients and discouraged levodopa as first-line therapy in younger subjects. This is also in line with the currently available U.S. guideline, which distinguishes between elderly and younger patients without declaring a special age threshold for separation (U.S. Department of Health and Human Services 2011). However, these recommendations are not based on results from randomized clinical trials or large treatment cohorts, but rather represent a consensus statement. Furthermore, such recommendations are not found in other guidelines (e.g., from the United Kingdom; NICE, The Royal College of Physicians, National Collaborating Centre for Chronic Conditions 2006). Nevertheless, these arguments support concerns to treat patients younger than 60 years with levodopa and favor a first-line therapy with dopamine agonists instead. Some authors (e.g., in the German guideline) recommend a specified age limit to guide treatment decisions, but the cutoff level remains arbitrary in the absence of specific data to define this threshold age. Thus, considerable criticism on a specified age limit exists (Silver 2006). The German guideline mentioned proposes 70 years as relevant age threshold. I do not support this approach but favor a decision in reflection of a geriatric and clinical assessment based on the patient's functionality and remaining life expectancy.

If late disease with fluctuations of motor function is present, additional therapy with a catechol-O-methyl transferase (COMT) inhibitor may improve the effectiveness of drug therapy. This is particularly indicated if dyskinesia is the predominant clinical problem. Amantadine, or special drug preparations with delayed drug release, are recommended to avoid akinesia early in the morning. However, such escalations of drug therapy will inevitably lead to polypharmacy and frequent drug-drug interactions (Csoti and Fornadi 2008). If these interventions do not result in acceptable symptom control, the subcutaneous application of apomorphine, duodenal levodopa application, and deep brain stimulation are further treatment options. Those are preserved for carefully selected patients with advanced disease or severe treatment problems and are not the topic of this chapter.

Special Pharmacotherapeutic Treatment Strategies

Levodopa

Since 1962, levodopa preparations have been given to control symptoms of Parkinson's disease. Today, combination with a peripherally active DOPA-decarboxylase inhibitor is obligatory to control for peripheral ADRs (see following discussion). Typically, biological half-life ranges from 1 to 3 h. However, the action of levodopa is very complex and still not completely understood. Therefore, biological half-life may not represent the pharmacodynamic effect (on phase) (Nutt 2003). Levodopa remains the drug with the strongest effect on symptom control, and its efficacy is well established (Fahn et al. 2004). Furthermore, levodopa is still considered as the drug with the most favorable risk-benefit ratio. Common ADRs are nausea, vomiting, and orthostatic hypotension, representing peripheral ADRs, and delirium and delusions as CNS ADRs. From a geriatric point of view, orthostatic hypotension and delirium are the most significant in the elderly.

ADRs caused by dopaminergic action are the following:
– Nausea and vomiting
– Dizziness
– Orthostatic hypotension
– Delirium
– Hallucination.

Elderly are at higher risk for delirium (see chapter "Pharmacotherapy and Special Aspects of Cognitive Disorders in the Elderly"). The initial dose of levodopa should not exceed 300 mg/day, and the dose may be stepwise titrated up to 600 mg/day.

Levodopa can be combined with all other antiparkinsonism drugs to control for symptoms. Some critical drug interactions have to be mentioned:
– Interaction with tramadol (decreases efficacy of levodopa)

- Interaction with highly dosed vitamin B_6 (decreases efficiency of levodopa)
- Interaction with anticholinergics (possible delay of effect onset due to reduced gastrointestinal motility)
- Interaction with baclofene (not approved by the Food and Drug Administration [FDA]; high risk of delirium; Chou et al. 2005).

Furthermore, the drug-drug interaction with St. John´s wort—a drug widely available over the counter—may be significant and often overlooked. This interaction (mediated via P-glycoprotein) may result in an increased effect of levodopa. On the other hand, a significant decrease may be seen if iron preparations are given simultaneously with levodopa. Iron preparations may form chelates and thereby decrease the amount of absorbed drug.

Iron preparations are not to be administered simultaneously with antiparkinsonism drugs.

MAO-B Inhibitors

The MAO-B inhibitors expose a lower efficacy for symptom control in Parkinson's disease than L-dopa. MAO-B inhibitors (e.g., rasagiline) sufficiently control symptoms in only 10% of patients if prescribed as monotherapy at disease onset. For later disease stages, data are also not conclusive; therefore, these drugs are not recommended as first-line therapy. Nevertheless, rasagiline may attenuate motor fluctuations in late disease (Rascol et al. 2005). ADRs are sleep disorders, delirium, and loss of appetite.

MAO-B inhibitors are strictly forbidden to be combined with antidepressants, especially selective serotonin reuptake inhibitors (SSRIs), serotonin norepinephrine reuptake inhibitors (SNRIs), and noradrenergic and specific serotonergic antidepressants (NaSSA) to avoid the risk of a serotonergic syndrome.

COMT Inhibitors

COMT inhibitors decrease the peripheral levodopa breakdown and thereby improve levodopa availability without increasing peak levels. In late disease with motor fluctuations, this may be helpful to increase the "on-phase" duration and improve symptom control (Brooks 2004). Unfor-

tunately, COMT inhibitors do not delay or prevent these complications even if administered early in a preventive approach.

The main indication for COMT inhibitors is late disease with motor fluctuations.

As tolcapone was associated with serious hepatologic ADRs and thus withdrawn from the market in some countries, entacapone is the preferred drug in this drug class. Severe restrictions apply to tolcapone according to the FDA approval. A frequent but harmless ADR of entacapone is a reddish discoloration of urine. More serious but less-frequent side effects are delirium, dyskinesia, nausea, and diarrhea. In general, entacapone is well tolerated and can be recommended for treatment in the vulnerable elderly patient. Entacapone interacts with selegiline—a MAO-B inhibitor—via the cytochrome P (CYP) 2D6 system in the liver. This may cause unexpected increases in serum levels, leading to dyskinesia. The same interaction may occur with other CYP2D6 inhibitors, such as fluoxetine, paroxetine, and sertraline. This has to be kept in mind if depressive symptoms are to be controlled in patients with late Parkinson's disease (see the following discussion). Similar to levodopa, iron preparations may form chelates with entacapone as well. As mentioned, iron preparations should not be administered together with antiparkinsonism drugs.

Centrally Acting Dopamine Agonists

Centrally acting dopamine agonists represent a heterogeneous group of drugs acting directly on pre- and postsynaptic dopaminergic neurons. Dopamine agonists are divided in two groups:

- Ergot-like dopamine agonists (bromocriptine, pergolide, cabergoline; lisuride, not FDA approved)
- Non-ergot-like dopamine agonists (ropinirole pramipexol, apomorphine; piribedil, not FDA approved)

There is an ongoing debate on a potentially beneficial neuroprotective effect of these drugs. This would have implications for the retardation of late disease. Although related results were mainly obtained in cell culture or animal studies,

Potential risk for ADR delirium

anticholinergics

MAO-B-inhibitors

amantadine

dopamine-agonists

COMT-inhibitors

L-DOPA

Fig. 1 Schematic risk for delirium as ADR of different antiparkinson drugs. *ADR* adverse drug reaction, *MAO* monoamine oxidase, *COMT* catechol-O-methyl transferase, *L-DOPA* levodopa

at least some human studies showed a lower prevalence of motor fluctuations in long-term treatment (Parkinson Study Group 2000). However, symptom control is inferior to that by levodopa, and there is a broad range of ADRs to be considered. Dopamine agonists are in general less well tolerated compared to levodopa (Fig. 1). They frequently induce delirium and hallucination and may also cause orthostatic hypotension, especially at high initial doses.

Dopamine agonists carry a high risk of orthostatic hypotension at treatment initiation.

In the elderly, therefore, dosing of these drugs should always be carefully performed (start low, go slow) to avoid these serious ADRs. They are of great clinical significance particularly in the elderly (delirium leading to falls). Another ADR seen for all dopamine agonists is fluid retention and the occurrence of edema.

With regard to ergot-like drugs, another rare ADR needs to be considered. These drugs may cause fibrosis of soft tissues, including the cardiac valves. Therefore, close echocardiographic monitoring of cardiac valve morphology and function is mandatory. Furthermore, in the presence of preexisting morphologic changes of heart valves, these drugs are contraindicated. As many elderly show subtle morphologic changes of heart valves (sclerosis, insufficient closing),

ergot-like drugs are generally not recommended for the elderly.

If a dopamine agonist is indicated in the elderly, a non-ergot-like drug should be prescribed.

Among non-ergot-like dopamine agonists ropinirole and pramipexole may present the best risk-benefit ratio. Besides the ADRs mentioned, these drugs may lead to unusual compulsive behavior like hypersexuality, compulsive gambling, and overeating.

A recently developed treatment strategy is the transdermal application of rotigotine (Jenner 2005), which allows for a continuous absorption of the drug. This simplifies the treatment in patients with difficulties adhering to complex schedules. In general, this application is well tolerated. However, there is only limited experience and few data, particularly in the elderly (Splinter 2007).

Amantadine

The antiparkinson effects of this drug are mainly explained by low-affinity antagonism at glutamate receptor sites. However, the range of actions is not fully understood. Amantadine is widely used in Parkinson treatment, and large clinical experience exists for this drug. Its effects to control Parkinson's disease symptoms are weaker compared to levodopa, but it has beneficial effects in controlling levodopa-induced dyskinesia. Moreover, amantadine showed some neuroprotective effects in cell culture experiments.

However, the risk for delirium and other dopaminergic ADRs is increased compared to levodopa (see Fig. 1), and additional anticholinergic ADRs like tachycardia, disturbances of accommodation, or bladder outlet obstruction may occur. Moreover, amantadine increases the risk of torsade de pointe due to QT prolongation. Although this is rare, QT time has to be monitored at the beginning of amantadine treatment. This is of special significance when other drugs potentially prolonging QT time have to be prescribed (e.g., class I antiarrhythmics, amiodarone, sotalol). In that case, amantadine is not the first choice to control Parkinson's disease symptoms.

When starting amantadine, QT time has to be controlled in the electrocardiogram (ECG).

Anticholinergics

Anticholinergics expose only limited effects on symptom control in Parkinson's disease but carry a high risk of ADRs, namely, gastrointestinal dysfunction, bladder outlet obstruction, and delirium (see Fig. 1). Therefore, they are generally not recommended for the elderly. In case of Parkinson's disease, they are also not drugs of first choice per se. Otherwise, poorly controlled tremor might be an indication for anticholinergics (biperiden, trihexyphenidyl, procyclidine; metixen, bornaprine [not FDA approved]). Finally, concomitant application of antidepressants may severely aggravate anticholinergic syndromes and particularly increase the risk of delirium.

Special Treatment Issues

Treatment of Depression in Patients with Parkinson's Disease

Depression is very common in patients with Parkinson's disease, and in the literature prevalence rates of up to 69% are reported (Starkstein et al. 1990). A minimal prevalence rate of 40% has to be expected. Depressive symptoms may precede Parkinson symptoms, and some authors classify depressive symptoms as a prodromal stage of Parkinson's disease (Santamaría et al. 1986). Conversely, depressive symptoms are often overlooked in patients with Parkinson's disease and misinterpreted as motor function disorder. In general, depression requires a targeted and specific antidepressive drug therapy. However, monotherapy should be preferred whenever possible to minimize polypharmacy and ADR issues. As depressive symptoms are often caused and aggravated by insufficient control of dopaminergic symptoms, an optimization of parkinsonian motor symptoms should always precede the initiation of antidepressive drug therapy. If depressive symptoms are strictly related to off phases, antidepressive drug treatment is not recommended.

Before adding antidepressive drugs, dopaminergic antiparkinson treatment should always be optimized.

The question of antiparkinson drugs with a profile preferable in depression cannot be answered at present as no conclusive data pointing to a differential effect are available.

Oppositely, data are also lacking to support the choice of antidepressants preferable in Parkinson's disease, leading to a differential treatment algorithm compared with that in depression alone (see chapter "Dementia"). Therefore, in elderly patient the ADR profile mainly determines the drug of choice; thus, the generally well-tolerated SSRI should be preferred, and tricyclics are not recommended. Mirtazapine is beneficial in patients with agitation and citalopram if adynamia is dominating.

The combination of SSRI and MAO-B-inhibitors is forbidden in Parkinson's disease as the risk of a serotonergic syndrome is inadequately high.

If in a patient receiving MAO-B inhibitors an antidepressant has to be given, discontinuing the MAO-B inhibitor has to be considered to control ADR risk. Finally, in rare cases a worsening of motor function control has been reported after establishing an antidepressant therapy with an SSRI (Dell'Ágnello et al. 2001). In this case, the SNRI reboxetine (not FDA approved) may be an alternative.

Dementia in Parkinson's Disease

A cognitive decline is frequent in Parkinson's disease. In about 40% of all patients with Parkinson's disease, dementia will occur (Aarsland et al. 2005). As mentioned, the presence of both motor symptoms and a cognitive decline requires the differentiation of primary Parkinson's disease from dementia with Lewy bodies. In primary Parkinson's disease, motor symptoms precede the cognitive decline by at least 1 year. If a cognitive decline is suspected in Parkinson patients, it has to be mentioned that common diagnostic instruments Mini-Mental-State (e.g., MMST) may not be adequate—cognitive function may fluctuate in dementia with Parkinson's disease—and special tools have to be used (Parkinson Neuropsychiatric Dementia Assessment).

In Parkinson patients with cognitive decline, improvement of motor function by optimized dopaminergic drug therapy may improve cognitive function.

The beneficial effects of antidementives, in particular inhibitors of cholinesterase, are not well studied in Parkinson's disease compared with Alzheimer's disease. There are some positive data concerning rivastigmine showing a moderate beneficial effect on the further development of cognitive function (Emre et al. 2004; Maidment et al. 2006). Furthermore, like in Alzheimer's disease, psychotic symptoms (e.g., hallucination) may be attenuated. Frequent ADRs of rivastigmine are nausea, vomiting, and both agitation and somnolence. Tremor may deteriorate in Parkinson's patients on cholinesterase inhibitors.

Delirium and Psychotic Symptoms

Psychotic symptoms, especially optical hallucinations, are frequent in Parkinson patients and can be expected in up to 50% of all patients, occurring at least once during the course of the disease (Holroyd et al. 2001). In principle, all antiparkinson drugs can cause psychotic symptoms and delirium, and these ADRs are dose dependent. Advancing age represents an additional risk factor for these complications, which are due to progressive morphological and functional changes in the brain. In most cases, delirium is precipitated by multiple factors. In any case, the correction for contributing factors like dehydration, infection, and hypoxia needs to be supplemented by a comprehensive assessment of the drug schedule. This aims at the discontinuation of drugs with high delirium risk or the attenuation of the risk by dose reduction. Among drugs with high delirium risk are anticholinergics, MAO-B inhibitors, and amantadine.

Unfortunately, drug discontinuation or dose correction does not always relieve psychotic symptoms, and short-time treatment with antipsychotic drugs may become necessary. As classical antipsychotics (e.g., haloperidol) act strongly on the dopaminergic system, atypical antipsychotics should be preferred. Among

those, useful data exist for clozapine. These show a sufficient effect to control psychotic symptoms but no influence on motor symptoms (Pollak et al. 2004). However, clozapine is associated with a rare but serious idiosyncratic ADR, agranulocytosis. Therefore, prescription of this drug has to be strictly accompanied by a close monitoring of (white) blood cell counts, and in some countries, including the United States, restrictive prescription terms are instituted. Olanzapine and risperidone are discussed as alternatives, although they are not free of negatively influencing motor symptoms even at low dosages. Therefore, their use is limited, especially in severe hallucinations or delirium (Goetz et al. 2000). Quetiapine revealed only very little influence on motor function (Reddy et al. 2002), but to date, this drug has been less studied in patients with Parkinson's disease than clozapine (Wood et al. 2010). Another important issue that has to be considered in this context is the frequent induction of orthostatic hypotension by all atypical antipsychotics, which carries a significant increase of fall risk. This may be clinically significant in particular in the frail elderly. Low-potency antipsychotics such as melperone (not FDA approved) or the benzodiazepine lorazepam may be considered as problematic treatment alternatives.

Orthostatic Hypotension

Orthostatic hypotension is very frequent in Parkinson patients, especially in the elderly. In up to two thirds of patients with late-stage disease, this is a significant clinical problem. Besides addressing all modifiable factors described, nonpharmacological measures should be preferred in the management of postural hypotension and fall risk. Adequate hydration, improving muscle strength by exercise, and compression stockings have to be mentioned in this context. Drug treatment for orthostatic hypotension has not been well established and mainly relies on clinical experience. It should only be considered if nonpharmacological treatment and modification of medication schemes are ineffective. Drugs discussed for this indication are fludrocortisone and midodrine (Wood et al. 2010).

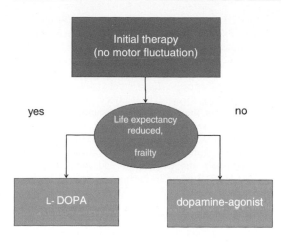

Fig. 2 Algorithm for the choice of initial antiparkinson treatments in the elderly. *L-DOPA* levodopa

Conclusion and Comprehensive Evaluation of Drug Therapy in Parkinson's Disease

In elderly Parkinson patients, adequate drug therapy is often complex and highly dependent on individual needs and resources. The main risks for treatment errors in this context are unnecessary treatment escalations resulting from misleading interpretations of a complex disease status and multimorbidity; missing ADRs is the other major pitfall area. Figure 2 provides an algorithm for the choice of initial drug treatment strategies in the elderly.

As control of motor symptoms is always demanding when these symptoms influence patients' self-management competence, antiparkinson therapy usually cannot be discontinued. However, within the variety of different drugs, evaluation according to the FORTA criteria provides some comprehensive clues for choosing the appropriate drug.

Classification of Drugs Against Parkinson's Disease According to Their Fitness for the Aged (FORTA)

In this classification of drugs against Parkinson's disease according to their Fitness for the Aged (FORTA), the same compounds may receive

alternative marks if applied in different indications (see chapter "Critical Extrapolation of Guidelines and Study Results: Risk-Benefit Assessment for Patients with Reduced Life Expectancy and a New Classification of Drugs According to Their Fitness for the Aged"); comments are included here.

Drug or drug group	Examples	Comments	FORTA
Levodopa		Drug of choice for initial treatment in the elderly	B
MAO-B inhibitor	Selegiline	Reduced effect, critical interaction with antidepressants	C
	Rasagiline		
COMT inhibitor	Entacapone	Useful as additive drug in case of motor fluctuations	B
Dopamine agonists (nonergot like)	Ropirinole	If comorbidities are minor and no frailty syndrome is present; ergot-like drugs are contraindicated in elderly	C
	Pramipexole		
	Rotigotine		
Amantadine		Useful as additive drug for dyskinesia; keep QT prolongation in mind	C
Anticholinergics		High ADR risk; may be indicated if tremor cannot be controlled otherwise	D

References

Aarsland D, Zaccai J, Brayne C (2005) A systematic review of prevalence studies of dementia in Parkinson's disease. Mov Disord 20:1255–1263

Bennett DA, Beckett LA, Murray AM, Shannon KM, Goetz CG, Pilgrim DM, Evans DA (1996) Prevalence of parkinsonian signs and associated mortality in a community population of older people. N Engl J Med 334:71–76

Brooks DJ (2004) Safety and tolerability of COMT inhibitors. Neurology 62(Suppl 1):S39–S46

Chou KL, Messing S, Oakes D, Feldman PD, Breier A, Friedman JH (2005) Drug-induced psychosis in Parkinson disease: phenomenology and correlations among psychosis rating instruments. Clin Neuropharmacol 28:215–219

Csoti I, Fornadi F (2008) Medikamentöse Interaktionen in der Parkinson-Therapie. NeuroGeriatrie 5:160–168

de Rijk MC, Launer LJ, Berger K (2000) Prevalence of Parkinson's disease in Europe: a collaborative study of population-based cohorts. Neurologic Diseases in the Elderly Research Group. Neurology 54(11 Suppl 5): S21–S23

Dell'Ágnello G, Ceravolo R, Nuti A et al (2001) SSRIs do not worsen Parkinson's disease: evidence from an open-label, prospective study. Clin Neuropharmacol 24:221–227

Emre M, Aarsland D, Albanese A et al (2004) Rivastigmine for dementia associated with Parkinson's disease. N Engl J Med 351:2509–2518

Fahn S, Oakes D, Shoulson I et al (2004) Levodopa and the progression of Parkinson's disease. N Engl J Med 351:2498–2508

German Society for Neurology (2009) Leitlinien der Deutschen Gesellschaft für Neurologie 2008. Parkinson-syndrome. Diagnostik und Therapie. http://www.dgn.org. Accessed 18 Dec 2009

Goetz CG, Blasucci LM, Leurgans S, Pappert EJ (2000) Olanzapine and clozapine: comparative effects on motor function in hallucinating PD patients. Neurology 55:789–794

Holroyd S, Currie L, Wooten GF (2001) Prospective study of hallucinations and delusions in Parkinson's disease. J Neurol Neurosurg Psychiatry 70:734–738

Janno S, Holi M, Tuisku K, Wahlbeck K (2004) Prevalence of neuroleptic-induced movement disorders in chronic schizophrenia in patients. Am J Psychiatry 161:160–163

Jenner P (2005) A novel dopamine agonist for the transdermal treatment of Parkinson's disease. Neurology 65(2 Suppl 1):S3–S5

Maidment I, Fox C, Boustani M (2006) Cholinesterase inhibitors for Parkinson's disease dementia. Cochrane Database Syst Rev CD004747

Mitchell SL, Sullivan EA, Lipsitz LA (1997) Exclusion of elderly subjects from clinical trials for Parkinson disease. Arch Neurol 54:1393–1398

National Collaborating Centre for Chronic Conditions (UK) (2006) Parkinson's disease: national clinical guideline for diagnosis and management in primary and secondary care. Royal College of Physicians (UK), London. National Institute for Health and Clinical Excellence: guidance. http://www.ncbi.nlm.nih.gov/pubmed/21089238. Accessed 17 Aug 2011

Nutt JG (2003) Long-term levodopa therapy: challenges to our understanding and for the care of people with Parkinson's disease. Exp Neurol 184:9–13

Parkinson Study Group (1993) Effects of tocopherol and deprenyl on the progression of disability in early Parkinson's disease. N Engl J Med 328:176–183

Parkinson Study Group (2000) A randomized controlled trial comparing pramipexole with levodopa in early Parkinson's disease: design and methods of the CALM-PD Study. Clin Neuropharmacol 23:34–44

Poewe WH, Wenning GK (1998) The natural history of Parkinson's disease. Ann Neurol 44(3 Suppl 1):S1–S9

Pollak P, Tison F, Rascol O et al (2004) Clozapine in drug induced psychosis in Parkinson's disease: a randomised, placebo controlled study with open follow up. J Neurol Neurosurg Psychiatry 75:689–695

Quinn N, Critchley P, Marsden CD (1987) Young onset Parkinson's disease. Mov Disord 2:73–91

Rascol O, Brooks DJ, Melamed E et al (2005) Rasagiline as an adjunct to levodopa in patients with Parkinson's disease and motor fluctuations (LARGO, Lasting effect in Adjunct therapy with Rasagiline Given Once Daily, study): a randomised, double-blind, parallel-group trial. Lancet 365(9463):947–954

Reddy S, Factor SA, Molho ES, Feustel PJ (2002) The effect of quetiapine on psychosis and motor function in parkinsonian patients with and without dementia. Mov Disord 17:676–681

Santamaría J, Tolosa E, Valles A (1986) Parkinson's disease with depression: a possible subgroup of idiopathic parkinsonism. Neurology 36:1130–1133

Silver D (2006) Impact of functional age on the use of dopamine agonists in patients with Parkinson disease. Neurologist 12:214–223

Splinter MY (2007) Rotigotine: transdermal dopamine agonist treatment of Parkinson's disease and restless legs syndrome. Ann Pharmacother 41:285–295

Starkstein SE, Preziosi TJ, Bolduc PL, Robinson RG (1990) Depression in Parkinson's disease. J Nerv Ment Dis 178:27–31

Stephen PJ, Williamson J (1984) Drug-induced parkinsonism in the elderly. Lancet 2(8411):1082–1083

U.S. Department of Health and Human Services. American Medical Directors Association (AMDA). Parkinson's disease. Columbia (MD). 2010 http://www.guideline.gov/content.aspx?id =9628&search = parkinson. Accessed Dec 2011

Wood LD, Neumiller JJ, Setter SM, Dobbins EK (2010) Clinical review of treatment options for select nonmotor symptoms of Parkinson's disease. Am J Geriatr Pharmacother 8:294–315

Therapy of Chronic Pain

Heinrich Burkhardt

Relevance for Elderly Patients, Epidemiology

Chronic pain is very frequent in the elderly, and the prevalence rate increases with advancing age. The main reason for this rise is an increasing incidence of musculoskeletal disorders, such as osteoarthritis and osteoporosis. Up to 70% of persons aged 70+ years complain about chronic pain (Brattberg et al. 1996). However, exact data depend on the assessment method, and prevalence rates in institutional care and specialized hospital departments may even exceed this value. If pain is recorded, one should distinguish between acute and chronic pain. Both variants are frequently found in the elderly (Ferrell et al. 1990). Chronic pain is of special interest in the context of pharmacotherapy as this condition almost always requires long-term drug treatment. Therefore, this chapter mainly refers to chronic pain. To define chronic pain and distinguish it from acute pain is somewhat arbitrary, and exact and consented criteria are lacking. A common definition describes chronic pain as pain lasting for at least 3 months (Charette and Ferrell 2007). However, this time frame may seem excessive and is thus a matter of dispute.

Pain, whether acute or chronic, severely influences quality of life and self-management competence. If pain remains poorly controlled, it may lead to disability. Disability may be inflicted by the limitation of locomotion and mobility, reduced muscle strength, and malnutrition due to loss of appetite. Furthermore, pain may result in behavioral changes, mood disturbances, cognitive decline, and anxiety.

An optimized control of pain is a high-priority therapeutic goal for every form of pain and in each patient. In elderly patients, however, an early and proper detection of pain might be difficult. This is of great importance as untreated pain may lead to the crippling chronic pain syndrome involving cerebral and spinal remodeling. These late pain syndromes are very difficult to treat.

An early detection and proper management of pain is demanding to avoid chronic pain syndromes.

Unfortunately, there are abundant data underpinning the fact that undertreatment of pain syndromes in the elderly is very common. In an analysis after surgery including elderly patients aged 65+ years, up to 62% of these patients reported severe postsurgery pain and gaps in the postoperative pain monitoring (Sauaia et al. 2005). Another cross-sectional study not only disclosed a high prevalence rate of pain among elderly in nursing homes (49%) but also showed that 25% of residents did not receive any pain medication (Won et al. 2004).

H. Burkhardt (✉)
IVth Department of Medicine, Geriatrics, University Medical Centre Mannheim, Theodor-Kutzer-Ufer 1-3, Mannheim 68167, Germany
e-mail: heinrich.burkhardt@umm.de

M. Wehling (ed.), *Drug Therapy for the Elderly*,
DOI 10.1007/978-3-7091-0912-0_14, © Springer-Verlag Wien 2013

In the elderly, pain is often undetected and undertreated.

Undertreatment of pain is clearly inacceptable and a serious marker of inadequate treatment quality. Improvement of this shortcoming is a major issue as it represents a keystone to improve quality of life and self-management in the elderly (Laurell et al. 2006).

Therapeutically Relevant Special Features of Elderly Patients

In the elderly, the underdiagnosing and undertreatment of pain may be partially explained by changes of pain perception accompanying the aging process. Data from standardized experimental settings show that elderly may experience increases in the pain perception threshold but develop a lower tolerance of chronic pain. Moreover, study data point to a change of pain quality perception in the elderly (McCleane 2008). Another reason for both altered pain perception and misdiagnosing may be an increasing prevalence of barriers in the elderly that impede pain perception and diagnosing. Among these barriers, a cognitive decline is the most significant one. Dementia patients in advanced disease stages are often incapable of describing and expressing pain by verbal communication. In these patients, discomfort, anxiety, and pain are often solely expressed by ambiguous behavioral changes (e.g., agitation, shouting) that may be misunderstood by family, nurses, and physicians. This further aggravates the undertreatment issue in elderly patients with dementia (Frondini et al. 2007).

A variety of assessment instruments have been established to detect and monitor pain in elderly patients, in particular elderly patients with dementia (Bruckenthal 2008). To meet this challenge in dementia patients, intense efforts and special instruments have to be employed (Zwakhalen et al. 2006).

Pain Treatment Always Mandates a Multimodal Approach

Though generally true for all pain patients, this is even much more significant in the elderly (Mattenklodt et al. 2008). Multimodal therapy means the implementation of nonpharmacological treatments alongside drug therapy, which is insufficient by itself. Nonpharmacological pain treatment may help to reduce dosages and complexity of drug schedules and minimize the risk of polypharmacy. Among nonpharmacological measures in this context, the following have to be mentioned:

- Measures of physical therapy (e.g., TENS, transcutanous electrical nerve stimulation)
- Thermal therapy (application of heat and cold)
- Exercise
- Occupational therapy
- Psychological measures (e.g., progressive relaxation or behavioral therapy).

Another important issue in chronic pain is patient education. This also covers in-depth counseling and history taking with regard to drug therapy. An important topic in patient education in that respect reflects the use of over-the-counter (OTC) drugs, namely NSAIDs (nonsteroidal anti-inflammatory drugs), as these drugs are the major culprits for adverse drug reactions (ADRs) associated with pain therapy. Many physicians are unaware of important aspects of drug schemes and dosages in a considerable fraction of their patients; this includes the lack of knowledge about not only the intake of relevant drugs such as NSAIDs, but also timing of applications, nonadherence issues, and drug sharing between friends and relatives. Another important aspect of patient education relates to ADRs of prescribed drugs, which have to be explained in advance regarding their detection and management. Patient education should cover at least

– Dosage schedule and dosing rules (time and dosage)
– Self-managed escalation options in case of pain exacerbation (dosing on demand)
– Potential ADRs
– Handling of OTC drugs.

Evidence-Based, Rationalistic Drug Therapy and Classification of Drugs According to Their Fitness for the Aged (FORTA)

General Treatment Goals and Strategies

The general treatment goal for all pain syndromes is to establish the best pain relief by the smallest drug burden. In this context, a World Health Organization (WHO) concept proposed originally for pain relief in cancer patients is most cited, the WHO "pain ladder" (WHO 1996; Nikolaus and Zeyfang 2004). It is a treatment strategy for medication escalation depending on severity of pain symptoms. Unfortunately, in many patients with severe pain or complex pain syndromes, pain control may only be achieved by polypharmacy. In this case, a particularly close monitoring for ADRs and an intense education of the patient are necessary. The WHO "pain ladder" does not distinguish with respect to classical drug classes, but rather categorizes drugs into four different groups, which may contain widely heterogeneous drugs:
– Nonopioid analgesics
– Weak opioids
– Strong opioids
– Adjuvant drugs.

The WHO treatment schedule recognized three categories of pain severity. However, this distinction remains rather arbitrary and is not well defined. It depends solely on clinical judgment. The three categories are
– Moderate pain
– Moderate-to-severe pain
– Severe pain.

If the suggested therapy does not work, proper escalation to the next level is recommended as depicted in Fig. 1.

For the assessment of pain severity, a visual analogue scale is widely used. It has to be kept in mind, though, that in chronic pain management additional symptoms such as emotional and functional impairment have to be considered as well (Waldvogel 1996). A proper clinical judgment therefore cannot entirely rely on results from visual analogue scaling, but rather has to build a complex clinical synopsis of those distinct dimensions mentioned. The scope of the visual analogue scale is limited to pain monitoring.

In principle, there are no reasonable arguments to skip the WHO recommendation in the elderly, although WHO is aware of differentiating views for different age groups (WHO 2007). The major conditions affecting the escalation strategy in the elderly are functional limitations and the risk of ADRs (e.g., risk of fall); this is highlighted in the special chapters on defined drug classes.

Further important conditions for drug choice are the suspected pain pathophysiology and pain location. Pain management due to bone disease such as osteoporosis may be different from that of pain resulting from neuropathy. Again, in the elderly the diagnosis of cause and the exact location of pain may be more difficult to determine than in younger adults as elderly tend to expose hypo- and asymptomatic forms of pain.

Figure 1 summarizes these arguments and their influence on drug choice in pain management. Resources and functionality may also be important for the patient's adherence to complex treatment schedules (e.g., exact timing of dosage). In elderly with advanced functional limitations, especially in advanced dementia, transdermal application systems may be preferable.

As in other fields, specific data on risk-benefit assessment are largely absent for pain management in the vulnerable population of elderly patients. This is astonishing as pain-relieving drugs are prescribed predominantly in this

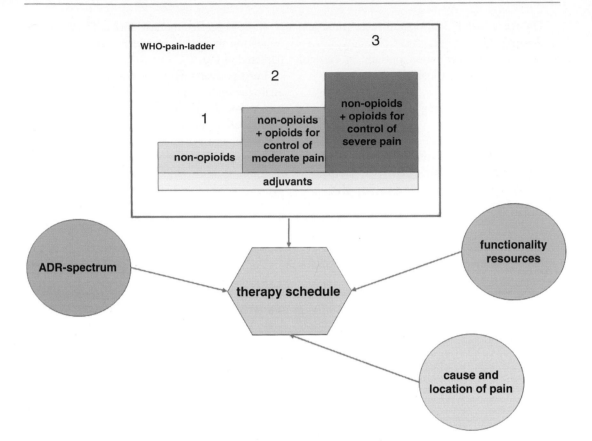

Fig. 1 Factors influencing a comprehensive drug therapy to control chronic pain. *ADR* adverse drug reaction, *WHO* World Health Organization

population; thus, serious questions remain unanswered. Therefore, the majority of views detailed in the following chapters is rather indirectly extrapolated from studies in younger adults or reflect the estimated ADR risk in the elderly.

Finally, some general rules concerning pain management in the elderly should be followed:

- Medication escalation according to the pain ladder schedule should be critically indicated.
- Maximum dosages should be avoided wherever possible.
- Functional limitations need to be considered.
- Symptoms and possible ADRs need to be regularly reevaluated.
- Medication with OTC drugs should always be questioned ("teased out").
- Timed drug schedules should always be given.
- Use of pain-relieving nonpharmacological measures is encouraged.

- Physical activity should be encouraged in pain patients.
- The least-invasive route should be favored (e.g., oral vs. intravenous route).

Special Pharmacotherapeutic Treatment Strategies

Nonopioid Analgesics
Acetylsalicylic Acid

Acetylsalicylic acid is recommended for relief of defined pain forms like tooth pain, acute headaches, or migraine. However, in the management of chronic pain syndromes, no indication exists due to the high risk of gastrointestinal ADRs. For pain relief, high dosages are needed (500–2,000 mg/day), thus largely increasing ADR risk.

Acetaminophen

The exact mechanism of action of acetaminophen remains unknown. Some data point to direct effects on central nervous system (CNS) function. It is recommended for mild-to-moderate pain syndromes and has some advantages compared to NSAIDs as incidence of ADRs is rather low, with particular reference to gastrointestinal and renal ADRs.

Hepatotoxicity of acetaminophen has to be kept in mind, which may occur at higher (3 g/ day and above) or—in the presence of hepatic dysfunction by disease or ethanol—even lower dosages.

The therapeutic range of this drug is fairly wide, and the slowly decreasing hepatic function associated with age (both hepatic perfusion and enzyme activity) does not matter. For unknown reasons, doses above 3 g/day have been associated with hepatic damage in the elderly and should thus be avoided. Unfortunately, its efficacy to control pain symptoms is rather low compared to NSAIDs, it lacks a major anti-inflammatory component, and there is a significant ceiling effect (dosage escalation does not improve pain control). A randomized study comparing acetaminophen and ibuprofen in patients with osteoarthritis detected no significant difference in pain relief (Bradley et al. 1991). However, this was found in adults aged less than 60 years, and the severity of pain at baseline remains unclear. An advantage of acetaminophen compared to NSAIDs is a lower rate of drug-drug interactions (Baxter 2008). In multimorbid elderly, this is obviously an important issue. The only exception seems to be the coadministration of oral anticoagulants; a dose adaption of these may be necessary (Van den Bemt et al. 2002).

Metamizole

The mechanism of action of metamizole is not completely understood. Both central and peripheral effects are discussed. This drug provides spasmolytic and strong antipyretic effects. The spasmolytic effect is especially beneficial to control for colic-like abdominal pain (e.g., biliary colic), and metamizole was widely used for this purpose up to the 1970s, when serious concerns were triggered by a particular ADR. This was the occurrence of agranulocytosis with and without idiosyncratic aplastic anemia, which caused some fatalities. Ever since, the risk-benefit ratio of this drug has been debated. To date, it is banned in over 30 countries, among those are the United States, Sweden, and several other European countries. However, in some countries (e.g., Brazil), it remains an OTC drug; in other countries, a renaissance of prescription could be observed in recent years (e.g., Germany). The true rate of this serious ADR remains unclear and may range from 1/5,000 to over 1/100,000 prescriptions. Moreover, there are unexplainable geographic differences in the estimated ADR rates. For example, in Sweden the rate for serious hematological changes had been found to be 1 per 439 prescriptions, and metamizole was banned again in Sweden in the 2000s in reflection of this figure (Hedenmalm and Spigset 2002). In countries where it is available, authorities recommend restrictive use (e.g., Germany). Nevertheless, metamizole remains a widely used drug when available, and its tolerability is quite fair. Compared to nonbanned NSAIDs, the rate of serious side effects is rather low. This causes some criticism about the rationale behind banning this drug. It is estimated that ADR mortality in elderly patients is 1/10 to 1/30 of that by NSAIDs (Andrade et al. 1998). Thus, serious attempts should be undertaken to reintroduce it to geriatric therapy in those countries where it is banned, including the United States. It is obvious that measures (frequent blood cell counts) have to be taken to detect the serious ADRs early and stop medication accordingly.

Another disadvantage that has to be mentioned is the rather short half-life of metamizole. To control for chronic pain, dosage interval should not exceed 4 h, which limits its practical use.

Nonsteroidal Anti-inflammatory Drugs

The NSAIDs are among the most prescribed analgesics, especially in an ambulatory setting. They are effective as drugs to control musculoskeletal pain. As the elderly show an increasing prevalence rate of osteoarthritis and other musculoskeletal problems associated with chronic pain, a considerable fraction of elderly persons regularly receive NSAIDs. An epidemiologic study in the United States among nursing home inhabitants found daily NSAID prescriptions in up to 10% (Lapane et al. 2001).

NSAIDs mainly act peripherally by a reversible inhibition of cyclooxygenases (COX) types I and II. In general, all NSAIDs are alike in this regard, explaining that the range of ADRs is similar for all (Yost and Morgan 1994):

– Gastrointestinal disorders, especially ulceration and bleeding.
– Worsening of renal perfusion in a hyperreninemic status (volume depletion, cardiac failure, sodium loss) and thereby worsening of renal function.
– Increase of blood pressure, increasing demand for antihypertensives in case of arterial hypertension or manifestation of hypertension in normotensives.
– Central nervous symptoms like dizziness, confusion, and depression associated with increased fall risk.
– Increased incidence of cardio- and cerebrovascular incidents.

The last two ADRs are less well understood but nevertheless significant in practice. In the elderly, especially the risk of confusion and dizziness (fall risk) may be aggravated compared to younger adults (see chapter "Fall Risk and Pharmacotherapy"). Unfortunately, there are few data concerning the risk-benefit ratio of these ADRs in the elderly, forcing its extrapolation from general data and clinical experience.

Gastrointestinal disorders (mainly ulceration and bleeding, but also loss of appetite and malnutrition) are still the most significant and frequent ADRs associated with NSAID.

With regard to this, elderly have a higher risk than younger patients, as shown in a survey from the United Kingdom (Hippisley-Cox et al. 2005). Among the elderly, risk is even more pronounced (factor 5–6) when frailty is present (Nikolaus and Zeyfang 2004). As for other symptoms, it has to be kept in mind that alerting signs for this ADR

are often misinterpreted or less well perceived in the elderly (Lapane et al. 2001).

Conflicting data exist concerning differences in ADR incidence with regard to different NSAIDs. In summary, nonselective COX inhibitors are associated with an overall rate of gastrointestinal disorders of up to 10% (Semla et al. 2003). Data reporting a lower risk associated with ibuprofen and diclofenac compared to indomethacin, piroxicam, and naproxen (Henry et al. 1996) have been criticized as dosages of the different drugs may not be comparable. COX-II inhibitors were primarily developed to lower the rate of gastrointestinal ADRs. Selective inhibition of the COX-II enzyme should reduce the rate of ulceration in the stomach as this was thought to depend mainly on COX-I inhibition. A study comparing naproxen with rofecoxib in a highly selected cohort of patients with rheumatoid arthritis confirmed this (Bombardier et al. 2000), but surprisingly few data support a lower rate of gastrointestinal ADRs associated with COX-II inhibitors compared to nonselective COX inhibitors in practice. An analysis of population-based data in the United Kingdom even failed to show superiority of COX-II inhibitors compared to nonselective NSAIDs concerning gastrointestinal ADRs in long-term treatment (Hippisley-Cox et al. 2005). Another study comparing diclofenac and ibuprofen with celecoxib was primarily based on overoptimistic short-term data, but failed in its long-term results to show a superiority of celecoxib (Jüni et al. 2002). With long-term prescription of NSAIDs, the prescription of a proton pump inhibitor (PPI) should be discussed (Kean et al. 2008), although not routinely performed if risk factors (history of gastrointestinal disorders, glucocorticoid medication, gastrointestinal symptoms) are absent and frequent ambulatory controls provided. The preventive effect of this comedication was found lowest if diclofenac had been prescribed (Hippisley-Cox et al. 2005).

Worsening of renal function is a significant ADR associated with all NSAIDs (Yost and Morgan 1994).

In most cases, changes of renal function are mild and fully reversible. However, in 5% of all prescriptions a clinically significant incident has to be expected, and aggravation of renal damage leading to acute renal failure requiring dialysis is possible. As renal function may already be impaired in a large portion of elderly subjects, elderly are more prone to this ADR than younger adults. Also, comorbidities leading to increased renal vulnerability may often be present (cardiac failure, volume depletion, low serum sodium level). There has been some discussion whether prescription of a COX-II inhibitor may decrease the rate of renal impairment, and in fact data showed lower renal ADR rates in younger adults. However, in the elderly this could not be confirmed (Ruoff 2002).

It is well known from former meta-analyses that prescriptions of NSAIDs cause an increase in blood pressure. Mean increments of 5 mmHg have been reported, although in individual patients even more pronounced increases may be clinically significant and render blood pressure control ineffective. Exact incidences are hard to obtain from epidemiological data due to methodological problems handling blood pressure data. The blood-pressure-increasing effect was found for all NSAIDs, including COX-II inhibitors (Chan et al. 2002). Bearing methodological shortcomings of available data in mind, results may indicate the most pronounced blood pressure increases associated with indomethacin and piroxicam. Finally, increasing blood pressure is certainly a reason for increased mortality associated with long-term prescription of NSAIDs (Andrade et al. 1998) which is increased by four- to fivefold compared to acetylsalicylic acid.

NSAIDs may cause delirium or other central nervous symptoms (dizziness, somnolence).

Central nervous symptoms also occur frequently under NSAID medication (up to 10%). The underlying mechanism of this type ADR is not well understood. It was found to be associated with all drugs in this group, but available data do support a ranking list for this type ADR.

Finally, there have been reports pointing to an increased risk of cardio- and cerebrovascular incidents associated with all NSAIDs. This effect was initially thought to be more pronounced for COX-II inhibitors; as a consequence, two COX-II inhibitors were removed from the market (rofecoxib and valdecoxib). The suspected cause besides effects on blood pressure (see previous discussion) is an upregulation of the COX-II enzyme in the endothelium under ischemic conditions followed by a local dysbalance of pro- and anticoagulatory eicosanoids (Schmedtje et al. 1997; Mukherjee et al. 2001). There is an ongoing debate whether these effects are inherent to all NSAIDs or if differences exist in the incidence of this ADR. A meta-analysis focusing on this issue found that among nonselective COX inhibitors diclofenac was associated with a considerable risk but, conversely, only a smaller risk increase with celecoxib (McGettigan and Henry 2006). A recent meta-analysis comparing seven NSAIDs (naproxen, diclofenac, ibuprofen, celecoxib, etoricoxib, rofecoxib, and lumiracoxib) identified naproxen as the least harmful with respect to cardiovascular incidents (Trelle et al. 2011), which is in line with previous data. Although the cardiovascular ADRs of NSAID have recently gained considerable attention, it has to be kept in mind that incidence rates are rather low compared with that of gastrointestinal or central nervous effects. However, in certain clinical conditions, aggravating cardiovascular risk may be fatal (e.g., coronary stent placement or acute cerebral ischemia), and this effect also definitively contributes to the increased cardiovascular mortality seen for all NSAIDs. Furthermore, it is fair to assume that as these clinical conditions are more frequent in the elderly, NSAIDs are particularly associated with increased prevalences and incidences of cardio- and cerebrovascular incidents in this age group. A special benefit of selective COX-II inhibitors in this respect has not been confirmed. As long as data are missing, this should be held true for the elderly as well. Prescription of COX-II inhibitors in the elderly has even been discouraged in some countries (e.g., Germany).

Selective COX-II inhibitors do not offer a more favorable risk-benefit ratio in the elderly compared to naproxen.

Table 1 Adverse drug reaction (ADR) spectrum of important nonsteroidal anti-inflammatory drugs (NSAIDs)

Drug	Gastrointestinal ADR	Cardiovascular incidents	Elevated blood pressure	Worsening of renal function	Central nervous effects	Comment
Diclofenac	++	#	*	+	++	Unfavorable risk-benefit ratio
Naproxen	++	−	*	+	++	Supposed to cause least-frequent cardiovascular incidents
Indomethacin	+++	No data	**	+	++	Supposed to cause most frequent gastrointestinal ADR
Piroxicam	++	−	**	+	++	
Ibuprofen	++	−	*	+	++	
Celecoxib	+	#	*	+	+	Selective COX2 inhibitors failed to show clear advantage compared with nonselective

+ 5–10 %, ++ 10–25 %, +++ over 25 %, * effect proven, ** effect clearly proven, − no elevated relative risk, # elevated relative risk (estimated incidence below 1/1,000)
COX cyclooxygenase

Important issues concerning different NSAIDs are summarized in Table 1.

All NSAIDs bear a high risk of several clinically significant ADRs in long-term treatment.

In the elderly, NSAIDs are even more cumbersome in long-term treatment than in younger patients. If they cannot be avoided, a careful monitoring for possible ADRs should take place. This includes blood pressure monitoring, monitoring of renal function, avoiding comedications that increase gastrointestinal risk, gastrointestinal symptom search, and optimization of ischemia management.

Opioids

Opioids are centrally acting drugs. In the escalating schedule provided by WHO, the different opioids are categorized as moderate and strong analgesics. In severe pain syndromes, there should be no hesitation to apply strong opioid analgesics (Mercadante and Arcuri 2007). Opioids can be categorized according to four dimensions:

− Strength of action
− Duration of action
− ADR spectrum
− Management in practice.

With regard to these dimensions, some drugs are provided as buccal or subcutaneous applications. This allows rapid absorption independent of the gastrointestinal function (e.g., in case of vomiting, nausea). Table 2 provides an overview concerning major aspects of common opioids. Regarding the efficacy of opioids in different pathophysiologies of pain consensus exists that opioids are effective to control pain in both cancer and musculoskeletal disease. Efficacy is lower in neuropathic pain (e.g., postzoster neuralgy) resulting in the requirement of higher doses to control symptoms.

The ADR spectrum of opioids covers several clinically significant symptoms and incidents:

− Nausea and vomiting
− Constipation
− Dizziness, delirium and somnolence
− Respiratory depression.

As for a majority of drugs, it is also true for opioids that data analyzing the benefit-risk ratio especially in the elderly are rare. Recommendations have to be mainly based on data

Table 2 Pharmacodynamic, pharmacokinetic parameters, and ADR spectrum of some opioids recommended for use in the elderly

Drug	Strength of action	Duration of action (h)	Nausea–vomiting (%)	Constipation (%)	Dizziness–sedation (%)	Confusion (%)	Comment
Tramadol (retarded drug release form available)	0.1–0.2	4–8	>10	>10	>10	1–10	Increased sedation, lowers seizure threshold
Tilidine (not FDA approved) (retarded drug release form available)	0.2	3–5	>10	—	1–10	—	Sedation rare, short duration of action
Buprenorphine (transcutaneous drug system available)	75–100	6–10	1–10	<1	>10	<1	Increased sedation, lower rate of confusion
Morphine (retarded drug release form available)	1	4–5	9	40	48	>10	Delayed elimination, frequent orthostatic hypotension
Hydromorphone (retarded drug release form available)	7.5–8	4–5	1–10	1–10	1–10	5–7	Preferable in impaired renal function, favorable to control pain exacerbation
Fentanyl (transcutaneous drug system available)	100	<1	>10	1–10	>10	1–10	Frequent orthostatic hypotension
Oxycodon (retarded drug release form available)	1.5–2	2–3	>10	1–10	>10	—	Prescribe only retarded drug release form

ADR adverse drug reaction

extrapolation. With regard to the strength of action and efficacy to control pain, no conclusive arguments support the assumption of a differential effect in the elderly. Categorizing opioids according to their risk-benefit ratio in the elderly will therefore mainly follow the ADR spectrum and management in practice (Table 2).

Nausea and vomiting are less frequent in elderly than in younger subjects (Mercadante and Arcuri 2007). Furthermore, these symptoms mainly occur within the first days of drug treatment and may be easily controlled by the short-term application of antiemetics (e.g., metoclopramide). Obstipation, however, may represent a more serious problem, especially in inactive or bedridden elderly with low fluid intake. Respiratory depression is the most serious ADR, but there are no reports pointing to an increased vulnerability of the elderly with regard to this ADR (Pergolizzi et al. 2008). Patients at risk are those with simultaneously prescribed CNS-affecting drugs or an underlying advanced pulmonary disease (e.g., emphysema). Respiratory depression is strictly dose dependent. Therefore, if the initial dosage is adequate (high initial dosage is discouraged), this ADR should be avoidable.

In the elderly, delirium and sedation are the most significant ADRs associated with opioids.

Both may increase the risk of falls and delirium in general, which are negative prognostic factors with regard to both morbidity and mortality. Contrary to respiratory depression, these ADRs are not strictly dose dependent and may occur even at low doses. If further risk factors for delirium are present (e.g., dementia, previous cerebral incident, fluid imbalance, anesthesia, etc.), dosing should be careful (low initial doses, slow dose escalation), and opioids with low risk of delirium induction should be preferred (see following discussion; Gaudreau et al. 2007). It should be noted that delirium may persist for days and even weeks after discontinuation of the incidental drug. Sedation is more dose dependent and recovers promptly after dosage reduction or discontinuation of the drug.

Retarded opioid preparations should not be prescribed in the initial treatment phase to minimize the risk of sedation. High doses are also discouraged in the initial treatment phase, and rapid dose escalations should be avoided if possible.

Initial dosing problems may be more pronounced in the elderly as most opioids are undergoing hepatic degradation, and hepatic blood flow and enzyme activity may decrease with age. Unfortunately, no bedside estimation of these hepatic parameters is available for an individual subject. Buprenorphine may be an exception as its duration of action is not found to be prolonged in the elderly (Pergolizzi et al. 2008).

Another aspect is the risk of opioid addiction. However, this is overemphasized, and epidemiologic data reveal that this problem is present only in a minority of patients on long-term opioid treatment (McQuay 1997). Increased tolerance to opioids may be avoided by constant dosing.

Pentazocine, pethidine (not approved by the Food and Drug Administration [FDA]), and dextropropoxyphene (taken off the markets in the United States and Europe) disclose an unfavorable benefit-risk ratio and are not recommended for use in the elderly (Pergolizzi et al. 2008). Pentazocine is associated with an increased psychotropic risk, and pethidine and dextropropoxyphene induce frequently toxic effects, resulting in agitation and tremor. Two other opioids with rather weak analgesic effect are not recommended for pain treatment in the elderly: codeine and methadone. To control moderate-to-severe pain, higher doses are necessary, resulting in an unfavorable benefit-risk ratio due to increased ADR frequency (e.g., sedation). Codeine is a weak opioid that is frequently used in pain treatment in combination with acetaminophen. In some countries, this combination is available over the counter, and criticism on facilitating dependency by this practice has been raised. Methadone as another weak opioid is now mainly recommended for the treatment of opioid dependency and addiction, but not for pain control.

Table 2 gives an overview on opioids that seem principally recommendable for the elderly.

Data on risk-benefit ratio variations between different opioids in the elderly from controlled studies are missing.

This also applies to the rates of certain ADRs in different age groups. Their estimation is only based on case reports, registries, and pharmacoepidemiologic reports.

Tramadol discloses an additional effect on noradrenaline reuptake and may therefore interact with antidepressants (risk of serotonergic syndrome). This phenomenon may be linked to the pronounced sedative effect that may be troublesome in the elderly as the risk of falls may be increased. Furthermore, a decreased seizure threshold has been reported. This fact is particularly important if other risk factors for seizures are present, such as preexisting epilepsy, alcoholism, or comedications that decrease the seizure threshold (e.g., antipsychotics). Tilidine—in Germany prescribed as fixed combination with naloxone to lower risk of misuse—has a minor sedative effect that may be helpful in elderly patients, in whom sedation needs to be avoided. The compound is illegal in the United States. A disadvantage of this drug is a rather short duration of action. This impairs drug management in practice (Nikolaus and Zeyfang 2004) as the patient has to be capable of taking the drug five times a day.

The ADR risk of opioids with regard to delirium is hard to assess. Prevalence and incidence rates of delirium are often inaccurate as hypoactive forms are frequently overlooked. According to available data, oxycodone, tilidine, and buprenorphine are associated with lowest delirium rates. This aspect qualifies them as preferable opioids in the elderly. Buprenorphine, however, shows a considerable sedative effect. Sedation may be troublesome if frailty, depression, dysthymia, or otherwise evoked adynamia is present. In this case, hydromorphone appears to be an alternative. Finally, oxycodone should only be given if an immediate-release preparation is available (such as Oxepta™ in the United States); otherwise, it should not be used for initial treatment (e.g., in Germany, no immediate-release preparation available).

If an effective dose has been established in the initial treatment phase, switching to retarded preparations may be helpful to maintain stable blood drug concentrations in most patients. Furthermore, treatment schedules can be simplified by retarded preparations and adherence improved. In this context, transcutaneous systems are especially helpful.

Transdermal Drug Delivery Systems in Geriatric Medicine

Dermal and transdermal therapy to treat local pathologies of the skin or subcutaneous structures are widely applied in dermatology, orthopedics, and surgery. Beside this, transdermal systems—patches—may also offer an option for systemic pharmacotherapy. For this purpose, they are frequently applied in geriatric medicine and palliative medicine to simplify pharmacotherapy and overcome shortcomings of orally administered drugs.

Administering drugs via the oral route may provide the best balance between reliability of resorption and serum drug level on the one hand and patient comfort and adherence on the other. Transdermal systems are advantageous in some special pharmacological situations (e.g., if there is a large first-pass effect by liver metabolism). Besides this, there are clinical circumstances in which an oral route may no longer be feasible. This is the case if serious problems with swallowing arise or gastrointestinal absorption is compromised (e.g., motility problems, obstruction, nausea, and vomiting). Moreover, functional limitations may limit self-management of oral drugs (e.g., loss of cognitive abilities). Due to the increased prevalence of cognitive decline and swallowing problems in elderly patients, transdermal systems may help to maintain pharmacotherapy in these situations. They are predominantly used in treatment of Parkinson's disease, pharmacotherapy of chronic pain, hormone replacement therapy, and recently, in pharmacotherapy of dementia. Unfortunately, transdermal systems are amenable only for a few drugs as this route depends highly on physicochemical drug properties (e.g., molecular weight less than 500 Da, hydro- or

Table 3 Commonly used drugs for transdermal application

	Half-life (transdermal) (h)	Comment
Fentanyl	20–27	Frequently used in control of chronic pain
Buprenorphine	20–24	No accumulation in case of renal failure
Lidocaine	24–48	Indicated in postherpetic neuropathic pain as local therapy
Scopolamine	10	Treatment of motion sickness
Selegiline		Treatment of major depression in nonresponders to SSRI/SNRI
Rotigotin	6–8	Treatment of Parkinson's disease
Rivastigmine	3–4	Treatment of Alzheimer's dementia
Oxybutinine	48	Control of overactive bladder syndrome
Nitroglycerine		Control of recurrent angina pectoris
Clonidine	17	Control of hypertension, treatment of withdrawal symptoms (e.g., alcohol), gradually discontinue to avoid withdrawal symptoms (hypertensive crisis)
Estradiol		Hormone replacement therapy
Testosterone		Hormone replacement therapy

SSRI selective serotonin reuptake inhibitor, *SSNRI* selective serotonin norepinephrine reuptake inhibitor

lipophilicity). Only low plasma levels are achievable by this route; therefore, it is only an option for highly potent drugs, for which low plasma levels result in significant systemic effects (Brown et al. 2006). Suitable and commonly used drugs are given in Table 3.

In addition, there are several strategies in development to improve transdermal application by electrical (iontophoresis), mechanical (microneedles), or ultrasound-based methods. In the future, this will allow transdermal pharmacotherapy for drugs that are not yet suitable for this route due to their chemical characteristics (Prausnitz and Langer 2008).

Besides these drug-related limitations, there are additional patient-related aspects that may impede reliable and constant drug delivery via the skin barrier and lead to a large interindividual variability of transdermal absorption. In an experimental setting done with skin probes of women undergoing reconstructive skin surgery, an interindividual variability of fentanyl absorption by more than 100% was found, whereas intraindividual variability between different regions of the skin (breast vs. abdominal region) was found to be below 20% (Larsen et al. 2003). Furthermore, intercurrent changes in skin physiology have to be mentioned (e.g. skin irritation, allergy, edema, sweating) as significant factors altering transdermal drug resorption.

Transdermal drug delivery systems should not be applied on areas with skin irritation or skin pathologies like erythema and edema. In addition, the application site has to be changed regularly to avoid irritation by the transdermal system itself.

There are several age-associated changes in skin physiology and ultrastructure potentially leading to age-related changes in absorption. This may be particularly important for hydrophilic substances, but to date no clinically significant age-related change of absorption has been demonstrated in studies based on clinical practice (Gupta et al. 2005). Therefore, no general recommendation for dose adaption in the elderly concerning transdermal drug delivery systems can be given (Kaestli et al. 2008). In summary, drug absorption by transdermal systems may vary widely between individuals, and this variability remains less predictable.

In case of chronic pain, transdermal systems should not regularly be used in the initial treatment phase. They are helpful to maintain pain control in the long run. As a further limitation, transdermal systems are to be avoided in treating acute pain or exacerbations of chronic pain. In patients with chronic pain, transdermal systems should not be prescribed without additional fast-acting substances that can be taken on demand as "escape medication" (e.g., buprenorphine or fentanyl for transbuccal treatment). As transdermal systems delivering fentanyl disclose both a long mean elimination half-life and a long time to reach peak concentrations after first dosing (20–27 h), it is necessary to start with low doses and to avoid escalation intervals shorter than 72 h.

In the initial phase, start with a low dose of transdermal opioid (dosing rule for transdermal fentanyl: Transdermal fentanyl dose = Daily dose of oral morphine/100). Do not escalate the dose of the transdermal system before 72 h.

Usually, the transdermal fentanyl system has to be replaced after 72 h. A minority of patients show loss of effectivity in pain control at day 3. If this is the case, the system has to be replaced every 48 h. These aspects render it essential to observe and monitor the patient carefully, especially in the initial treatment phase to avoid overdosing and treatment errors.

Adjuvants in the Treatment of Chronic Pain

Adjuvants may help to control chronic pain and are prescribed as comedication to analgesics. They are not analgesics per se but are able to modulate pain perception. They should be routinely considered if reduced efficacy of classical analgesics is expected (e.g., neuropathic pain) or if an additional drug effect is to be utilized (e.g., bisphosphonates for bone pain in cancer or skeletal disease). The major field for the prescription of adjuvants is neuropathic pain. However, an unreflected administration of these drugs has to be discouraged as ADRs and drug-drug interactions are relevant.

There is a great variety of different adjuvants. Because of low efficacy and high ADR rates, the following drugs are not recommended for the elderly:

– Antihistaminics
– Memantine
– Mexiletine
– Clonidine
– Lidocaine.

Antihistaminics and memantine are associated with high rates of delirium, and the class

I antiarrythmic lidocaine exposes a negative risk-benefit ratio in long-term treatment due to its proarrythmic potential; in general, such drugs are discouraged for use in the elderly.

In the following, the focus is on the treatment of neuropathic pain. Prescription of adjuvants in bone pain treatment (bisphosphonates and calcitonin) is not considered in this chapter. For these special drugs, no arguments exist at present to deviate from the recommendations valid for younger adults. Finally, steroids and neuroleptics may be given as adjuvants. These also are not mentioned in this chapter (see chapter "cognitive disorders special aspects" for steroids and chapter "Immobility" for neuroleptics).

Adjuvants in Neuropathic Pain

Following accepted definitions, painful neuropathy requires a central or peripheral lesion in the neural system (Cruccu et al. 2004). Although exact prevalence rates are missing, it is assumed that neuropathy is among the more frequent causes of chronic pain. The prevalence in the total population was estimated to range from 1% to 1.5% (Vadalouca et al. 2006). Main causes are postzoster pain, diabetic neuropathy, and traumatologic lesions of the peripheral nervous system. Neuropathy may also follow stroke and trauma of the spine. All together, neuropathy reflects a wide variety of different diseases, rendering highly standardized treatments difficult and inadequate. In principle, two major drug classes are prescribed as adjuvants in painful neuropathy:

– Antidepressants
– Gabapentin.

Current recommendations categorize different treatment options as follows (Dworkin et al. 2003):

– First-line adjuvants:
  – Gabapentin
  – Tricyclic antidepressants (amitriptyline, nortriptyline, desipramine)
  – Local treatment with lidocaine.
– Second-line adjuvants:
  – Other anticonvulsants (lamotrigine, carbamazepine, etc.)

– Other antidepressants (paroxetine, citalopram, venlafaxine).

Unfortunately, these categories do not take
special issues in the elderly into account and
have to be commented. Drugs listed in the
"first-line" category have been analyzed in several controlled studies and proved their efficacy,
whereas drugs in the "second-line" category are
supported by limited data only.

Antidepressants Used as Adjuvants in Chronic Pain Treatment

Tricyclic antidepressants—mostly amitriptyline—have been prescribed as adjuvants in
chronic pain syndromes for decades and are
rather well analyzed. However, the paucity of
studies specially designed to examine the risk-
benefit ratio in the elderly is astonishing (Giron
et al. 2005). It is well known that amitriptyline
shows an unacceptably high rate of ADRs and
should be avoided in this population (see chapter
"Depression"). Frequent anticholinergic actions
(Fig. 2), cardiotoxicity, increased orthostatic
hypotension, and risk of fall are most troublesome; mortality in long-term treatment is
increased twofold (Cohen et al. 2000).

**Data do not allow for the exact description
of risk-benefit ratios concerning different
antidepressants in adjuvant pain therapy.**

Although this paucity of controlled studies
precludes evidence-based recommendations,
modern antidepressants should be preferred to
tricyclics as the risk of major ADRs is reduced.
Efficacy in neuropathic pain has been shown for
citalopram, paroxetine, bupropion, and venlafaxine, but the data still do not support comprehensive recommendations based on efficacy and
ADR risk (Barber and Gibson 2009). As venlafaxine increases anticholinergic risk only
slightly, this drug is supposed to provide the
most favorable risk-benefit ratio (Tasmuth et al.
2002). In general, more recent treatment recommendations favor modern antidepressants (selective serotonin reuptake inhibitors [SSRIs] or
serotonin norepinephrine reuptake inhibitors
[SNRIs]) and discourage tricyclics not only
for antidepressant therapy (see also in chapter

Anticholinergic potential of antidepressants

paroxetine

citalopram

bupropion

venlafaxine

mirtazapine

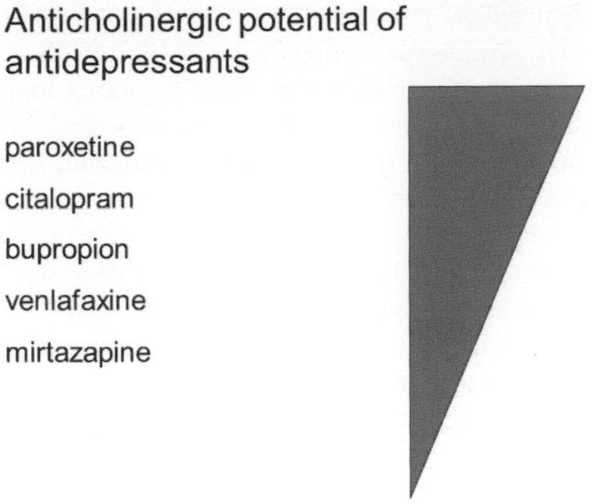

Fig. 2 Potential for anticholinergic ADRs (adverse drug
reactions) for different antidepressants

"Depression") but also for adjuvant pain control
(Namaka et al. 2004).

**Modern antidepressants (SSRIs, SNRIs)
should be used in adjuvant pharmacotherapy
to control pain in the elderly; tricyclics are no
longer recommended.**

For all antidepressants, the onset of the pain-
modulating effect is supposed to precede the
antidepressant effect. A single and low initial
dose is recommended, and dose escalation
should take place at 1- to 2-week intervals. At
the latest, a pain-modulating effect can be
expected after 4 weeks of treatment.

Anticonvulsants Used as Adjuvants in Chronic Pain Treatment

Among all forms of neuropathic pain, antiepileptics show the best efficacy in trigeminal neuropathy (Attal et al. 2006). Nevertheless, to a lesser
extent they are also effective in all other forms
(Finnerup et al. 2005). Although they are often
prescribed in neuropathic pain, their efficacy
compared to that of antidepressants remains
unclear. Collins et al. (2000) found in their extensive review and meta-analysis comparable
efficacy for both drug classes. Therefore, the
decision about adding an antidepressant or an
anticonvulsant should be based on the ADR risk
estimate for the individual patient.

Although special data on the elderly are rare,
three relevant issues for the differentiation of

Table 4 ADR spectrum of anticonvulsants used as adjuvants in chronic pain treatment

Drug	Hyponatremia (%)	Somnolence (%)	Cognitive dysfunction	Comment
Carbamazepine	1–10	29	Frequent cause of delirium	Frequent drug-drug interactions (CYP3A4)
Oxcarbazepine	6	>10	1–10 %	Drug-drug interactions (CYP3A4)
Gabapentin	<1	20	2 %	Rare drug-drug interaction, accumulation in reduced renal function
Pregabalin	—	>10	1–10 %	No drug-drug interactions
Lamotrigine	—	12	3 %	Sleep disorders, accumulation in reduced renal function

ADR adverse drug reaction, *CYP* cytochrome P

drugs may be identified: the ADR spectrum of the drug, the rate of ADRs, and the width of the therapeutic range. For anticonvulsants, the last issue is more critical than for antidepressants and is the main reason for the requirement of particularly close treatment monitoring. Furthermore, anticonvulsants show frequent drug-drug interactions and therefore are more problematic in patients with multimorbidity.

ADR rates in long-term treatment with anticonvulsants are high and discontinuation of drug treatment frequent. There are reports that up to 42% of all patients on carbamazepine stopped this treatment because of ADRs (Brodie et al. 1999). In the elderly, the most significant ADRs associated with anticonvulsants are

– Hyponatremia
– Sedation
– Cognitive impairment.

Table 4 gives an overview for anticonvulsants commonly used in pain management.

Studies comparing the risk-benefit ratio of different anticonvulsants are mainly done in the context of seizure control and not for pain therapy. These studies show the highest ADR and interaction rates for carbamazepine. Furthermore, carbamazepine disclosed the smallest therapeutic range among all anticonvulsants and is therefore the least-favorable drug of all mentioned. More favorable aspects were found for pregabalin and lamotrigine (Leppik 2005). More data exist for pregabalin with regard to pain control (Haslam and Nurmikko 2008);

thus, this drug is preferable as an adjuvant for pain control, especially in multimorbid or frail elderly.

Concluding Remarks

Table 5 summarizes the aspects mentioned and comments on different drug classes used for pain control in the elderly. Although polypharmacy has to be avoided, this will not be possible in many cases as in patients with chronic pain drugs cannot be skipped unless this therapeutic goal is met. However, within this essential framework of drug therapy a differential approach considering efficacy and ADR rates of different drugs is possible for optimization. The following classification according to the FORTA (Fitness for the Aged) criteria may be helpful for the choice and prioritization of drugs.

Classification of Drugs for Chronic Pain Treatment According to Their Fitness for the Aged (FORTA)

In this classification of drugs for chronic pain treatment according to their Fitness for the Aged (FORTA), the same compounds may receive alternative marks if applied in different indications (see chapter "Critical Extrapolation of Guidelines and Study Results: Risk-Benefit Assessment for Patients with Reduced Life Expectancy and a New Classification of Drugs According to Their Fitness for the Aged")

Table 5 Drugs for chronic pain control in the elderly: general remarks and characteristics

Drug group	Drug	Comment
	Acetaminophen	Well tolerated but less effective
	Metamizole	Rare but serious side effects (aplastic anemia)
NSAID	Naproxen	In general unfavorable risk-benefit ratio, lowest risk assumed with naproxen
	Celecoxib	No strict advantage compared to nonselective NSAID in the elderly proven
Opioids	Buprenorphin	Low risk of confusion
	Morphine	High risk of confusion
Tricyclic antidepressants	Amitriptyline	Highest ADR rate of all antidepressants
SSRI	Venlafaxine	Low anticholinergic potential
Anticonvulsants	Carbamazepine	Frequent hyponatremia, low therapeutic range
	Pregabalin	Low risk of hyponatremia, wider therapeutic range

ADR adverse drug reaction, *NSAID* nonsteroidal anti-inflammatory drug, *SSRI* selective serotonin reuptake inhibitor

Drug class	Drug	FORTA
	Acetaminophen	A
	Metamizole (not FDA approved)	B
NSAID	Naproxene	D
	Celecoxib	D
Opioids	Buprenorphine	B
	Tilidine (not FDA approved)	B
	Morphine	C
Antidepressants	Amitriptyline	D
	Venlafaxine	B
Anticonvulsants	Carbamazepine	D
	Pregabalin	C

References

Andrade SE, Martinez C, Walker AM (1998) Comparative safety evaluation of non-narcotic analgesics. J Clin Epidemiol 51:1357–1365

Attal N, Cruccu G, Haanpaa M et al (2006) EFNS guidelines on pharmacological treatment of neuropathic pain. Eur J Neurol 13:1153–1169

Barber JB, Gibson SJ (2009) Treatment of chronic non-malignant pain in the elderly: safety considerations. Drug Saf 32:457–474

Baxter H (ed) (2008) Stockley's drug interactions 2008. Pharmaceutical Press, London

Bombardier C, Laine L, Reicin A et al (2000) Comparison of upper gastrointestinal toxicity of rofecoxib and naproxen in patients with rheumatoid arthritis. VIGOR Study Group. N Engl J Med 343:1520–1528

Bradley JD, Brandt KD, Katz BP, Kalasinski LA, Ryan SI (1991) Comparison of an antiinflammatory dose of ibuprofen, an analgesic dose of ibuprofen, and acetaminophen in the treatment of patients with osteoarthritis of the knee. N Engl J Med 325:87–91

Brattberg G, Parker MG, Thorslund M (1996) The prevalence of pain among the oldest old in Sweden. Pain 67:29–34

Brodie MJ, Overstall PW, Giorgi L (1999) Multicentre, doubleblind, randomised comparison between lamotrigine and carbamazepine in elderly patients with newly diagnosed epilepsy. The UK Lamotrigine Elderly Study Group. Epilepsy Res 7:81–87

Brown MB, Martin GP, Jones SA, Akomeah FK (2006) Dermal and transdermal drug delivery systems: current and future prospects. Drug Deliv 13:175–187

Bruckenthal P (2008) Assessment of pain in the elderly adult. Clin Geriatr Med 24:213–236

Chan FK, Hung LC, Suen BY et al (2002) Celecoxib versus diclofenac and omeprazole in reducing the risk of recurrent ulcer bleeding in patients with arthritis. N Engl J Med 347:2104–2110

Charette SL, Ferrell BA (2007) Rheumatic diseases in the elderly: assessing chronic pain. Rheum Dis Clin North Am 33:109–122

Cohen HW, Gibson G, Alderman MH (2000) Excess risk of myocardial infarction in patients treated with antidepressant medications: association with use of tricyclic agents. Am J Med 108:2–8

Collins SL, Moore MA, McQuay HJ et al (2000) Antidepressants and anticonvulsants for diabetic neuropathy and postherpetic neuralgia: a quantitative systematic review. J Pain Symptom Manage 20: 449–458

Cruccu G, Anand P, Attal N et al (2004) EFNS guidelines on neuropathic pain assessment. Eur J Neurol 11:153–162

Dworkin RH, Backonja M, Rowbotham MC et al (2003) Advances in neuropathic pain: diagnosis, mechanisms, and treatment recommendations. Arch Neurol 60:1524–1534

Ferrell BA, Ferrell BR, Osterweil D (1990) Pain in the nursing home. J Am Geriatr Soc 38:409–414

Finnerup NB, Otto M, McQuay HJ, Jensen TS, Sindrup SH (2005) Algorithm for neuropathic pain treatment: an evidence based proposal. Pain 118:289–305

Frondini C, Lanfranchi G, Minardi M, Cucinotta D (2007) Affective, behavior and cognitive disorders in the elderly with chronic musculoskelatal pain: the impact on an aging population. Arch Gerontol Geriatr 44 (Suppl 1):167–171

Gaudreau JD, Gagnon P, Roy MA, Harel F, Tremblay A (2007) Opioid medications and longitudinal risk of delirium in hospitalized cancer patients. Cancer 109:2365–2373

Giron MS, Fastbom J, Winblad B (2005) Clinical trials of potential antidepressants: to what extent are the elderly represented: a review. Int J Geriatr Psychiatry 20:201–217

Gupta SK, Hwang S, Southam M, Sathyan G (2005) Effects of application site and subject demographics on the pharmacokinetics of fentanyl HCl patient-controlled transdermal system (PCTS). Clin Pharmacokinet 44(Suppl 1):25–32

Haslam C, Nurmikko T (2008) Pharmacological treatment of neuropathic pain in older persons. Clin Interv Aging 3:111–120

Hedenmalm K, Spigset O (2002) Agranulocytosis and other blood dyscrasias associated with dipyrone (metamizole). Eur J Clin Pharmacol 58:265–274

Henry D, Lim LL, Garcia Rodriguez LA et al (1996) Variability in risk of gastrointestinal complications with individual nonsteroidal anti-inflammatory drugs: results of a collaborative meta-analysis. BMJ 312:1563–1566

Hippisley-Cox J, Coupland C, Logan R (2005) Risk of adverse gastrointestinal outcomes in patients taking cyclo-oxygenase-2 inhibitors or conventional non-steroidal anti-inflammatory drugs: population based nested case-control analysis. BMJ 331:1310–1316

Jüni P, Rutjes AW, Dieppe PA (2002) Are selective COX 2 inhibitors superior to traditional non steroidal anti-inflammatory drugs? BMJ 324:1287–1288

Kaestli LZ, Wasilewski-Rasca AF, Bonnabry P, Vogt-Ferrier N (2008) Use of transdermal drug formulations in the elderly. Drugs Aging 25:269–280

Kean WF, Rainsford KD, Kean IR (2008) Management of chronic musculoskeletal pain in the elderly: opinions on oral medication use. Inflammopharmacology 6:53–75

Lapane KL, Spooner JJ, Mucha L, Straus WL (2001) Effect of nonsteroidal anti-inflammatory drug use on the rate of gastrointestinal hospitalizations among people living in longterm care. J Am Geriatr Soc 49:577–584

Larsen RH, Nielsen F, Sorensen JA, Nielsen JB (2003) Dermal penetration of fentanyl: inter- and intraindividual variations. Pharmacol Toxicol 93:244–248

Laurell H, Hansson LE, Gunnarsson U (2006) Acute abdominal pain among elderly patients. Gerontology 52:339–344

Leppik IE, Epilepsy Foundation of America (2005) Choosing an antiepileptic. Selecting drugs for older patients with epilepsy. Geriatrics 60:42–47

Mattenklodt P, Ingenhorst A, Wille C et al (2008) Multimodale Gruppentherapie bei Senioren mit chronischen Schmerzen. Schmerz 22:551–5561

McCleane G (2008) Pain perception in the elderly patient. Clin Geriatr Med 24:203–211

McGettigan P, Henry D (2006) Cardiovascular risk and inhibition of cyclooxygenase: a systematic review of the observational studies of selective and nonselective inhibitors of cyclooxygenase 2. JAMA 296.1633–1644

McQuay HJ (1997) Opioid use in chronic pain. Acta Anaesthesiol Scand 41(1 Pt 2):175–183

Mercadante S, Arcuri E (2007) Pharmacological management of cancer pain in the elderly. Drugs Aging 24: 761–776

Mukherjee D, Nissen SE, Topol EJ (2001) Risk of cardiovascular events associated with selective COX-2-inhibitors. JAMA 286:954–959

Namaka M, Gramlich CR, Ruhlen D, Melanson M, Sutton I, Major J (2004) A treatment algorithm for neuropathic pain. Clin Ther 26:951–979

Nikolaus T, Zeyfang A (2004) Pharmacological treatment for persistent non-malignant pain in older persons. Drugs Aging 21:19–41

Pergolizzi J, Boger RH, Budd K et al (2008) Opioids and the management of chronic severe pain in the elderly: consensus statement of an International Expert Panel with focus on the six clinically most often used World Health Organization Step III opioids (buprenorphine, fentanyl, hydromorphone, methadone, morphine, oxycodone). Pain Pract 8:287–313

Prausnitz MR, Langer R (2008) Transdermal drug delivery. Nat Biotechnol 26:1261–1268

Ruoff GE (2002) Challenges of managing chronic pain in the elderly. Semin Arthritis Rheum 32(3 Suppl 1):43–50

Sauaia A, Min SJ, Leber C, Erbacher K, Abrams F, Fink R (2005) Postoperative pain management in elderly patients: correlation between adherence to treatment guidelines and patient satisfaction. J Am Geriatr Soc 53:274–282

Schmedtje JF Jr, Ji YS, Liu WL, DuBois RN, Runge MS (1997) Hypoxia induces cyclooxygenase-2 via the NF-kappaB p65 transcription factor in human vascular endothelial cells. J Biol Chem 272:601–608

Semla TP, Beizer JL, Higbee MD (2003) Geriatric dosage handbook, 9th edn. Lexi Comp, Hudson

Tasmuth T, Hartel B, Kalso E (2002) Venlafaxine in neuropathic pain following treatment of breast cancer. Eur J Pain 6:17–24

Trelle S, Reichenbach S, Wandel S et al (2011) Cardiovascular safety of non-steroidal anti-inflammatory drugs: network meta-analysis. BMJ 342:c7086

Vadalouca A, Siafaka I, Argyra E, Vrachnou E, Moka E (2006) Therapeutic management of chronic neuropathic pain: an examination of pharmacologic treatment. Ann N Y Acad Sci 1088:164–186

Van den Bemt PM, Geven LM, Kuitert NA, Risselada A, Brouwers JR (2002) The potential interaction between oral anticoagulants and acetaminophen in everyday practice. Pharm World Sci 24:201–204

Waldvogel HH (1996) Analgetika, Antinozizeptiva, Adjuvantien. Handbuch fur die Schmerzpraxis. Springer, Berlin

Won AB, Lapane KL, Vallow S, Schein J, Morris JN, Lipsitz LA (2004) Persistent nonmalignant pain and analgesic prescribing patterns in elderly nursing home residents. J Am Geriatr Soc 52:867–874

World Health Organization (WHO) (1996) Cancer pain relief with a guide to opioid availability, 2nd edn. WHO, Geneva

World Health Organization (WHO) (2007) Normative guidelines on pain management. Geneva, WHO. http://www.who.int/medicines/areas/quality_safety/Tagelphi_study_pain_guidelines.pdf. Accessed 27 Dec 2009

Yost JH, Morgan CJ (1994) Cardiovascular effects of NSAIDs. J Musculoskelet Med 11:22–34

Zwakhalen SM, Hamers JP, Abu-Saad HH, Berger MP (2006) Pain in elderly people with severe dementia: a systematic review of behavioural pain assessment tools. BMC Geriatr 6:3

Dementia

Stefan Schwarz and Lutz Frölich

Relevance for Elderly Patients, Epidemiology

Dementia is a clinical syndrome characterized by various symptoms, such as memory and concentration difficulties, behavioral abnormalities, language and perception difficulties, as well as problems with the ability of comprehension and judgment.

The clinical diagnosis of dementia can be established when the following three criteria apply:

1. Newly incurred cognitive deficits
2. Duration over at least half a year
3. Impairment in the activities of the daily life due to cognitive deficits.

The diagnosis of dementia cannot be established in the absence of impairments in the activities of daily living.

Mild cognitive impairment (MCI) has to be delimited from dementia. This syndrome, like clinically defined dementia, also includes cognitive deficits; these deficits, however, are less marked and therefore do not lead to relevant impairments of the daily routine activities. People with mild cognitive disorders carry a high risk of developing dementia in the foreseeable future and should therefore be observed closely not to miss the right time for an intervention.

Dementia is a clinical syndrome with a heterogeneous etiology. The most frequent cause for a dementia is Alzheimer's disease (approximately 60% of all dementia disorders). The terms *Alzheimer's disease* and *dementia* are often used synonymously, but this is incorrect. In fact, a large number of other disorders can cause dementia. Primary dementia, most commonly resulting from neurodegenerative disorders, can be roughly partitioned from secondary dementia as a complication of other diseases. The most frequent neurodegenerative dementia disorders are

– Alzheimer's disease
– Group of frontotemporal dementias
– Lewy-body dementia
– Dementia associated with Parkinson's disease.

The most frequent dementia diseases that cannot be traced back to neurodegenerative processes are

– Vascular dementia
– Dementia after stroke, including multi-infarct dementia.

In addition, a large number of dementia syndromes result from infectious, inflammatory, toxic, endocrine, and metabolic causes, with significant regional differences. For example, in Southern Africa, HIV infection is one of the most frequent causes for dementia, whereas in industrialized countries, HIV-associated dementia only plays a minor role.

Dementia is a clinical syndrome with a heterogeneous etiology.

S. Schwarz (✉) · L. Frölich
Central Institute of Mental Health, Medical Faculty
Mannheim/Heidelberg University, Square J 5, 68159
Mannheim, Germany
e-mail: stefan.schwarz@zi-mannheim.de;
lutz.froelich@zi-mannheim.de

M. Wehling (ed.), *Drug Therapy for the Elderly*,
DOI 10.1007/978-3-7091-0912-0_15, © Springer-Verlag Wien 2013

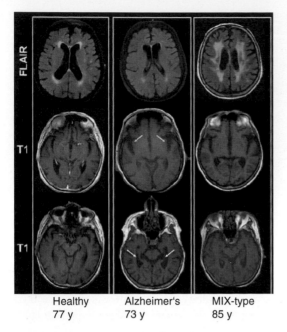

Healthy   Alzheimer's   MIX-type
77 y   73 y   85 y

Fig. 1 Typical MRT findings for Alzheimer's and mixed dementia (neurodegenerative plus vascular components). *MRT* magnetic resonance tomography (From F. Hentschel, Central Institute of Mental Health, Mannheim, Germany)

Pathological studies demonstrated that the majority of patients with dementia display different concurrent etiologies (e.g., features typical for Alzheimer's plus vascular changes; Fig. 1). This is one of the reasons why an unequivocal classification of dementia is difficult in many patients. Although neurodegenerative dementias show typical result constellations, a distinct classification of dementia is mostly impossible on clinical grounds without additional use of biomarkers.

Due to the etiological heterogeneity of dementia, a standard therapy for the clinical syndrome of dementia is not possible. The therapy should rather focus on the cause of the disease. Therefore, prior to treating dementia, a thorough differential diagnostic classification in terms of psychological and technical examinations has to be implemented. A careful clinical-neurological examination, cerebral imaging, and lab tests are obligatory parts of the diagnosis. Several dementias are causally treatable and curable, for instance, those due to infectious, inflammatory,

or endocrine causes. Yet, for the treatment of neurodegenerative dementias, which present by far the largest group of all dementia disorders worldwide, no causal therapies are available up to now.

The treatment of dementia has to focus on the underlying disorder or causes.

Dementia is one of the most frequent illnesses, with considerable health and economic impacts worldwide. Globally, the prevalence of dementia was estimated around 24 million people in the year 2001, whereas this number is supposed to increase to 81 million people until the year 2040 (Ferri et al. 2005; Reitz et al. 2011). The expected increase of the prevalence of dementia, especially in the industrialized countries, is explained by the dynamics of age development; the prevalence of dementia rises with an increasing life span. Among people over 65 years of age, the prevalence of dementia is estimated at 5–8%, with the incidence significantly increasing at higher age (Lobo et al. 2000). While among 65-year-old people, the prevalence of dementia amounts to approximately 1%, more than a third of all 90-year-old people fulfill the criteria for the diagnosis of dementia. In a study on centenarians, the majority of the examined persons suffered from dementia (Andersen-Ranberg et al. 2001). In several countries in Europe, in China, in the United States, and in the developing countries in the Western Pacific where the populations are rapidly aging, it is estimated that the present share of people over 65, or about one fifth or less of the population, will increase over one third until the year 2060. This problem is even aggravated by the fact that in most industrialized countries the majority of those over 80 years old are living alone. Considering the high prevalence of dementia of over 20% in this age group, significant consequences for society and the social security nets are inevitable.

Due to demographic changes, the prevalence of dementia will increase significantly in most industrialized and developing countries during the next years.

Women have a higher total prevalence of dementia than men, which is mainly credited to the higher life expectation of women. In a Dutch study, the lifetime risk for dementia was estimated at around 34.5% for women and around 16% for men (Ott et al. 1998). Dementia is one of the diseases that affect quality of life almost immediately. Surveys showed that elderly people fear the development of a dementia more than most other illnesses.

Dementia will attain an increasing economic relevance. Dementia causes the highest total costs of all illnesses for the social and health systems in general. In the industrialized countries, the direct and indirect costs of dementia are significantly higher than the costs for cardiac diseases, stroke, or cancer (Craig and Birks 2006).

Dementia causes the highest total costs of all illnesses.

The high total costs of dementia emerge from the comparably long duration of the illness, often leading to years-long need for help and care. The mean duration of illness amounts to 6–10 years, with a highly individual variability. A clearer prognosis of the individual case is not possible currently. Dementia is one of the most frequent causes for the loss of independence in the aged population and the most frequent cause for the referral to a residential care home for the elderly.

Regarding the increase of prevalence of dementia in the foreseeable future, the financial and structural support of appropriate medical and nursing care of dementia patients has not been properly addressed.

Therapeutically Relevant Special Features of Elderly Patients

For a complex illness such as dementia that significantly impedes the functional and social abilities of a patient, therapeutic interventions have to be multimodal. Besides medical interventions, social and psychotherapeutic measures in a wider sense are necessary. An isolated pharmacological approach to dementia treatment is not appropriate. As caregivers and relatives in the vicinity of dementia patients are often under considerable stress, an appropriate therapeutic approach may have to include these persons as well. In this context, the family doctor plays a major and central role, which also involves collaboration and support of social workers, psychologists, and nursing staff.

The treatment of dementia is multidimensional and includes pharmacological, social, and psychotherapeutic measures.

Since dementia mainly occurs at advanced age, drug treatment studies should aim at elderly people. In the majority of important clinical studies for the treatment of dementia, a lower age limit (e.g., 50 years) was defined. Thus, in contrast to most other diseases, the results from studies on dementia almost exclusively refer to elderly individuals. In turn, it may be questionable whether these results could also be applied to younger patients with dementia onset before 50 years of age since in this age group particular conditions frequently apply (e.g., genetically determined forms of dementia such as Huntington's disease or inherited forms of Alzheimer's disease).

Within the group of elderly people, no convincing studies on possible differences of drug reactions in correlation to increasing age exist. It could be assumed that efficacy and especially the rate of side effects may differ between elderly and very old, especially frail, patients. The available studies do not provide any clear references to different adverse effect rates in dementia patients within different age groups as they usually do not specifically pursue this issue.

In contrast to most other groups of drugs, antidementive medications were mainly studied in elderly people.

Most of the large clinical studies relate to the most frequent form of dementia, Alzheimer's disease. Pharmacological therapies are approved only for dementia in association with Parkinson's disease and Alzheimer's disease. For most other forms of dementia, the available evidence is not sufficient for solid recommendations, and large studies are not available.

The validity of most clinical studies is limited due to the regular exclusion of multimorbid individuals or patients with severe comorbidities such as tumors or cerebrovascular or cardiac diseases in approval studies. Thus, only patients with isolated dementia but without significant comorbidity were included in those studies. The fraction of dementia patients to be recruited for a drug trial is usually only about 10% of all screened patients. This leads to the fact that for the large number of multimorbid or severely frail patients with dementia even approved medications have not been evaluated sufficiently.

Due to numerous exclusion criteria, only a small proportion of all dementia patients were included in clinical studies for antidementive medications.

Evidence-Based, Rationalistic Drug Therapy and Classification of Drugs According to Their Fitness for the Aged (FORTA)

Causal Therapy of Dementia, General Problems of Antidementive Therapies

The causal therapy for secondary dementia diseases is the treatment of the primary disease. If no irreversible damages have developed, in theory, cognitive deficits could be reduced by applying an effective therapy of the underlying causes.

Up to now, for primary neurodegenerative dementias, no causal therapies that positively influence or reverse the underlying pathological processes are available. There are, however, a few medications with proven efficacy, but also a large number of medications with uncertain efficacy, to symptomatically influence the deterioration of cognitive performance.

A causal therapy for the vast majority of neurodegenerative dementias is not available.

According to the European Medicines Agency (2009), an effective antidementive medication requires evidence of efficacy using psychometric test procedures at a minimum of two levels:
– At the cognitive level
– At the functional level (activities of daily life)

– At the global level (clinical overall impression).

In addition, the evidence of positive effects in the following areas is useful:
– Behavioral disorders
– Strain for relatives
– Costs of illness.

For only some available medications was a positive effect for at least two of the first three sections proven.

In Table 1, the individual medications are specified regarding the mechanism of action, fitness for the aged (FORTA classification; see chapter "Critical Extrapolation of Guidelines and Study Results: Risk-Benefit Assessment for Patients with Reduced Life Expectancy and a New Classification of Drugs According to Their Fitness for the Aged") and approved indications. An overview of the therapeutic recommendations for the different forms of dementia is shown in Table 2.

Antidementive medication has proven efficacy on cognitive function. It is a matter of debate how relevant these beneficial effects are for the patient's quality of life or functional abilities, which are not only driven by medical but also by health economy aspects.

The benefit of the approved antidementive medications for cognitive performances is well documented. The clinical relevance of this therapeutic effect, however, is still controversial.

All antidementive medications were mainly tested in patients with Alzheimer's disease since this is the most common form of dementia and related insights into pathophysiology are most comprehensive. There are only a few convincing studies on the efficacy of antidementive medications for other forms of dementia. Patients with concurrent etiology, as, for example, the common mixed form of vascular and Alzheimer's disease, were excluded from most studies.

As with all chronically progressive diseases, the implementation of controlled studies over several years proved to be obstructively troublesome and expensive. Most of the controlled drug studies only had a short observation period, from a few months up to 1 year. In contrast, most dementia patients experience a course of several years.

Table 1 Medications specified regarding the mechanism of action, fitness for the aged (FORTA classification; see chapter "Critical Extrapolation of Guidelines and Study Results: Risk-Benefit Assessment for Patients with Reduced Life Expectancy and a New Classification of Drugs According to Their Fitness for the Aged") and approved indications

Mechanism of action	Substance	FORTA classification	Approved indications
Acetylcholinesterase inhibitors	Donepezil	B	Mild, moderate, severe[a] Alzheimer's dementia
	Galantamine	B	Mild-moderate Alzheimer's dementia
	Rivastigmine	B	Mild-moderate Alzheimer's dementia and dementia associated with Parkinson's disease
	Tacrine	—	Mild-moderate Alzheimer's dementia
NMDA (glutamate) antagonist	Memantine	B	Moderate-severe Alzheimer's disease
Calcium channel blocker	Nimodipine	C	Not approved for dementia[b]
Antioxidants, inhibition of platelet aggregation	Gingko biloba	C	Not approved[b]
α-Adrenergic and 5-HT agonistic	Ergolin derivates (nicergoline)	C	Not approved for dementia[b]
Antioxidants	Piracetam	C	Not approved for dementia[b]
Impact on cerebral metabolism	Pyritinol	C	Not approved[b]
Antioxidants	Vitamin E, selenium, vitamin C, etc.	C	Not approved for dementia
Diverse phytotherapeutics	Ginseng, e.g.	C	Not approved
Hormone compounds	DHEA, testosterone, e.g.	C	Not approved for dementia
MAO inhibitor antioxidant	Selegiline	C	Not approved for dementia
Antiphlogistics	Indomethacin, e.g.	D	Not approved for dementia
Cholesterol lowering	Simvastatin, e.g.	C	Not approved for dementia
Chelating agent	Desferrioxamine	C	Not approved for dementia

[a]In Europe, donepezil is approved for mild and moderate Alzheimer's disease only
[b]In some countries approved for various types of dementia despite lack of scientific evidence

Therefore, the beneficial effects of antidementive medications are well documented for a short observation period only. Potential long-term effects can only be assumed from the results of uncontrolled cohort studies but have not been firmly ascertained yet.

As a consequence, the optimal duration for an antidementive therapy with approved drugs is unknown. Most authors recommend continuing antidementive therapy as long as the medication is well tolerated and as long as the therapy proves to have a (putative) benefit. However, the latter point is difficult to evaluate in the individual patient and often missed in reality.

The individual case observation may be rather inappropriate concerning the ssessment of efficacy of a medication since the core therapeutic effect of most antidementive medications is to slow progression of the disease. Therefore, in most patients only a short-term improvement of symptoms can be expected at best. Since the spontaneous course of dementia is usually not predictable, the individual therapeutic effect of a medication cannot be sufficiently assured. Therefore, the "therapy efficiency review" claimed to be necessary by several authorities may hardly be provided in practice; only in cases of rapid aggravation of dementia symptoms despite medication can the inefficacy of the therapy

Table 2 Evidence-based pharmacotherapy of dementia: overview

	Alzheimer's disease	Vascular dementia	Frontotemporal dementia	Lewy body dementia	Dementia associated with Parkinson's disease
Antidementive medication	*Mild-moderate*	Galantamine ↔	Cholinesterase inhibitors ↔/↓	Rivastimine ↔	Rivastigmine ↑↑
	Galantamine ↑↑	Donepezil ↔	Trazodone ↔		Donepezil ↑
	Rivastigmine ↑↑	Rivastigmine ↔	Paroxetine/SSRI ↔		Memantine ↔
	Donepezil ↑↑	Memantine ↔	Moclobemide ↔		
	Memantine ↓				
	Moderate-severe				
	Memantine ↑↑				
	Acetylcholinesterase inhibitors ↔/↑				
	Combination therapy of memantine plus acetylcholinesterase inhibitors ↔/↑				
Behavioral abnormalities	Antipsychotics ↔,/↓		Men with sexual inhibition: leuproreline ↑	Psychotic symptoms: Clozapine ↑	Psychotic symptoms: Clozapine ↑↑
				Quetiapine ↔	Olanzapine ↑
				Conventional antipsychotics ↓	Quetiapine ↔
					Conventional antipsychotics ↓
Parkinsonism				Levodopa ↑	Conventional Parkinson medication

SSRI selective serotonin reuptake inhibitor
↑↑ Efficacy supported by several valid clinical studies. Positive statement well documented
↑ Efficacy supported by at least one valid clinical study. Positive statement well documented
↔ No secured study results. Lack of adequate studies or contradictory results
↓ Negative statement on efficacy well documented

be assumed. The practitioner is in fact obliged to document the course of the disease, but no obligation exists to carry out a successful control for the individual patient as this is hardly feasible.

The benefit of antidementive therapies is difficult to assess in the individual patient.

Moreover, medication effects may depend on the stage of dementia. Most clinical studies were implemented for patients with mild or moderate dementia. It seems questionable that these findings can also be assigned to other states of dementia. Some studies suggest a benefit of antidementive treatment on cognitive parameters in patients with severe dementia, but the clinical relevance of the therapeutic effect remains controversial in this group of patients.

Many patients with dementia have a multifactorial etiology and a complex pathophysiology.

Therefore, in theory, it seems useful to administer not only a single compound but also a combination of medications with different mechanisms of action. There are some indications from clinical studies that the combination of acetylcholinesterase inhibitors (e.g., donepezil) with memantine may be beneficial (Atri et al. 2008; Lopez et al. 2009). In practice, these two substance groups are often prescribed in combination, although this procedure cannot be unequivocally recommended due to insufficient data.

Prevention

Neurodegenerative dementias only become symptomatic when degenerative processes have led to significant damage in the brain over a long period of time. Therefore, effective approaches for prevention at an early stage would be highly preferable.

Unfortunately, medications for the prevention of dementia illnesses are not available. There is an ongoing controversial debate on the value of certain therapeutic approaches, such those involving vitamin B, antioxidants, or specific immune therapies. In epidemiological studies, the intake of antihypertensives, nonsteroidal antiphlogistics, alcohol, estrogens, and statins are correlated with a lower incidence of dementia. Therapeutic recommendations cannot be derived at present; intervention studies with vitamin E as well as statins turned out to be disappointing so far. An actual large study with gingko biloba extract could not show any positive preventive effect (Snitz et al. 2009).

In patients with mild cognitive dysfunctions (MCI), no therapies to halt the progression of a dementia disease are established so far. A few studies have tested acetylcholinesterase inhibitors in patients with MCI. The results from these studies have been disappointing so far, presumably since in this group of patients no obvious deficit of neurotransmitters is assumed to have occurred.

At present, no specific medications for the prevention of dementia or for MCI can be recommended (Ballard et al. 2011). Obviously, any contribution by vascular processes should be the target of the typical interventions, including treatment of arterial hypertension, hyperlipemia, and diabetes mellitus, for which antidementia effects have been suggested considering evidence from observational studies (Davies et al. 2011; Wehling and Groth 2011).

For the prevention of dementia and MCI, no pharmacological interventions are available at present.

Therapy of Alzheimer's Disease

All acetylcholinesterase inhibitors are approved for the treatment of mild-to-moderate Alzheimer's disease (Mini-Mental State Examination [MMSE], 10–26 points), and donepezil and memantine are approved for the treatment of moderate-to-severe Alzheimer's disease (MMSE ≤ 22 points). Memantine is not effective in patients with mild Alzheimer's disease (Schneider et al. 2011). In Europe, donepezil is approved for mild-to-moderate Alzheimer's disease only. Previously, it was thought that acetylcholinesterase inhibitors are not effective in patients with severe Alzheimer's disease. However, results from newer studies have challenged this view, and accordingly, donepezil is now approved for all stages of Alzheimer's dementia in the United States (Winblad et al. 2006; Cummings et al. 2010; Burns et al. 2009). All antidementive medications offer only moderate disease-modifying therapeutic effects and do not causally influence the main pathological mechanisms in Alzheimer's disease (Kavirajan and Schneider 2007). The clinical effect relates to improved signal transmission on the cholinergic respective to the glutamatergic synapses.

Besides effects on cognitive function, antidementive treatment may improve the ability to perform activities of daily living, behavioral symptoms, and quality of life of the patient and reduce caregiver stress; concomitantly, it may result in cost savings, partly due to delayed referral to nursing homes (Getsios et al. 2010; Kiencke et al. 2011).

There is no clear preference among the different acetylcholinesterase inhibitors. Recent data do not show any superiority of any compound despite differing pharmacological features, so that these medications are regarded as equivalent concerning their efficacy (Hogan et al. 2004).

There is also no convincing study comparing memantine with acetylcholinesterase inhibitors. Approval studies on these substances show similar therapy effects, so that the decision for the administration of one of the medications has to be done according to their side-effect profile and to personal experiences. Frequent contraindications for the use of acetylcholinesterase inhibitors in elderly patients are bradycardic arrhythmias and cardiac conduction disorders, a history of gastric ulcers, or obstructive pulmonary diseases and for memantine severe renal insufficiency.

Memantine and acetylcholinesterase inhibitors are approved for the treatment of Alzheimer's dementia.

Besides the antidementive therapy, it is essential for the treatment of patients with Alzheimer's dementia to discontinue medications with central nervous system (CNS) depressive or anticholinergic effects and—if truly indicated and alternatives are available—to replace them with other compounds. These problematic drugs are, among others, not only tricyclic antidepressants but also urospasmolytics, asthma medications, sedatives, neuroleptics, or opioid analgesics, which are used most frequently.

Drugs with anticholinergic effects have to be avoided in patients with dementia.

Overview of Compound Details
Acetylcholinesterase Inhibitors

Acetylcholine is a pivotal neurotransmitter in the CNS and plays an important role for the ability of learning, memory, attention, and vigilance. The cholinergic hypothesis of Alzheimer's disease postulates that the disease leads to a cholinergic deficit in certain brain areas that is mainly responsible for the clinical manifestations. The extent of the cholinergic deficit in the brain correlates with the severity of dementia and with the amount of amyloid plaques and neurofibrillary tangles. The relative specificity of cholinergic neurotransmitter degeneration indicates a dysfunction in the metabolism of the presynaptic neuron prior to synaptic degeneration—probably as a consequence of this presynaptic dysfunction.

The pharmacologically induced increase of the functional activity of the cholinergic neurotransmitter system is currently the most effective therapy for Alzheimer's disease, although not representing a causal therapy. Different approaches were pursued to increase the activity of the cholinergic system in the CNS. In clinical practice, only the acetylcholinesterase inhibitors prevailed. These substances increase the concentration of acetylcholine in the brain by inhibiting the enzymes acetylcholinesterase and butyrylcholinesterase, responsible for the hydrolysis of acetylcholine.

Due to their comparable mode of action, the most important therapeutic principles equally apply to all available acetylcholinesterase inhibitors and are discussed here. Comparisons between the different substances did not lead to any clear superiority of a specific acetylcholinesterase inhibitor concerning efficacy or side effects (Hansen et al. 2008). Tacrine is no longer marketed due to unacceptable rates of side effects and only remains of historical relevance as the first available acetylcholinesterase inhibitor.

It is essential to begin acetylcholinesterase inhibitor treatment with a small dose and slowly increase it to reduce adverse effects and thereby support compliance. In some patients, a dose increase even slower than recommended by the manufacturer may be useful. Cholinergic gastrointestinal intolerances in terms of nausea, vomiting, or diarrhea frequently occur on treatment initiation. In addition, bradycardia, vertigo, and orthostatic dysregulation may occur temporarily due to systemic cholinergic effects. Patients have to be informed that these side effects are reversible and often spontaneously recede during the course of treatment. However, acetylcholinesterase inhibitors have been associated with an increased incidence of syncope and falls. Gastric and duodenal ulcers represent a relative contraindication.

Prior to acetylcholinesterase inhibitor therapy, electrocardiographic (ECG) screening is mandatory. In patients with sick sinus syndrome, bradycardia, higher-grade conduction abnormalities, or prolonged QT interval, acetylcholinesterase inhibitors should not be prescribed at all or only after careful consideration of the risk-benefit ratio. The same holds true for patients with bronchial asthma and obstructive bronchitis, which could deteriorate due to the cholinergic properties of the substances. For patients with preexisting cardiac disorders, a second ECG should be performed after initiation of therapy to identify bradycardia or other complications. Since galantamine and recently also donepezil were discussed to be associated with excess mortality in controlled studies (although performed for off-label indications), cardiac contraindications should be carefully excluded prior to start of therapy with acetylcholinesterase inhibitors.

Main contraindications of acetylcholinesterase inhibitors are bradycardia, cardiac arrhythmias,   atrioventricular   block,

bronchial asthma/obstructive bronchitis, and a history of gastric ulcer.

Donepezil. Initially, a single dose of 5 mg is given at night. After 4 weeks, the dose is increased to 10 mg. The dose can be administered as a single dose in the evening or can be split into two doses. Donepezil is available as a tablet or lozenge. Systemic cholinergic side effects under donepezil are rather rare in comparison with other oral acetylcholinesterase inhibitors.

Rivastigmine. Therapy starts with a total daily dose of 3 mg, split into two doses of 1.5 mg each. This dose is increased by 1.5 mg biweekly, aiming at a final dose of 6–12 mg/day, split into two doses. For patients with dysphagia, rivastigmine is also available as solution. Rivastigmine has a lower potential for drug-drug interactions than other acetylcholinesterase inhibitors and is therefore useful, for example, for patients on oral anticoagulants. Rivastagmine as a transdermal patch is preferred for patients with dysphagia or aversion against tablets. The rate of gastrointestinal side effects is comparable to that of donepezil and— due to a steadier release—lower than for the oral administration of rivastigmine. In some patients, however, skin irritations can lead to discontinuation of the patch medication. Treatment with the transdermal patch is started with the smaller patch used daily over 4 weeks (4.6 mg/24 h); then, the larger patch (9.5 mg/24 h) is applied.

Galantamine. The drug is started at 8 mg o.d. in the morning. Galantamine is available as an extended-release formulation, so that dose splitting is not necessary. The dose is increased every 4 weeks by 4–8 mg up to a dose of 16–24 mg o.d. For patients with difficulties swallowing, it is also available as a solution. The solution should be administered in two doses per day, in the morning and in the evening.

Memantine. Memantine mainly acts by enhancing glutamatergic neurotransmission via the NMDA (*N*-methyl-D-aspartate) receptor. Compared to acetylcholinesterase inhibitors, it is relatively well tolerated. Relevant cholinergic side effects are not expected (and have not been observed). After discontinuation, reversible side effects of the CNS, such as agitation, disorientation, epileptic seizures, vertigo, and sometimes even psychotic symptoms, may occur. In patients with insufficiently controlled epilepsy, memantine is contraindicated.

Memantine is not nephrotoxic, but is eliminated via the kidney and cumulates in patients with renal failure. In patients with mild-to-moderate renal dysfunction, the maximal dose is limited to 10 mg/day. For patients with severe renal dysfunction (creatinine clearance <9 ml/min), memantine is contraindicated. Since medications such as amantadine, ranitidine, and procaine use the same renal cation transport system, an increase of the plasma level can occur if used concomitantly. Hydrochlorothiazide, frequently prescribed in elderly patients with high blood pressure, can also accumulate in the presence of memantine. Under simultaneous application of dopaminergic and anticholinergic substances, additive effects may occur; thus, the risk of a drug-induced psychosis is increased.

In patients with impaired renal function the dose of memantine must be adapted.

Memantine is started at a dose of 5 mg o.d. in the morning and then uptitrated by 5 mg/day over a week to a maximum dose of 20 mg/day. The dose can be administered as a total dose in the morning or split into two single doses in the morning and in the evening. In cases of difficulties swallowing, memantine is also available as solution.

The following overview shows a dose comparison; Table 3 is a comparison of significant pharmacological/clinical features:

Dosage Schedule of Antidementive Medications

Donepezil
- Start with 5 mg in the evening.
- If well tolerated, increase after 4 weeks to 10 mg in the evening.
- Maximum dosage is 10 mg/day.

Galantamine
- Use the retarded compound as a single dose.
- Start with 8 mg in the morning.
- If well tolerated, increase at 4-week intervals by 4–8 mg/day.

Table 3 Comparison of donepezil, rivastigmine, and galantamine

	Donepezil	Rivastigmine oral	Galantamine
Class	Piperidine	Carbamate	Tertiary alkaloid
Mechanism	Reversible, competitive and not competitive AChE inhibitor	Pseudoirreversible AChE/BuChE inhibitor	Reversible competitive AChE inhibitor and allosteric modulator of nicotinergic receptors
Pharmacokinetics	Fast uptake, high protein binding, hepatic metabolism (P450 isoenzymes 2D6 and 3A4)	Fast uptake, delayed by food, hydrolysis by esterases, duration of CNS effect approximately 10 h	Faster uptake, delayed by food, hepatic metabolism (P450 isoenzymes 2D6 and 3A4)
Biological half-life	70 h	1–2 h	5–7 h
Protein binding	93–96%	40%	18–34%
Bioavailability	43%	40%	85–100%
Interactions	Medications metabolized by P450 isoenzymes, medications acting on the cholinergic system	Medications acting on the cholinergic system	Medications, metabolized over P450 isoenzymes, medications acting on the cholinergic system
Start dosage	5 mg at night	1.5 mg twice daily	8 mg once daily (extended release)
Dose escalation	Increase after 4 weeks to 10 mg	Increase biweekly by 1.5 mg	Increase monthly by 4–8 mg
Maximum dose	10 mg once daily	6 mg twice daily	24 mg once daily
Main side effects	Nausea, diarrhea, vomiting, insomnia, muscle cramps, weight loss	Nausea, vomiting, diarrhea, stomachache, weight loss	Nausea, diarrhea, vertigo, vomiting, weight loss

Source: Modified from Hogan and Patterson 2002
AChE acetylcholinesterase, *BuChE* butyrylcholinesterase, *CNS* central nervous system

– Maximum dosage is 24 mg/day.

Rivastigmine oral
– Start with 1.5 mg in the morning and in the evening.
– If well tolerated, increase at 2-week intervals by 1.5 mg/day.
– Maximum dose is 12 mg/day, split into two single doses.

Rivastigmine transdermal patch
– Start with the smaller patch (4.6 mg/day).
– If well tolerated, increase after 4 weeks to the larger patch (9.5 mg/day).

Memantine
– Start with 5 mg as a single dose in the morning.
– Increase weekly by 5 mg.

– Maximum dose is 20 mg as a single dose or 10 mg twice daily.

Other Antidementive Medications for the Treatment of Alzheimer's Disease

Only for memantine and the acetylcholinesterase inhibitors, a clear therapeutic effect has been demonstrated in clinical studies.

Therefore, no other antidementive drugs are first-choice medications but could be prescribed in cases in which first-line drugs are not well tolerated or relevant contraindications are present. Fortunately, this only rarely applies.

Except for memantine and acetylcholinesterase inhibitors, no other compound has a proven antidementive effect.

Many patients take additional medications on their own, mainly vitamins or herbal medicines. As far as the scientifically evidenced therapy is maintained, this usually will not cause problems.

A discontinuation of such medications may not always be encouraged unless the medication is of dubious origin or very expensive. Usually, these compounds are tolerated quite well, but depending on the ingredients, side effects may also occur. For example, bleeding complications have been repeatedly discussed for the concomitant use of gingko products and anticoagulants.

Therapy Monitoring, Combination Therapy, Therapy Change, Therapy Duration

The problem of therapy monitoring for efficacy has already been discussed in detail.

If a proven diagnosis has been established, follow-up studies of cognitive functions usually do not lead to therapeutic consequences under a continued pharmacotherapy if no particular aspects prevail.

The same difficulty is also relevant when a change to another antidementive medication is considered due to obvious ineffectiveness. For this procedure, only few data from valid studies exist (Gardette et al. 2010). If a change from one medication to another is deemed necessary, this is usually done as an individual attempt ("trial and error").

If a compound has to be exchanged due to intolerable side effects, another acetylcholinesterase inhibitor can be administered and might be well tolerated despite a similar mode of action. In this case, the second substance should be carefully increased in small steps. Due to the different side-effect profiles, the change from an acetylcholinesterase inhibitor to memantine or vice versa may also be successful.

The appropriate duration of an antidementive therapy remains an unsolved problem. In approval studies for the available medications, the drug was usually investigated for 6–12 months. For the long-term effects of the treatment—mean survival after the diagnosis of dementia is 6–10 years—no findings from large randomized trials are available. Cohort studies suggested that it might be useful to continue the treatment over a longer period of time. It should be kept in mind that discontinuation of antidementive medication has been found to be associated with a rapid decline of cognitive function (Doody et al. 2001).

The optimal therapy duration for antidementive medications is unknown.

The benefit of a combination therapy of an acetylcholinesterase inhibitor with memantine is not proven. However, several studies demonstrated small-to-moderate benefits from a combination of different antidementive drugs (Atri et al. 2008). For patients with mild dementia, a combination therapy is not recommended; if necessary, an add-on therapy with memantine on top of donepezil may be considered only for patients with moderate-to-severe dementia (Tariot et al. 2004).

The treatment indication for antidementive medications in patients with severe and very severe dementia is discussed controversially. Even in patients living in a care or nursing home due to severe dementia, antidementive medications may have an attested effect on cognitive functions and cause significant improvements on neuropsychological scales (Winblad et al. 2006; Burns et al. 2009; Cummings et al. 2010). The extent of the clinical relevance, however, is subject to debate (Hogan 2006). Subjective quality of life and the presumed interest of the patients are critical aspects for the decision against or for an antidementive medication in this situation. Surveys among elderly people revealed that the vast majority of patients do not wish any life-prolonging medical measures if substantial care dependency cannot be prevented or is even facilitated by the intervention.

Therapy of Dementia in Association with Parkinson's Disease

The majority of patients with idiopathic Parkinson's disease develop a dementia in the course of the disease (Aarsland et al. 2003). In cross-sectional studies, the prevalence of dementia in all patients with Parkinson's disease amounts to approximately 25% (Fuchs et al. 2004).

For the treatment of cognitive deficits, acetylcholinesterase inhibitors proved to be successful, mainly donepezil, tacrine, and rivastigmine (Camicioli and Fisher 2004). In reflection of a large randomized trial (Emre et al. 2004), rivastigmine at a dosage of 6–12 mg is approved for the treatment of dementia associated with Parkinson's disease. During the treatment with rivastigmine, a clinically relevant improvement of approximately 15% of patients can be expected (Maidment et al. 2006). Yet, a relatively high rate of cholinergic side effects is observed, as demonstrated by the high rate of dropouts in the active arm of the approval study. The results of the study have not been replicated in another study up to now. In addition, it was criticized that the sponsor of this study was responsible for the data analysis.

Rivastigmine is the only medication approved for dementia in association with Parkinson's disease and is thus the first choice in this situation if well tolerated. The application as a patch is not approved for this indication; there are, however, no good reasons arguing against the application in patients with Parkinson's disease.

Rivastigmine is the only medication approved for dementia at Parkinson's disease.

Two current studies yielded controversial results on the efficacy of memantine in patients with dementia in association with the Parkinson's disease (Aarsland et al. 2009; Emre et al. 2010). In the light of these data, memantine cannot be recommended for this indication at present.

Vascular Dementia

Up to now, no proven beneficial therapy of vascular dementia exists. One of the reasons relates to the diagnostic problem of differentiating the mixed forms of Alzheimer's disease as well as the differentiation in etiologically distinct subgroups, such as multi-infarct dementia, subcortical vascular encephalopathy, or dementia after stroke. During recent years, several studies of the treatment of vascular dementia with donepezil, galantamine, and memantine were published (Bowler 2005). A Cochrane analysis could not identify enough valid studies to implement a meta-analysis on the data for rivastigmine; data from smaller studies with rivastigmine for vascular dementia, however, seemed to be comparable with the results for donepezil and galantamine (Craig and Birks 2005). A current large clinical trial did not show any apparent advantage of donepezil treatment (Roman et al. 2010). Presently, no pharmacological treatment of cognitive or functional defects can be recommended for vascular dementia.

A beneficial effect of antidementive medications has not been convincingly demonstrated for vascular dementia.

Lewy Body Dementia

The available data on the therapy of Lewy body dementia are limited, which can be explained—besides the relatively low incidence of the disease compared to Alzheimer's disease—with the diagnostic problems inherent to this disease (McKeith et al. 2005). Large controlled therapy studies are lacking. Two smaller randomized studies showed an improvement of cognitive performance by acetylcholinesterase inhibitors at the same doses administered in Alzheimer's dementia; an uncontrolled study suggested an even better effect of donezepil in comparison to Alzheimer's dementia (Samuel et al. 2000). This is not surprising since distinct cholinergic deficits have been repeatedly shown in patients with Lewy body dementia. Long-term effects of acetylcholinesterase inhibitors have not been investigated so far. According to these data, treatment of patients with Lewy body dementia with acetylcholinesterase inhibitors can be recommended, although this represents an off-label use. Positive data from two recent studies of patients with Lewy body dementia are also available for memantine (Aarsland et al. 2009; Emre et al. 2010).

In the presence of Parkinson's motor symptoms, treatment with levodopa should be attempted. However, only a small fraction of patients responds to this therapy, and the beneficial effects are much less pronounced than in patients with Parkinson's disease. Levodopa should be carefully titrated (starting with 100 mg/day, then increase by about

50–100 mg/day every 3–4 days) and administered at the lowest possible dose to avoid psychotic side effects, which may escalate to a pharmacologically induced, full-blown dopaminergic psychosis. If levodopa does not show clear treatment success, the medication should be discontinued.

Except for quetiapine and clozapine, no antipsychotics should be prescribed in Lewy body dementia since these medications may cause severe deterioration of the motor symptoms.

Patients with Lewy body dementia typically show marked intolerance against antipsychotic drugs except for clozapine and quetiapine.

Frontotemporal Dementia

No therapy for frontotemporal dementia beyond symptomatic measures is established. Only a few valid clinical studies exist. The main problem concerning clinical studies for frontotemporal dementia is the heterogeneity of the disease, congregated under the umbrella term, and the substantial diagnostic difficulties. Due to pathological and positron emission tomographic (PET) findings suggesting abnormalities in the metabolism of serotonin, some small studies with serotonergic compounds were undertaken. The results of smaller studies with trazodone, moclobemide, and paroxetine were ambiguous and do not allow derivation of any recommendations (Adler et al. 2003; Neary et al. 2005). Although no clear indications for a cholinergic deficit in frontotemporal dementia exist, studies of acetylcholinesterase inhibitors, especially rivastigmine, were performed but did not produce any clear indications for the efficacy of these substances.

In clinical practice, SSRIs (selective serotonin reuptake inhibitors), MAO-A (monoamine oxidase type A) inhibitors, and, sometimes, acetylcholinesterase inhibitors are prescribed. Yet, these drugs are only individual and to some extent experimental therapeutic attempts; in the case of side effects or obviously absent efficacy, they have to be discontinued.

An effective pharmacotherapy for frontotemporal dementias is not known.

Treatment of Behavioral Abnormalities

In particular at an advanced stage of dementia, behavioral symptoms often dominate the clinical picture and typically represent an enormous strain for relatives and caregivers. The treatment of behavioral symptoms in dementia is often difficult. No generally established pharmacological treatment approaches are available. In Table 4, pragmatic therapeutic suggestions are summarized.

Prior to symptomatic therapy, an adequate pharmacological antidementive therapy should be implemented; clinical studies indicated that the approved antidementive medications discussed not only positively influence the cognitive symptoms in dementia but also may improve behavioral symptoms.

For many patients, the symptomatic therapy of behavioral symptoms is unavoidable, especially if restlessness, aggressive behavior, and productive psychiatric symptoms become clinically prominent. In selected cases, sedative medications such as neuroleptics should be administered only short term and at the smallest dose possible.

Sedative drugs and antipsychotics have to be avoided for the treatment of behavioral symptoms.

Depression in Patients with Dementia

Patients with dementia often suffer from a depressive syndrome. Characteristically, at early stages of the disease, differentiation of depression from dementia can be challenging. Unfortunately, no large clinical trials exist for the treatment of depression with concurrent dementia as dementia usually represents an exclusion criterion in studies of antidepressants. The medical treatment thus focuses on pragmatic considerations. The benefit of antidepressants in dementia patients is uncertain. In addition to pharmaceutical treatment, an

Table 4 Pragmatic therapy of dementia-associated syndromes

Symptoms	Drug group/medications (FORTA classification)	Remarks
Depression	SSRI (e.g., citalopram/escitalopram, fluoxetin in usual dosages) (B)	
	Venlafaxine/duloxetine (B)	Useful for escalation after failure of SSRI, higher adverse event rate
	Nortriptyline (75–150 mg/day) (B)	Anticholinergic effects, adjust dose according to serum concentrations
	Mirtazapine (15–45 mg/day) (C)	In a recent study, both drugs have not been effective
	Sertraline (50–100 mg/day) (C)	
Psychosis	Haloperidol (start with 0.5 mg/day, up to 3 mg/day) (D)[a]	High rate of motor side effects
	Risperidone (start with 0.5–1 mg/day, max. 2 mg/day) (D)[a]	High rate of motor side effects
	Aripiprazole (2–15 mg/day) (D)[a]	
	Quetiapine (25–200 mg/day) (D)[a]	Low rate of motor side effects
	Clozapine (10–50 mg/day) (D)[a]	Lowest rate of motor side effects, particular prescription requirements apply
Restlessness, agitation	Risperidone (start with 0.5–1 mg/day, max. 2 mg/day) (D)[a]	High rate of motor side effects
	Quetiapine (25–200 mg/day) (D)[a]	
	Trazodone (50–200 mg/day) (C)[a]	
	Melperone (not FDA approved, 25–100 mg/day) (D)[a]	Motor side effects
Insomnia	Zopiclone (3.75–7.5 mg) (C)	Addictive potential
	Doxepin (25–50 mg) (C)	Anticholinergic side effects
	Mirtazapine (15–30 mg) (C)	
	Extended-release melatonin (2–4 mg) (C)	Not FDA approved, in the United States available as a supplement

FDA Food and Drug Administration, *FORTA* Fit for the Aged, *SSRI* selective serotonin reuptake inhibitor
[a]Due to cardiovascular and metabolic side effects and increased mortality, antipsychotics should not be prescribed to elderly people. This also holds true for sedatives due to the increased risk of falls. In emergency situations (delirium, restlessness, aggression, etc.), short-term administration is sometimes unavoidable

optimization of social aspects, especially regarding care and provision, should be sought.

Due to their pronounced anticholinergic and other systemic side effects, tricyclic antidepressants should be avoided in elderly patients. Serotonin reuptake inhibitors seem to be more appropriate (e.g., citalopram/escitalopram, fluoxetine). However, a recent controlled study did not show any beneficial effects of mirtazapine and sertraline in patients with depression in association with dementia but demonstrated an increased risk of adverse effects (Banerjee et al. 2011). As a consequence, these two substances should be avoided as well. If tricyclic antidepressants are prescribed, secondary amines (nortriptyline) should be preferred to other medications.

Generally, medications for elderly patients should be administered carefully at low doses. After 6–8 weeks, the effect and the indication of the antidepressant should be carefully examined, and if without measurable effect or in the presence of side effects, the medication should be discontinued.

Psychosis and Agitation

If in patients with marked subjective discomfort or with severe symptoms of psychosis or agitation medication is inevitable, antipsychotics with low or absent anticholinergic effects should be preferred. An actual overview of controlled studies on antipsychotics in dementia patients was given in the review by Schneider et al. (2006).

In recent years, antipsychotics, mainly atypical ones such as olanzapine and risperidone, have repeatedly been linked to increased mortality. The risk of cerebrovascular complications is particularly pronounced for olanzapine; this drug should thus be avoided in patients with dementia. Meta-analyses suggested a small but significant increase of mortality in dementia patients on antipsychotics (Herrmann and Lanctot 2005). This finding was clearly confirmed by a recent well-conducted controlled study Trial (Ballard et al. 2009). Presumably, in addition to cardiac side effects, a higher incidence of pneumonia contributes to the less-favorable prognosis of patients on antipsychotics (Trifiro et al. 2010). Therefore, a careful risk-benefit assessment for the application of these drugs is indispensable. Patients with cerebrovascular risk factors are of particular concern. However, the use of antipsychotics may reduce caregiver stress, and this certainly constitutes an important reason for their (probably too) frequent use. However, the use of antipsychotics in patients with dementia is generally not approved by the Food and Drug Administration (FDA).

Mortality is increased in dementia patients on atypical antipsychotics.

Older high-potency antipsychotics should also be avoided if possible in elderly patients as the rate of extrapyramidal and sedative adverse effects is increased in the elderly. If unavoidable, they should only be administered at the lowest possible doses (e.g., haloperidol; start with 0.5 mg/day up to 3 mg/day). Despite their association with increased mortality, many clinicians prefer atypical antipsychotics due to a generally more favorable side-effect profile. Risperidone is approved for this indication in several countries but not in the United States (start with 0.5–1 mg/day up to 2 mg/day). Quetiapine is an alternative, in particular, since extrapyramidal adverse effects are almost absent (start with 25 mg/day up to 200 mg/day). In dementia patients with psychotic symptoms, aripiprazole may also be administered at doses of 2–15 mg/day. In patients with Parkinson's disease or Parkinson syndromes due to other disorders, clozapine is administered at a low dosage of 10–50 mg/day. Quetiapine is an alternative due to its generally better tolerability, but its efficacy has not been well established for this indication. As mentioned, the use of antipsychotics in patients with dementia is off label but may be unavoidable in some patients.

In patients with psychosis in association with Parkinson's disease, low-dose clozapine is recommended.

Restlessness, Milling Around, and Disturbances of the Circadian Rhythm

Mainly in progressed states of the disease, the symptoms of restlessness, milling around, and circadian rhythm disturbances frequently occur. Besides the atypical antipsychotics (risperidone, start with 0.5–1 mg/day up to 3 mg/day; quetiapine, start with 25 mg/day up to 200 mg/day); melperone (start 25 mg/day up to 150 mg/day; not FDA approved) may be applied successfully if medication is unavoidable.

Benzodiazepines should be avoided due to the risk of falls and the addictive potency of this class of drugs. In patients in whom hypnotics are inevitable, an attempt with a nonbenzodiazepine benzodiazepine receptor agonist (e.g., eszopiclone up to 2 mg/day) or extended-release melantonin (2–4 mg/day; not FDA approved but available as a supplement in the United States) or ramelteon (8 mg) can be undertaken. In clinical practice, the sedative side effects of some antidepressants are utilized in some cases (e.g., 7.5–15 mg/day mirtazapine), although these drugs are only approved for depression but not for insomnia. In everyday practice, tri- or tetracyclic compounds such as trazodone, doxepine, or opipramol (not FDA labeled) are frequently prescribed, although these drugs have numerous adverse effects, mainly due to their anticholinergic properties. Moreover, these compounds are not approved for insomnia. In patients with predominant disturbances of the circadian rhythm and problems falling asleep, extended-release melatonin may also be tried (2–4 mg/day). Extended-release melatonin has the advantage of overall very good tolerability (Buscemi et al. 2006; Cardinali et al. 2002).

Benzodiazepines and other sedative drugs have to be avoided in patients with dementia.

Apathy

Apathy is one of the most frequent symptoms in patients with dementia. Many patients actually do not subjectively suffer from apathy. However, apathy typically contributes to caregiver stress. The differentiation to depression can be quite difficult. Large controlled studies for the treatment of apathy in patients with dementia do not exist. Smaller case studies and individual case reports suggest a positive effect of amantadine, amphetamines, bromocriptine, bupropion, methylphenidate, and selegiline (off-label use; Boyle and Malloy 2004). Several publications indicated the benefit of cholinergic therapy. Besides the initiation of an antidementive treatment, it may be useful to try to administer antidepressants with pronounced stimulatory effects (e.g., venlafaxine, citalopram/escitalopram, bupropion). As always when prescribing antidepressants, the risk-benefit ratio has to be critically reassessed after 6–8 weeks, particularly in the case of off-label use in demented patients with apathy. For the use of other drugs, the evidence accumulated so far is not sufficient to derive any recommendations.

Classification of Drugs for Prophylaxis and Therapy of Dementia According to Their Fitness for the Aged (FORTA)

In this classification of drugs for prophylaxis and therapy of dementia according to their Fitness for the Aged (FORTA), the same compounds may receive alternative marks if applied in different indications (see chapter "Critical Extrapolation of Guidelines and Study Results: Risk-Benefit Assessment for Patients with Reduced Life Expectancy and a New Classification of Drugs According to Their Fitness for the Aged").

Principle	Example	FORTA
Acetylcholinesterase inhibitors	Donepezil	B
	Galantamine	B
	Rivastigmine	B
	Tacrine	—
NMDA-(glutamate-) antagonist	Memantine	B
Calcium channel blocker	Nimodipine	C

(continued)

Antioxidants, antiplatelet drugs	Gingko biloba	C
α-Adrenergic and 5-HT agonist	Ergoline derivates	C
Antioxidants	Piracetam	C
Influence on cerebral metabolism	Pyritinol	C
Antioxidants	Vitamin E, selenium, vitamin C, etc.	C
Diverse phytotherapeutics	Ginseng preparations	C
Hormone preparations	DHEA, testosterone	C
MAO inhibitor	Selegiline	C
Antiphlogistics	Indomethacin	D
Cholesterol reduction	Statins	C
Chelating agent	Desferrioxamine	D

DHEA dehydroepiandrosterone, *MAO* monoamine oxidase, *NMDA* N-methyl-D-aspartate

References

Aarsland D, Andersen K, Larsen JP, Lolk A, Kragh-Sorensen P (2003) Prevalence and characteristics of dementia in Parkinson disease: an 8-year prospective study. Arch Neurol 60:387–392

Aarsland D, Ballard C, Walker Z et al (2009) Memantine in patients with Parkinson's disease dementia or dementia with Lewy bodies: a double-blind, placebo-controlled, multicentre trial. Lancet Neurol 8:613–618

Adler G, Teufel M, Drach LM (2003) Pharmacological treatment of frontotemporal dementia: treatment response to the MAO-A inhibitor moclobemide. Int J Geriatr Psychiatry 18:653–655

Andersen-Ranberg K, Vasegaard L, Jeune B (2001) Dementia is not inevitable: a population-based study of Danish centenarians. J Gerontol B Psychol Sci Soc Sci 56:152–159

Atri A, Shaughnessy LW, Locascio JJ, Growdon JH (2008) Longterm course and effectiveness of combination therapy in Alzheimer disease. Alzheimer Dis Assoc Disord 22:209–221

Ballard C, Hanney ML, Theodoulou M et al (2009) The dementia antipsychotic withdrawal trial (DART-AD): long-term follow-up of a randomised placebo-controlled trial. Lancet Neurol 8:151–157

Ballard C, Gauthier S, Corbett C, Aarsland D, Jones E (2011) Alzheimer's disease. Lancet 377:1019–1031

Banerjee S, Hellier J, Dewey M et al (2011) Sertraline or mirtazapine for depression in dementia (HTA-SADD): a randomised, multicentre, double-blind, placebo-controlled trial. Lancet 378:403–411

Bowler JV (2005) Vascular cognitive impairment. J Neurol Neurosurg Psychiatry 76(Suppl 5):v35–v44

Boyle PA, Malloy PF (2004) Treating apathy in Alzheimer's disease. Dement Geriatr Cogn Disord 17:91–99

Burns A, Bernabei R, Bullock R et al (2009) Safety and efficacy of galantamine (reminyl) in severe Alzheimer's disease (the SERAD study): a randomized, placebo-controlled, double blind trial. Lancet Neurol 8:39–47

Buscemi N, Vandermeer B, Hooton N et al (2006) Efficacy and safety of exogenous melatonin for secondary sleep disorders and sleep disorders accompanying sleep restriction: meta-analysis. BMJ 332:385–393

Camicioli R, Fisher N (2004) Progress in clinical neurosciences: Parkinson's disease with dementia and dementia with Lewy bodies. Can J Neurol Sci 31:7–21

Cardinali DP, Brusco LI, Liberczuk C, Furio AM (2002) The use of melatonin in Alzheimer's disease. Neuro Endocrinol Lett 23(Suppl 1):20–23

Craig D, Birks J (2005) Rivastigmine for vascular cognitive impairment. Cochrane Database Syst Rev 2: CD004744

Craig D, Birks J (2006) Galantamine for vascular cognitive impairment. Cochrane Database Syst Rev 1: CD004746

Cummings J, Jones R, Wilkinson D et al (2010) Effect of donepezil on cognition in severe Alzheimer's disease: a pooled data analysis. J Alzheimers Dis 21:843–851

Davies NM, Kehoe PG, Ben-Shlomo Y, Martin YM (2011) Association of anti-hypertensive treatments with Alzheimer's disease, vascular dementia, and other dementias. J Alzheimers Dis 26:699–708

Doody RS, Geldmacher DS, Gordon B et al (2001) Open-label, multicenter, phase 3 extension study of the safety and efficacy of donepezil in patients with Alzheimer's disease. Arch Neurol 58:427–433

Emre M, Aarsland D, Albanese A et al (2004) Rivastigmine for dementia associated with Parkinson's disease. N Engl J Med 351:2509–2518

Emre M, Tsolaki M, Bonuccelli U et al (2010) Memantine for patients with Parkinson's disease dementia or dementia with Lewy bodies: a randomised, double-blind, placebo-controlled trial. Lancet Neurol 9:969–977

European Medicines Agency (2009) Committee for medicinal products for human use. Guidelines on medicinal products for the treatment of Alzheimer's disease and other dementias. http://www.ema.europa.eu/pdfs/human/ewp/055395en.pdf. Accessed 11 Jan 2010

Ferri CP, Prince M, Brayne C et al (2005) Global prevalence of dementia: a Delphi consensus study. Lancet 366:2112–2117

Fuchs GA, Gemende I, Herting B et al (2004) Dementia in idiopathic Parkinson's syndrome. J Neurol 251(Suppl 6):VI/28–VI/32

Gardette V, Andieu S, Lapeyre-Mestre M et al (2010) Predictive factors of discontinuation and switch of choline esterase inhibitors in community-dwelling patients with Alzheimer's disease: a 2-year prospective, multicentre, cohort study. CNS Drugs 24:431–442

Getsios D, Blume S, Ishak KJ et al (2010) Cost effectiveness of donepezil in the treatment of mild to moderate Alzheimer's disease: a U.K. evaluation using discrete-event simulation. Pharmacoeconomics 28:411–427

Hansen RA, Gartlehner G, Webb AP et al (2008) Efficacy and safety of donepezil, galantamine, and rivastigmine for the treatment of Alzheimer's disease: a systematic review and meta-analysis. Clin Interv Aging 3: 211–225

Herrmann N, Lanctot KL (2005) Do atypical antipsychotics cause stroke? CNS Drugs 19:91–103

Hogan DB (2006) Donepezil for severe Alzheimer's disease. Lancet 367:1031–1032

Hogan DB, Patterson C (2002) Progress in clinical neurosciences: treatment of Alzheimer's disease and other dementias—review and comparison of the cholinesterase inhibitors. Can J Neurol Sci 29:306–314

Hogan DB, Goldlist B, Naglie G, Patterson C (2004) Comparison studies of cholinesterase inhibitors for Alzheimer's disease. Lancet Neurol 3:622–626

Kavirajan H, Schneider LS (2007) Efficacy and adverse effects of cholinesterase inhibitors and memantine in vascular dementia: a meta-analysis of randomised controlled trials. Lancet Neurol 6:782–792

Kiencke P, Daniel D, Grimm C, Rychlik R (2011) Direct costs of Alzheimer's disease in Germany. Eur J Health Econ 12:533–539

Lobo A, Launer LJ, Fratiglioni L et al (2000) Prevalence of dementia and major subtypes in Europe: a collaborative study of population-based cohorts. Neurologic diseases in the elderly research group. Neurology 54: S4–S9

Lopez OL, Becker JT, Wahed AS et al (2009) Long-term effects of the concomitant use of memantine with cholinesterase inhibition in Alzheimer disease. J Neurol Neurosurg Psychiatry 80:600–607

Maidment I, Fox C, Boustani M (2006) Cholinesterase inhibitors for Parkinson's disease dementia. Cochrane Database Syst Rev 1:004747

McKeith IG, Dickson DW, Lowe J et al (2005) Diagnosis and management of dementia with Lewy bodies: third report of the DLB Consortium. Neurology 65:1863–1872

Neary D, Snowden J, Mann D (2005) Frontotemporal dementia. Lancet Neurol 4:771–780

Ott A, Breteler MM, van Harskamp F, Stijnen T, Hofman A (1998) Incidence and risk of dementia. The Rotterdam Study. Am J Epidemiol 147:574–580

Reitz C, Brayne C, Mayeux R (2011) Epidemiology of Alzheimer disease. Nat Rev Neurol 7:137–152

Roman GC, Salloway S, Black SE et al (2010) Randomized, placebo-controlled, clinical trial of donepezil in vascular dementia: differential effects by hippocampal size. Stroke 41:1213–1321

Samuel W, Caligiuri M, Galasko D et al (2000) Better cognitive and psychopathologic response to donepezil in patients prospectively diagnosed as dementia with

Lewy bodies: a preliminary study. Int J Geriatr Psychiatry 15:794–802

Schneider LS, Dagerman K, Insel PS (2006) Efficacy and adverse effects of atypical antipsychotics for dementia: meta-analysis of randomized, placebo-controlled trials. Am J Geriatr Psychiatry 14:191–210

Schneider LS, Dagerman KS, Higgins JP, McShane R (2011) Lack of evidence for the efficacy of memantine in mild Alzheimer disease. Arch Neurol 68:991–998

Snitz BE, O'Meara ES, Carlson MC, Ginkgo Evaluation of Memory (GEM) Study Investigators et al (2009) Ginkgo biloba for preventing cognitive decline in older adults: a randomized trial. JAMA 302:2663–2670

Tariot PN, Farlow MR, Grossberg GT et al (2004) Memantine treatment in patients with moderate to severe Alzheimer disease already receiving donepezil: a randomized controlled trial. JAMA 291:317–324

Trifiro G, Gambassi G, Sen EF et al (2010) Association of community-acquired pneumonia with antipsychotic drug use in elderly patients: a nested case-control study. Ann Intern Med 152:418–425

Wehling M, Groth H (2011) Challenges of longevity in developed countries: vascular prevention of dementia as an immediate clue to tackle an upcoming medical, social and economic stretch. Neurodegener Dis 8:275–282

Winblad B, Kilander L, Eriksson S et al (2006) Donepezil in patients with severe Alzheimer's disease: double-blind, parallel group, placebo-controlled study. Lancet 367:1057–1065

Depression

Stefan Schwarz and Lutz Frölich

Relevance for Elderly Patients, Epidemiology

Depression in older people often presents with atypical symptoms. In the elderly, depression is frequently associated with physical and cognitive impairment. Compared with younger patients, older patients experiencing a depressive episode often show predominantly somatic symptoms. They frequently mislead physicians to concentrate initially on patients' organic symptoms in particular if the patient has no history of psychiatric disorders.

Older persons often refuse to accept the fact that they are suffering from depression. Among elderly individuals, the diagnosis of depression, and other mental disorders in general, is often met with considerable negative prejudice. In everyday life, this attitude often causes elderly patients to reject the diagnosis of depression vehemently. Instead of undergoing psychiatric treatment, elderly patients with depression frequently continue to request additional diagnostic procedures for suspected somatic disease and insist on extended medical treatment of their organic symptoms. As older people in particular refrain from the consultation of psychiatrists when suffering from depressive symptoms, general practitioners play an important role in diagnosing depressive disorders.

In the elderly, the clinical picture of depression is often primarily characterized by somatic symptoms.

Due to the aforementioned factors, the diagnosis of depression in older patients is typically delayed, and adequate treatment frequently is initiated rather late in the course of the disease. Particularly in the presence of an organic illness that is associated with pain, physical disability, or cognitive impairment, the possibility of comorbid depression is frequently overlooked. Keeping this in mind, it is of utmost importance to consider the differential diagnosis of depression early on when treating older patients with unexplained physical ailments or otherwise inexplicable symptoms.

Older patients frequently suffer from a number of disorders. Faced with this situation, geriatric specialists or general practitioners often do not focus on the patient's depression but concentrate primarily on the organic disorder relating to their specialty. In addition, the argument that the patient's depression is related to the patient's organic disorder and advanced age and is, thus, certainly understandable or even "normal" is often cited. This attitude is false and misleading as it denies the need for treatment and thereby precludes any chance for therapeutic success. This therapeutic nihilism is in clear contradiction to the fact that the majority of older patients clearly benefit from appropriate treatment, as do younger patients.

S. Schwarz (✉) · L. Frölich
Central Institute of Mental Health, Medical Faculty Mannheim/Heidelberg University, Square J 5, 68159 Mannheim, Germany
e-mail: stefan.schwarz@zi-mannheim.de; lutz.froelich@zi-mannheim.de

M. Wehling (ed.), *Drug Therapy for the Elderly*,
DOI 10.1007/978-3-7091-0912-0_16, © Springer-Verlag Wien 2013

In elderly patients, depression is frequently overlooked, diagnosed with considerable delay, and treated inadequately.

Regarding patients' quality of life depression often plays an important role which in fact may be by far more prominent than somatic/organic disorders. In addition to having an impact on patients' quality of life, depression promotes social isolation, inactivity, and dependence.

At any age, depression is the most common cause for suicide. In elderly people, the suicide rate increases with advancing age; overall, the suicide rate among older persons is approximately twice that of adults of middle age. Studies of suicide in the elderly clearly point to the importance of the diagnosis of depression: More than three quarters of all older persons who commit suicide had visited their family physician during the month preceding their suicide (Hawton and van Heeringen 2009). The majority of these patients had experienced a depressive episode that had either not been recognized or inadequately treated.

Suicide rates strongly increase in older age. Depression is the most common cause for suicide.

Despite the particular circumstances and manifestations of depression in the elderly, there are no established age-specific diagnostic criteria thus far (see "Summary" that follows).

Criteria for Major Depressive Episodes (Diagnostic Criteria After the *Diagnostic and Statistical Manual of Mental Disorders*)

The criteria for major depressive episodes, modeled after the criteria in the fourth edition of the *Diagnostic and Statistical Manual of Mental Disorders* (*DSM-IV*; 1994) as follows:
A. Five (or more) of the following symptoms have been present during the same 2-week period and represent a change from previous functioning; at least one of the symptoms is either (1) depressed mood or (2) loss of interest or pleasure:

1. Depressed mood most of the day, nearly every day as indicated by either subjective report (e.g., feels sad or empty) or observation made by others (e.g., appears tearful)
2. Markedly diminished interest or pleasure in all, or almost all, activities most of the day, nearly every day
3. Significant weight loss when not dieting or weight gain (e.g., a change of more than 5% of body weight in a month) or decrease or increase in appetite nearly every day
4. Insomnia or hypersomnia nearly every day
5. Psychomotor agitation or retardation nearly every day
6. Fatigue or loss of energy nearly every day
7. Feeling of worthlessness or excessive or inappropriate guilt (which may be delusional) nearly every day (not merely self-reproach or guilt about being sick)
8. Diminished ability to think or concentrate, or indecisiveness, nearly every day
9. Recurrent thoughts of death (not just fear of dying), recurrent suicidal ideation without a specific plan, or a suicide attempt or a specific plan for committing suicide

B. The symptoms do not meet criteria for a mixed episode (i.e., symptoms of both mania and depression)
C. The symptoms cause clinically significant distress or impairment in social, occupational, or other important areas of functioning
D. The symptoms are not due to the direct physiological effects of a substance (e.g., a drug of abuse, a medication) or a general medical condition (e.g., hypothyroidism)
E. The symptoms are not better accounted for by bereavement (i.e., after the loss of a loved one), the symptoms persist for longer than 2 months or are characterized by marked functional impairment, morbid preoccupation with worthlessness, suicidal ideation, psychotic symptoms, or psychomotor retardation

Geriatricians, internists, or general practitioners should be able to diagnose depressive episodes in uncomplicated cases with a sufficient degree of certainty and thus initiate adequate treatment. For the confirmation of the diagnosis and for differential treatment indications in complicated cases, or, at the latest, when initial treatment approaches fail, patients with a clinically relevant depression should be seen by a psychiatrist. In addition to depressive episodes and recurrent affective disorders, there are a number of related psychiatric disorders, such as dysthymia, mixed states occurring under the influence of premorbid personality disorders, or adjustment disorders, that require differential treatment strategies and are not always easy to diagnose.

A major diagnostic problem is the use of psychometric scales, which had generally been developed for and evaluated in young adults without organic comorbidity. With some of these scales, for example, symptoms of organic disorders such as apathy or weight loss frequently found in elderly persons may easily be misinterpreted as signs of depression. Although specific scales for diagnosing depression in older persons are available that properly address these problems, most clinical studies still use the more common scales that fail to take the specific issues of older people into account.

Prior to psychiatric treatment, possible organic causes of depression must always be ruled out or treated (see the "Summary" that follows).

Frequent Organic Causes or Cofactors of Depression (Selection)

- Medication
  - Sedatives, hypnotics, antipsychotics
  - Opiates
  - Beta-blockers
  - Clonidine
  - Anti-Parkinson drugs
  - Steroids
  - Antiestrogenes/antiandrogens
  - Interferons
- Viral infection
- Tumors
- General weakness, cachexia, weight loss
- Cerebrovascular disorders
  - Stroke
  - Vascular encephalopathy

- Neurodegenerative disorders
  - Parkinson's disease
  - Dementias
- Metabolic disorders
  - Malnutrition
  - Vitamin B deficiency
- Endocrine disorders
  - Thyroid hypo- or hyperfunction
  - Hyperparathyroidism
  - Cushing's syndrome
- Alcohol addiction and other addiction disorders.

Frequent causes or cofactors of depression particularly in the elderly:
- Hypothyreosis
- Stroke
- Malnutrition
- Vitamin B deficiency
- Various medications that can cause or increase a depressive syndrome.

Organic causes or cofactors of depression are frequently found in older patients and have to be carefully ruled out.

Prevalence figures on depression in older age vary greatly. This is mainly due to methodological aspects as the different studies employed varying diagnostic procedures and criteria. It is therefore not surprising that data on the point prevalence of major depression in persons older than 65 years of age range from 1% to 20% (Alexopoulos 2005). Compared to younger adults, the entire group of older persons has a lower incidence of depression; persons aged 75 + years, however, show a marked increase of the incidence of depression. This is most likely due to organic comorbidity, loss of socioeconomic status, and impaired cognitive abilities. As an additional important stress factor, the loss of the spouse or life partner is a frequent event in this age group, particularly for older women, who generally outlive their partners.

Compared to major depression, an equally large or even larger number of individuals present with subsyndromal and "minor depression," being at great risk for developing a major depressive episode in the near future (Meeks et al. 2011; Heok and Ho 2008). In addition, the proportion of older patients with recurrent unipolar or bipolar depression is steadily increasing due to the increasing life expectancy.

Thus far, studies have not been able to provide unanimously accepted data on the prevalence of depression among the elderly. Investigations on the topic consistently show that depression represents an important health problem for a large subgroup of older persons in the general population, but also that this is even more relevant for patients in hospitals, nursing homes, or other institutions.

Therapeutically Relevant Special Features of Elderly Patients

It is of particular importance for older patients that successful treatment not only will improve individual health and quality of life while lowering suicide rates, but also will have an attenuating effect for family members and other caregivers and will lower the overall medical costs in this population (Alexopoulos et al. 2001).

Treatment goals are thus:
1. Improving depressive symptoms
2. Preventing relapse
3. Improving quality of life and level of functioning
4. Improving overall health and particularly patient mortality
5. Reducing health care costs.

In the elderly, the treatment of depression follows the same basic rules that apply for younger adults.

In principle, the treatment of depression in the elderly follows the guidelines established for treating depression in general. There are, however, several aspects that are of particular importance when treating older people:
– Older patients are frequently multimorbid, which may have a negative effect on the tolerability of antidepressants.
– Many older patients take other medication that may interact with antidepressants.

– The pharmacokinetic and toxic properties of antidepressants may be different in older patients.
– Stress factors beyond patients' control, such as reduced physical and mental abilities, social descent, as well as somatic comorbidity, are frequent problems and complicate treatment success.

Translating the results of clinical studies on depression treatment in younger adults to older people poses a problem as most clinical trials on antidepressants explicitly exclude patients with comorbidity. Many clinical trials of antidepressants even explicitly excluded older persons to keep the risk of complications as low as possible. To date, sufficient data on pharmacokinetics and drug tolerance with special reference to older patients are limited. As a consequence, current therapy guidelines for depression barely differentiate treatment of younger adults from that of the large group of geriatric patients. Therapeutic recommendations for antidepressant treatment of older persons are thus largely based on cohort studies, which are hardly representative of geriatric patients, originate from unproven theoretical considerations, or reflect small, methodologically vulnerable studies and the personal clinical experiences of investigators.

Most clinical studies of the effectiveness of antidepressants were conducted in young, healthy adults. Translating their results to the treatment of geriatric patients is thus highly problematic.

Pharmacotherapy of Geriatric Depression

The benefits of antidepressant drug therapy have clearly been demonstrated for moderate-to-severe major depression, and the clinical relevance of this therapeutic effect has been unanimously recognized. In contrast, clinical studies have not been able to show unambiguous advantages of antidepressive pharmacotherapy compared to placebo in mild depression (Kirsch et al. 2008). These findings are in sharp opposition to the fact that the biggest share of antidepressants is prescribed to patients with mild depression, although beneficial effects are not well established in this patient group. Particularly for older patients, it thus holds that in minor depression pharmacological therapy with antidepressants is generally not indicated.

However, pharmacotherapy of depression is only one component within the overall treatment strategy, which always also has to take social aspects into consideration and should include psychotherapeutic treatment approaches in many patients. To simply prescribe antidepressants to most patients as solitary treatment intervention does not represent adequate treatment of their depressive episode.

Pharmacotherapy of geriatric depression constitutes an important aspect of treatment that, however, has always to take social and psychological measures into consideration as well.

In the elderly, benefits of psychotherapy are also well documented (Pinquart et al. 2007), with treatment effects being at least equal to those achieved with pharmacotherapy alone (Pinquart et al. 2006). For this group of patients, behavioral or cognitive therapies are generally preferred over analytical psychotherapeutic approaches. For minor depressive episodes, treatment with psychotherapy alone is frequently effective and sufficient. Combination of medication and psychotherapy is more effective in major depressive episodes than treatment with pharmacotherapy or psychotherapy alone.

In patients with major, therapy-resistant depression, treatment with electroconvulsive therapy (ECT) may be indicated. However, ECT may also be discussed in patients for whom antidepressants are contraindicated or who require complex combination therapies. Contrary to the frequently voiced prejudice that ECT poses a risk to patients, this approach is in fact very safe even in older patients and represents the treatment of choice in selected patients with comorbidities given the potential side effects of antidepressants (Tess and Smetana 2009; Hausner et al. 2011). Under the following circumstances, ECT may be indicated:

– Depression with psychotic symptoms
– Therapy-resistant, major depression
– Continued risk for suicide
– Life-threatening malnutrition caused by insufficient food or fluid intake due to depression.

Major concerns about ECT in elderly individuals are transient disturbances of episodic memory and other cognitive symptoms (Goodman 2011). However, ECT may be safely performed even in patients with mild cognitive impairment or mild dementia (Hausner et al. 2011). Repetitive transcranial magnetic stimulation (rTMS) may constitute an alternative to ECT with fewer cognitive side effects and better tolerability. However, clinical experience in elderly patients is limited for this method (Jalenques et al. 2010).

In the elderly, depressive episodes are frequently caused or sustained by external factors such as somatic disorders, pain, social isolation, or financial problems. Any thorough medical history must aim at identifying these aspects of depression. In many patients, depressive symptoms subside surprisingly fast whenever the underlying problem can be solved in cooperation with family members, experts from other disciplines, or where applicable, by improving the social conditions or nursing care.

Evidence-Based, Rationalistic Drug Therapy and Classification of Drugs According to Their Fitness for the Aged (FORTA)

Drug Groups and Their Efficacy at Old Age

Antidepressants belong to a heterogeneous group of psychotropic drugs that act on different symptoms of depression. From a psychiatric point of view, the substances are preferably grouped according to their point of action in the central nervous system; the more traditional classification according to their chemical structure is nonetheless still used in everyday practice.

Definite proof pointing to the superior efficacy of a particular group of compounds has not been demonstrated thus far. However, drugs not only differ with regard to their pharmacological efficacy but also show substantially distinct patterns of adverse effects. Thus, comorbidity and individual indications and contraindications play an important role for the choice of an antidepressant (Bauer et al. 2007).

In general, antidepressants are associated with many adverse outcomes, including falls, hyponatremia, fractures, and seizures, all of which are especially relevant for the elderly. Therefore, the risks and benefits of different antidepressants should be carefully evaluated when these substances are prescribed to elderly patients (Coupland et al. 2011). However, due to considerable methodological problems of most studies linking antidepressants with many adverse outcomes, it is often unclear if the relationship between adverse outcome and antidepressant use is causal.

The present chapter cannot offer a complete presentation of the numerous individual antidepressants. Reference compounds of the individual drug groups are listed in Table 1. The selection of these reference compounds is based on their prescription rate in geriatric patients and not on scientific data; that is to say, that drugs not explicitly listed in the table are not necessarily inferior.

Selective Serotonin Reuptake Inhibitors

The selective serotonin reuptake inhibitors (SSRIs; e.g., sertraline, citalopram/escitalopram, fluoxetine, fluvoxamine, paroxetine) represent a heterogeneous group of drugs whose common main effect is the inhibition of serotonin reuptake at the synaptic cleft, thus increasing the effect of serotonin. In addition to their serotonergic main effect, some drugs have an impact on other transmitter systems, explaining different tolerability spectra.

Most authors consider SSRIs as antidepressants of first choice in older patients based on their relatively good tolerability (Rodda et al. 2011). There are, however, only a few studies comparing antidepressants from different groups particularly in older persons with depression. Thus, the claimed superiority of SSRIs in terms of associated side effects is based on experience and theoretical considerations rather than conclusive data. A Cochrane review concluded that

SSRIs and tricyclic antidepressants have similar efficacy, but tricyclic drugs were associated with more adverse effects (Mottram et al. 2006). Data from recent studies and meta-analyses, however, no longer support the view that SSRs are superior to older tricyclic antidepressants with respect to efficacy as well as tolerability (Kok et al. 2011; Gribbin et al. 2011; Coupland et al. 2011).

Due to their supposedly favorable tolerability, SSRIs are the drug group of first choice in older patients.

Within the group of SSRIs, there is no clear preference. Citalopram and the S-enantiomer escitalopram, both with highly selective serotonergic action, and sertraline, which also has a dopaminergic component, are the drugs most frequently used in elderly patients. Among SSRI treatment, costs are highest for escitalopram; cheaper generic drugs are available for all other drugs. The advantage of escitalopram over citalopram is disputed and arguably does not justify the substantial difference in costs.

Serious, life-threatening adverse effects under SSRIs are rare. Even after ingestion of extremely high doses in attempted suicides, there are generally no life-threatening complications. Adverse effects urging patients to discontinue medication predominantly produce unspecific symptoms, such as

– Gastrointestinal intolerance
– Sleep disorders
– Anxiety
– Dizziness
– Headaches.

The potentially life-threatening serotonergic syndrome represents a serious, however very rare complication, which is primarily seen almost only with combination therapy. Very frequent side effects are reduced libido and erectile dysfunction, which patients often do not report. Accordingly, physicians must explicitly ask patients about these possible adverse effects.

SSRIs frequently cause hyponatremia, which in turn may cause patients to stop this medication. Particularly older patients are prone to experience this side effect, especially in the presence of diuretics, which is very common in this age group. After several weeks of medication

Table 1 Antidepressants (ADs) frequently used for the treatment of older patients

Compounds	Compound group	Dosages used for older patients	FORTA	Comments
Sertraline	Serotonin reuptake inhibitor	50 mg, possible dose increase to 150 mg	B	Low interaction potential. Good tolerability. Hyponatremia possible
Citalopram	Serotonin reuptake inhibitor	20 mg (maximum dose in persons > 60 years)	B	Low interaction potential. Good tolerability. Hyponatremia possible. Contraindications: Heart failure, bradyarrhyhtmia
Escitalopram	Serotonin reuptake inhibitor	10 mg	B	S-Enantiomer of citalopram. Greater efficacy compared with citalopram is disputed. Costs considerably higher compared with citalopram generics
Nortriptyline	Tricyclic AD	Initially 3 × 10 mg, slow dose increase to 75–150 mg	C	Numerous contraindications. Anticholinergic effects. Assessment of serum concentrations after reaching the steady state (60–120 µg/l). ECG controls
Mirtazapine	Noradrenergic and serotonergic AD	15 mg, possible dose increase to 45 mg	C	Sedative side effects. Weight increase. Frequent orthostatic dysregulation
Venlafaxine	Serotonin/norepinephrine reuptake inhibitor	Initially 25–75 mg, dose increase to 75–225 mg/day	C	Frequent gastrointestinal side effects. Sleep disorders and anxiety. Blood pressure increase possible. Frequent hyponatremia
Duloxetine	Serotonin/norepinephrine reuptake inhibitor	Initially 30 mg/day, dose increase to 60–120 mg	C	Frequent gastrointestinal side effects, insomnia, and anxiety. Blood pressure increase possible. Possible advantages in cases with associated pain symptoms
Moclobemide	MAO inhibitor	2 × 150 mg, possible dose increase to 600 mg/day	C	No combination with SSRI and other serotonergic substances
Reboxetine	Norepinephrine reuptake inhibitor	2 × 2 mg, possible dose increase to 10 mg	D	Not FDA approved. Frequent tachycardia, dry mouth, in male patients urinary retention. Dose reductions in patients with kidney and liver failure. Risk-benefit ratio unfavorable
Bupropion	Norepinephrine/dopamine reuptake inhibitor	150 mg/day, possible dose increase to 300 mg/day	C	Frequent blood pressure increase, regular blood pressure controls necessary. Increased risk for epileptic seizures
Agomelatine	Melatonergic and serotonergic AD	25 mg at night, possible dose increase to 50 mg	–	Not FDA approved. Drug with good tolerability. Possible advantages in patients with associated sleep disorders. To date no extensive experience with older patients, thus no classification is given

The listed reference compounds are those frequently used in everyday clinical practice for the treatment of depression in elderly patients. Their greater efficacy in comparison to substances not listed here has not been shown. The references concerning their FORTA classification refer to moderate-to-severe depressive episodes. With mild depressive episodes, all drugs receive the FORTA classification C.

ECG electrocardiogram, *FDA* Food and Drug Administration, *FORTA* Fit for the Aged, *MAO* monoamine oxidase, *SSRI* selective serotonin reuptake inhibitor.

with SSRIs or with the onset of related clinical symptoms, determination of patients' serum sodium levels is mandatory.

Hyponatremia is a frequent complication associated with SSRIs.

Several SSRIs impair glucose tolerance, although this rarely poses a clinically relevant problem. In particular in overdose, QT interval prolongation has been associated with use of citalopram and other SSRIs. Because of post-marketing reports of QT interval prolongation and Torsade de Pointes associated with Citalopram, the FDA recently issued a Drug Safety Communication warning against the use of Citalopram in persons with heart failure or bradyarrhythmia and limited the maximum dose of Citalopram in persons over 60 years of age to 20 mg/d. However, the risk of a clinically relevant long-QT syndrome from SSRI use seems to be small (Alvarez and Pahissa 2010).

Compared with other antidepressants, SSRIs show a small interaction potential with other drugs. Due to the risk of developing a serotonergic syndrome, comedication with monoamine oxidase (MAO) inhibitors is strictly contraindicated. Comedication with lithium also increases this risk, but to a much smaller extent.

An important advantage of SSRIs is the fact that there is no need for intricate dose adjustments since most SSRIs can be started with their respective therapeutic dose. SSRIs are generally taken in the morning in a single dose. Unspecific withdrawal symptoms only occur after long-term use and are rarely clinically relevant. In case of SSRI intolerance or lack of efficacy, serum levels should be determined as there are strong interindividual differences in the metabolism of SSRIs.

Tri- and Tetracyclic Antidepressants

Tricyclic antidepressants are imipramine derivatives whose chemical structure is characterized by three rings of atoms. The different side chains explain differences in efficacy and tolerability. Today, tetracyclic antidepressants (e.g., mianserine, maprotilin) are hardly ever the drug of first choice. Although based on its chemical structure mirtazapine also belongs to the group of tetracyclic antidepressants, it is rarely listed in this group due to its different pharmacological profile.

Overall, the antidepressive effect of tricyclic antidepressants is well documented. There are in fact several studies indicating that their therapeutic efficacy is superior to that of newer antidepressants.

As with all antidepressants, the onset of the therapeutic effect of tri- and tetracyclic antidepressants is delayed by 2–3 weeks.

Tricyclic antidepressants are associated with several adverse effects that render them less desirable particularly for use in older patients. Most relevant side effects are caused by their strong anticholinergic and $\alpha 1$-adrenergic actions.

Among the elderly, the susceptibility for peripheral and central anticholinergic symptoms is increased due to the degenerative decrease in cholinergic reserves associated with advanced age, explaining the increased tendency for anticholinergic side effects in this age group. In older patients, anticholinergic side effects in fact often already occur with standard dosages and at relatively low serum levels.

The most important cardiac adverse effect is the slowing of cardiac conduction. Preexisting bradycardia, prolongation of the QT_c interval, and comedication with QT_c-prolonging drugs thus represent important contraindications. In general, any preexisting cardiac damage represents a relative contraindication, substantially limiting the use of this drug group in the elderly. As therapy with tricyclic antidepressants may increase the risk for cardiac infarction, a thorough cardiac workup is mandatory before beginning treatment with tricyclic antidepressants and needs to be repeated after several weeks of medication. Special attention should be paid to QT_c intervals in the course of treatment and possible tachycardia, which is frequently caused by the α-adrenergic effect of tricyclic antidepressants.

Another age-related anticholinergic complication is urinary bladder dysfunction, particularly in older men with preexisting prostate hypertrophy. Erectile dysfunction and impotence are frequent adverse side effects.

As with many other antidepressants, tricyclic antidepressants are associated with substantial weight gain.

Within the central nervous system, the anticholinergic effect of tricyclic antidepressants may increase cognitive deficits. This is a frequent observation in patients with Alzheimer's dementia or mild cognitive impairment (MCI). Independent of cognitive deficits, patients frequently experience sedative effects, which may be desirable in patients with agitated depression or insomnia but are seen as adverse effects in other patients, triggering the discontinuation of the medication. With some patients, and as a rule in association with overdoses, tricyclic antidepressants may cause mental confusion or delirious states.

Particularly in older patients, orthostatic dysregulation is a frequent finding especially at the beginning of treatment. Due to this effect, doses of tricyclic antidepressants must be increased slowly. Typically, patients initially receive 25 mg/day before slowly increasing to effective doses of 100–150 mg/day. With older patients, the target dose should be reached after 7–14 days depending on how well the drug is tolerated. Faster dose increases very often lead to intolerable side effects and discontinuation of therapy.

Due to numerous side effects, tricyclic antidepressants are only second-choice medications in older people.

The therapeutic index of tricyclic antidepressants is narrow. Especially in the elderly, anticholinergic side effects in the central nervous system are frequently already seen at therapeutic doses. Thus, great care must be exercised to assess and promote patients' compliance, which is often poor among older patients. In association with accidental overdoses or overdoses with suicidal intention, patients quickly suffer life-threatening cardiac arrhythmias, agitation, delirium, and epileptic seizures. Such toxic doses are often lethal despite adequate intensive medical care, and triyclic antidepressants are among the most frequent drugs to cause lethal intoxications, both incidental and intentional ones.

Due to the danger of overdosage, serum concentrations should be assessed after reaching the steady state or in case of suspected overdose.

These limitations and associated risks render the use of tricyclic antidepressants in older patients problematic. Yet, there are no sound head-to-head studies comparing the tolerability of early and modern antidepressants in older patients to prove superiority. For some drug groups, however, such as SSRIs, clinical experience from daily practice suggests this to be the case even if large clinical studies are missing to confirm this observation. Surprisingly, however, studies of patients with depression in association with Parkinson's disease found no difference in the rate of adverse side effects between nortriptyline and sertraline.

In clinical practice, tricyclic antidepressants are generally only used second line when other medications have failed. Since nortriptyline has relatively fewer anticholinergic and α1-adrenergic effects, it is favored for use in older patients (Bondareff et al. 2000). As in older patients the bulk of available data is on nortriptyline, meta-analyses have advocated this compound if a tricyclic antidepressant is needed.

Nortriptyline offers the best tolerability of all tricyclic antidepressants in the elderly.

In a number of countries, general practitioners frequently prescribe opipramol (not FDA approved) to treat depression. As this drug produces all side effects tricyclic antidepressants have and is not approved for the treatment of depression, it cannot be recommended in this context.

Occasionally, the sedative side effect of tricyclic antidepressants (e.g., doxepin, opipramol, trimipramine) at low doses is utilized to treat sleep disorders. As more tolerable hypnotics are available, this practice is disadvantageous, particularly in older patients.

Mirtazapine

Mirtazapine is a noradrenergic and serotonergic antidepressant with α2-adrenoreceptor antagonistic action. Its efficacy in moderate-to-major depression is well documented. Compared with other antidepressants, the risk of sexual dysfunction is lower. Due to its sedative effect, mirtazapine is frequently used in patients with insomnia or for treating patients with agitated depression. Unfortunately, it is generally associated with increased appetite, impaired glucose tolerance, and weight gain, which is quite problematic particularly with long-term use. A rare complication is the reversible bone marrow depression caused by mirtazapine. Patients with severe liver and kidney dysfunction should not receive mirtazapine.

A frequent side effect, especially at the beginning of therapy, is orthostatic dysregulation, making the use in this patient group problematic. In older patients, it may be advisable to begin with a subtherapeutic evening dose of 7.5 mg to improve tolerability. In a recent large observational study, mirtazapine was associated with a higher adverse event rate than other antidepressants (Coupland et al. 2011).

Selective Serotonin and Norepinephrine Reuptake Inhibitors

Compounds in this drug group are venlafaxine and duloxetine. As venlafaxine has been marketed for some time already, there is more extensive clinical experience regarding its use, and inexpensive generic drugs are available. Compared with other antidepressants, venlafaxine is assumed to have a slightly better efficacy. Both compounds, but especially duloxetine, are possibly advantageous in patients with comorbid pain syndromes (Raskin et al. 2007).

Particularly in older patients, the tolerability of venlafaxine and duloxetine is worse than that of pure SSRIs. Especially at the beginning of therapy, patients frequently experience
- Gastrointestinal symptoms
- Increased anxiety
- Agitation
- Headaches.

Autonomic dysregulation is frequent. As a consequence, medication should begin at low doses that are slowly increased. Due to their better tolerability, extended-release formulations should be preferred. Especially at higher doses, patients occasionally experience an increase in blood pressure, calling for regular blood pressure controls.

Due to their poorer tolerability compared with pure SSRIs, selective serotonin norepinephrine reuptake inhibitors (SSNRIs) are generally not used as a first choice for older patients. Owing to their possibly superior antidepressant efficacy, they may nonetheless be administered in case of nonresponse to standard medication. In cases of intolerance or lack of response, serum concentrations should be determined.

MAO Inhibitors

Today, the relatively old substance tranylcypromine is rarely used due to its numerous adverse effects and the necessity for keeping a tyramine-reduced diet. In this drug group, moclobemide is the only medication administered to elderly patients. Compared with tricyclic antidepressants, moclobemide causes fewer anticholinergic and autonomous side effects. It also does not have sedative effects. At regular doses, pronounced hypertensive reactions should not be expected following ingestion of food rich in tyramine. Nonetheless, patients should refrain from eating certain cheeses (e.g., Cheddar or Stilton) that contain high levels of tyramine. It should be mentioned, however, that the cheeses cited in the literature are rarely consumed worldwide. Moclobemide should by no means be combined with SRIs or 5-HT1 agonists such as sumatriptane or related migraine medications as this is associated with an increased risk for serotonin syndromes. In patients with liver failure, moclobemide may only be administered in substantially reduced doses, if at all.

As data on moclobemide medication in the elderly is limited, it cannot be recommended as a drug of first choice in this group of patients. However, data generated in smaller studies suggest relatively good tolerability.

Norepinephrine Reuptake Inhibitors

The only compound in the group of norepinephrine reuptake inhibitor drugs is reboxetine (not FDA approved). In older patients, autonomic side effects, including tachycardia and low blood pressure, are frequently seen. Compared with other antidepressants, there is a relatively high incidence of urinary retention, particularly in older men, forcing the discontinuation of this medication. In patients with liver or kidney failure, the dose must be reduced. Meta-analyses comparing different antidepressants point to lower efficacy and poorer tolerability of reboxetine in comparison with other antidepressants (Cipriani et al. 2009). A recent meta-analysis concluded that reboxetine is an "overall ineffective and potentially harmful" antidepressant (Eyding et al. 2010). Accordingly, the use of reboxetine must be discouraged.

Bupropion

Bupropion is a selective norepinephrine dopamine reuptake inhibitor. Its efficacy has primarily been shown in patients with anhedonia and apathy. Bupropion has no sedative side effects. At the beginning of therapy, however, agitation, anxiety, and sleeplessness are common side effects. Particularly problematic in older patients, bupropion may cause rather marked blood pressure increases. Regular blood pressure controls are thus mandatory. An additional problem associated with bupropion is the lowering of the cerebral seizure threshold. Accordingly, epilepsy and cerebral disorders predisposing patients for epileptic seizures are contraindications. In patients with kidney and liver failure, bupropion should not be administered.

For these reasons, bupropion is only a drug of second choice for use in older patients. However, a recent small study on bupropion in elderly patients found good tolerability and efficacy of this drug (Bergman et al. 2011).

Melatonergic Substances

Agomelatine (not FDA approved), a melatonergic substance with additional serotonergic characteristics, has only recently been approved in the European Union for use in the treatment of depression. To date, there are no comprehensive insights or research data on its use in older patients. The only placebo-controlled study in elderly patients did not demonstrate a significant benefit for agomelatine. Nonetheless, the substance is included here as clinical experiences so far have shown very good tolerability so that it might play a future role in the treatment of depression in older patients. On the other hand, the cumulated data to now led to the conclusion that the antidepressive potency of agomelatine may not be high since several studies did not demon-

strate superiority over placebo (Howland 2011). However, its comparably high price despite the absence of a proof of superior efficacy poses a problem.

Pragmatic Aspects of Pharmacological Treatment of Depression

Initial Drug Therapy of Depression

With patients who had either been treated with a specific drug in the past or who are presently undergoing treatment, the decision on how to proceed has to be made on an individual basis. Whenever patients' current medication is either nonsensical or confusing, it is recommended that all medication should be discontinued and treatment be restarted with a different substance. In principle, antidepressant therapy is individualized with special emphasis on comorbidities and the predominant clinical picture (agitated, inhibited, reduced drive, etc.).

The respective procedures are summarized in a diagram (Fig. 1).

In everyday practice, physicians frequently commit avoidable mistakes when treating depressed patients.

The most frequent mistakes during pharmacotherapy of depression are (also see "Summary")

– Premature switch of medication:

As most antidepressants do not take effect before 1–3 weeks into treatment, medication should not be changed before at least 2–3 weeks have passed.

– Inefficient dose:

All medication should always be given at the highest possible doses first or until adverse side effects are noted before switching to a new medication.

– Use of medication not indicated for the particular clinical picture:

As a case in point, sometimes general practitioners frequently prescribe opipramol (in Europe; not FDA approved) or depot antipsychotics although they are neither approved nor suitable for the treatment of depression.

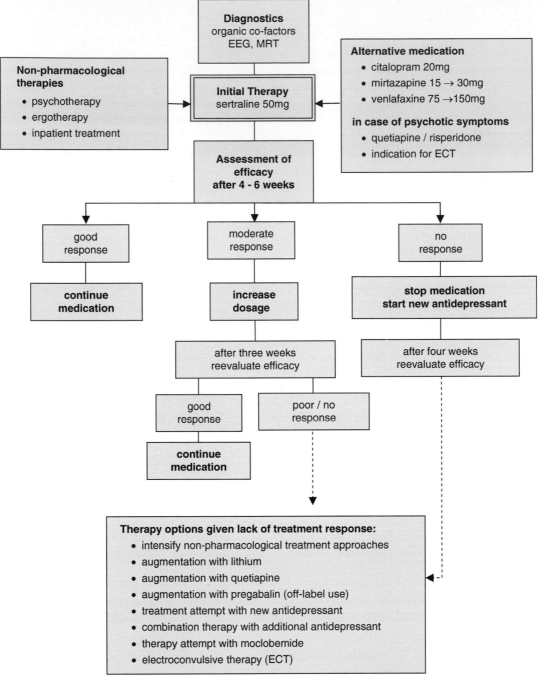

Mannheim scheme for the treatment of geriatric depression
The recommendations provided are based on current guidelines. Due to a lack of data in older patients the selection and preference of the listed substances and treatment details are based on clinical experience and local treatment practices and do not persistently reflect proven scientific evidence.

Fig. 1 Mannheim scheme for the treatment of geriatric depression. The recommendations provided are based on current guidelines. Due to a lack of data in older patients, the selection and preference of the listed substances and treatment details are based on clinical experience and local treatment practices and do not persistently reflect proven scientific evidence. *EEG* electroencephalogram, *MRT* magnetic resonance tomography

– Nonsensible treatment combinations:

As a rule, antidepressant combination therapies are rarely evidence based. If combination therapy is to be implemented at all, the first drug should at least have shown some effect before introducing the second compound.

– Disregard/neglect of nonpharmacological measures:

Pharmacotherapy is only one element in the treatment of depression. Psychotherapeutic or sociotherapeutic approaches should not be neglected.

– Uncritical use of sedatives:

As a rule, benzodiazepines or other sedatives should not be used for the treatment of depression in older patients. If this turns out to be unavoidable due to severe agitation or suicidal tendencies, for example, benzodiazepines may only be used for a short period and at the lowest possible dose.

– Failing to recognize dementia:

Particularly in the early stages of dementia, the disorder may falsely be diagnosed as depression. Thus, each older patient with depression should also be screened for dementia. Moreover, depression in association with dementia may not respond to antidepressants (see discussion in the chapter on dementia).

Summary

Frequent mistakes in the pharmacotherapy of depression are

- Premature switch of medication
- Use of inappropriate medication (e.g., depot antipsychotics)
- Nonsensible combination therapies
- Disregarding nonpharmacological treatment approaches
- Overlooking diagnosis of dementia

In patients with psychotic symptoms, antipsychotics should be given in addition to standard antidepressants. Quetiapine, the only antipsychotic drug explicitly approved to treat depression together with an antidepressant, appears to be the drug of first choice for older patients, at a typical starting dose of 25 mg at night and subsequent dose increases depending on efficacy and possible side effects. As an alternative, patients may be given risperidone, generally beginning with a dose of 0.5 mg twice daily and dose increases depending on efficacy and side effects. Haloperidol and other older antipsychotics should generally be avoided. This recommendation against older antipsychotics, however, is largely based on general consensus, not on reliable research results.

In the elderly, benzodiazepines are not recommended mainly due to the associated risk of falls and the danger of paradoxical reactions, including delirium and the development of tolerance. If this is unavoidable, patients should be given lorazepam in the lowest effective dose and for as short a period as possible. In patients on lorazepam, physicians should evaluate daily whether the drug can be discontinued.

In patients suffering from insomnia in association with depression, benzodiazepines should be avoided. If a hypnotic drug is unavoidable, newer hypnotics such as eszopiclone can be temporarily employed.

As a rule, benzodiazepines are not indicated. In patients with suicidal tendencies or with severe agitated depression, short-term use of lorazepam as an exception may be useful.

Recommendations on Management of Initial Treatment Failure

Two to four weeks after initiation of drug treatment, the response will be assessed based on clinical criteria and the results of depression scales and categorized as "good," "moderate," or "no effect."

The traditional dogma of a mandatory 4- to 6-week waiting period before the assessment of efficacy of initial therapy has been revised by recent works that were able to demonstrate that patients' response to medication may be evaluated 2 weeks after onset of therapy (Szegedi et al. 2009). In individual patients with severe depression, changes in therapy may thus already be considered after 2–3 weeks of therapy if the initial treatment does not show any noticeable benefit.

Given a satisfactory response to the initial treatment regime, patients' antidepressant medication should be continued without any change.

If the initial therapy induces a beneficial response but sufficient efficacy is not reached, the dose of the antidepressant medication will be increased in the presence of proper monitoring of serum concentrations (therapeutic drug monitoring, TDM) if necessary and of specific side effects. Reassessment should take place approximately 2 weeks after each dose increase. In addition, nonpharmacological methods should be intensified whenever possible.

Extended-release quetiapine (150–300 mg/day) has been recently approved for adjunctive treatment of a major depressive episode with inadequate response to antidepressant monotherapy in adults (Bauer et al. 2010).

Whenever anxiety or insomnia are prominent, pregabalin could be tested, beginning with 50 mg/day and increasing the dose to 150 mg/day after 1 week of treatment. It should be noted, though, that pregabalin is not approved for this indication (off-label use).

Whenever initial therapy shows absolutely no effect following 4 weeks of treatment, antidepressants should be discontinued and an alternative medication from a different drug group should be prescribed. Again, reevaluation should take place after 2–3 weeks of treatment.

Recommendations on Management of Initial Treatment Failure and Lack of Improvement After Adequate Dose Increase or First Medication Change

While even for younger patients data on the topic of management of initial treatment failure and lack of improvement after adequate dose increase or first medication change are already sparse, there are certainly no data for older patients that allow for reliable recommendations.

In addition to the search for appropriate medications, this situation calls for increased efforts into examination of nonpharmacological therapies depending on the indication.

With nonresponse to antidepressant medication, physicians should always examine drug concentrations in serum (TDM) to recognize noncompliance or an abnormal drug metabolism.

Whenever the present medication does not produce any response despite sufficient dose or serum concentrations, it is generally useful to stop this medication and to initiate an alternative, new treatment strategy.

Overall, the following additional pharmacological options are available (listed in hierarchical order):

Augmentation with lithium: In younger patients, the benefit of lithium augmentation of antidepressant medications is well documented. In older patients, however, physicians must carefully consider the numerous contraindications for lithium therapy (especially kidney failure, thyroid dysfunction, and concomitant diuretics). Dosing and the control of serum concentrations follow the same scheme as in younger patients.

Lithium is the standard medication for therapy augmentation in depression and for relapse prevention in recurrent depressive disorders. In older patients, there are often contraindications to lithium and a higher rate of adverse events. Close monitoring during therapy is absolutely essential.

In recent years, off-label use of lamotrigine has increasingly been employed as an alternative to lithium, particularly due to its greater tolerability. Unfortunately, lamotrigine requires a rather long phase of slow dose increases (with a target dose of 200 mg/day) before therapeutically effective serum concentrations are achieved. Particularly in older patients, clinical data on lamotrigine are very sparse.

Augmentation with quetiapine: In patients who do not sufficiently respond to monotherapy with an antidepressant, quetiapine (150–300 mg/day) has been approved together with an antidepressant.

Augmentation with pregabalin: In clinical practice, off-label use of pregabalin as an augmentation drug is often found, particularly in cases of comorbid anxiety or sleep disorders. After an initial dose of 50 mg at night for the first week, the administered dose is increased to a total of 150 mg/day given in two single doses; a maximum dose increase to 225 mg/day would be possible.

Renewed therapeutic attempt with a different antidepressant: In such an attempt, the present antidepressant is discontinued before a new substance with different mechanisms of action is introduced. As nortriptyline and venlafaxine are traditionally considered to be among the more effective antidepressants, they are often the drugs of choice under these particular circumstances, although there is no clear scientific evidence to underscore this opinion.

Combination therapy using a second antidepressant: To date, information on antidepressant combination therapies is insufficient; accordingly, solid recommendations are not possible. The additional medication should have a different mechanism of action.

Whenever patients fail to respond to standard medication with citalopram (or any other SSRI), it is theoretically possible to add bupropion (beginning with 150 mg/day for the first week before increasing the dose to 300 mg/day) or nortriptyline (or vice versa) as a combination drug.

Therapeutic attempt with moclobemide: Based on empirical data, moclobemide may be a viable alternative in patients in whom standard antidepressants showed no effect. Due to the risk of developing a serotonergic syndrome, all other serotonergic medication must be discontinued before switching to moclobemide. In older patients, the recommended maximum daily dose should be between 150 and 300 mg/day.

The combination of moclobemide with a serotonergic compound is absolutely contraindicated.

Electroconvulsive therapy: In patients who failed to respond to different pharmacological treatment approaches, ECT may be indicated. Individual decisions on the use of ECT should not be delayed unnecessarily as ECT is often highly effective and generally associated with a much smaller risk than prolonged treatment with a combination of different antidepressants.

Whenever pharmacological therapy fails, ECT may be indicated.

Duration of Drug Therapy

Although it is generally recognized that continuous treatment with antidepressants in elderly patients is efficacious compared with placebo in preventing relapses and recurrences, there are no conclusive recommendations for the optimal duration of antidepressant therapy (Kok et al. 2011). In many older patients, depression constitutes a recurrent disorder. Within the framework of a study by Alexopoulos et al. (2002), 90% of all older patients with major depression who were receiving placebo suffered another depressive episode within 3 years as compared with only 20% or 43% of those undergoing psychotherapy or continuous pharmacological treatment, respectively. Accordingly, medication should not be discontinued too quickly after remission of symptoms. After remission has been achieved, therapy should be continued for at least 12 months, although many authors recommend longer treatment periods. In patients who have already suffered several depressive episodes, antidepressive treatment should certainly be continued for at least 3 years. In patients with depression and psychotic symptoms, antipsychotics should be administered for at least 6 months after remission (Alexopoulos 2005).

Prophylactic Treatment in Bipolar Affective Disorders

In the elderly, indication and practical procedures for bipolar affective disorders are analogous to those in younger adults. While lithium is still regarded as the drug of choice by many physicians, the numerous contraindications in older patients must be considered carefully.

As alternatives, patients can be given quetiapine (with a standard target dose of 150–300 mg/day), valproic acid (with a standard dose of 1,000 mg/day), or lamotrigine (with a standard target dose of 200 mg/day).

Carbamazepine, on the other hand, is only drug of second choice in elderly patients due to its negative effect on cognitive functions and overall high rate of adverse effects, in particular falls.

Classification of Drugs for Relapse Prevention and Therapy of Depression According to Their Fitness for the Aged (FORTA)

In this classification of drugs for relapse prevention and therapy of depression according to their Fitness for the Aged (FORTA), the same compounds may receive alternative marks if applied in different indications (see chapter "Critical Extrapolation of Guidelines and Study Results: Risk-Benefit Assessment for Patients with Reduced Life Expectancy and a New Classification of Drugs According to Their Fitness for the Aged").

Drug group	Drug	FORTA
Serotonin reuptake inhibitors	Sertraline	B
	Citalopram	B
	Escitalopram	B
Tricyclic antidepressants	Nortriptyline	C
Noradrenergic and serotonergic antidepressants	Mirtazapine	C
Serotonin norepinephrine reuptake inhibitors	Venlafaxine	C
	Duloxetine	C
MAO inhibitors	Moclobemide	C
Norepinephrine reuptake inhibitors	Reboxetine	D
Norepinephrine dopamine reuptake inhibitors	Bupropion	C
Melatonergic and serotonergic antidepressants	Agomelatine	C

References

Alexopoulos GS (2005) Depression in the elderly. Lancet 365:1961–1970

Alexopoulos GS, Katz IR, Reynolds CF 3rd, Carpenter D, Docherty JP (2001) The expert consensus guideline series. Pharmacotherapy of depressive disorders in older patients. Postgrad Med Spec No Pharmacotherapy :1–86

Alexopoulos GS, Borson S, Cuthbert BN (2002) Assessment of late life depression. Biol Psychiatry 52:164–174

Alvarez PA, Pahissa J (2010) QT alterations in psychopharmacology: proven candidates and suspects. Curr Drug Saf 5:97–104

American Psychiatric Association (1994) Diagnostic and statistical manual of mental disorders, 4th edn. American Psychiatric Association, Washington, DC

Bauer M, Bschor T, Pfennig A et al (2007) World Federation of Societies of Biological Psychiatry (WFSBP) guidelines for biological treatment of unipolar depressive disorders in primary care. World J Biol Psychiatry 8:67–104

Bauer M, El-Khalili N, Datto C, Szamosi J, Eriksson H (2010) A pooled analysis of two randomised, placebo-controlled studies of extended release quetiapine fumarate adjunctive to antidepressant therapy in patients with major depressive disorder. J Affect Disord 127:19–30

Bergman J, Miodownik C, Palatnik A, Lerner V (2011) Efficacy of bupropion XR in treatment-resistant elderly patients: a case series study. Clin Neuropharmacol 34:17–20

Bondareff W, Alpert M, Friedhoff AJ et al (2000) Comparison of sertraline and nortriptyline in the treatment of major depressive disorder in late life. Am J Psychiatry 157:729–736

Cipriani A, Furukawa TA, Salanti G et al (2009) Comparative efficacy and acceptability of 12 new-generation antidepressants: a multiple-treatments meta-analysis. Lancet 373:746–758

Coupland C, Dhiman P, Morriss R, Arthur A, Barton G, Hippisley-Cox J (2011) Antidepressant use and risk of adverse outcomes in older people: population based cohort study. BMJ 343:d4551. doi:10.1136/bmj.d4551

Eyding D, Lelgemann M, Grouven U et al (2010) Reboxetine for acute treatment of major depression: systematic review and meta-analysis of published and unpublished placebo and selective serotonin reuptake inhibitor controlled trials. BMJ 341:c4737

Goodman WK (2011) Electroconvulsive therapy in the spotlight. N Engl J Med 364:1785–1787

Gribbin J, Hubbard R, Gladman J, Smith C, Lewis S (2011) Serotonin-norepinephrine reuptake inhibitor antidepressants and the risk of falls in older people: case–control and case-series analysis of a large UK primary care database. Drugs Aging 28:895–902

Hausner L, Damian M, Sartorius A, Frölich L (2011) Efficacy and cognitive side effects of electroconvulsive therapy (ECT) in depressed elderly inpatients with coexisting mild cognitive impairment or dementia. J Clin Psychiatry 72:91–97

Hawton K, van Heeringen K (2009) Suicide. Lancet 373:1372–1381

Heok KE, Ho R (2008) The many faces of geriatric depression. Curr Opin Psychiatry 21:540–545

Howland RH (2011) A benefit-risk assessment of agomelatine in the treatment of major depression. Drug Saf 34:709–731

Jalenques I, Legrand G, Vaille-Perret E, Tourtauchaux R, Galland F (2010) Efficacité et tolérance de la stimulation magnétique transcrânienne (SMTr) dans le traitement des dépressions chez le sujet âgé: revue de la littérature. Encéphale 36(Suppl 2):D105–D118

Kirsch I, Deacon BJ, Huedo-Medina TB et al (2008) Initial severity and antidepressant benefits: a meta-analysis of data submitted to the Food and Drug Administration. PLoS Med 5:e45

Kok RM, Heeren TJ, Nolen WA (2011) Continuing treatment of depression in the elderly: a systematic review and meta-analysis of double-blinded randomized controlled trials with antidepressants. Am J Geriatr Psychiatry 19:249–255

Meeks TW, Vahia IV, Lavretsky H, Kulkarni G, Jeste DV (2011) A tune in "a minor" can "b major": a review of epidemiology, illness course, and public health implications of subthreshold depression in older adults. J Affect Disord 129:126–142

Mottram P, Wilson K, Strobl J (2006) Antidepressants for the elderly. Cochrane Database Syst Rev 1:CD003491

Pinquart M, Duberstein PR, Lyness JM (2006) Treatments for later-life depressive conditions: a meta-analytic comparison of pharmacotherapy and psychotherapy. Am J Psychiatry 163:1493–1501

Pinquart M, Duberstein PR, Lyness JM (2007) Effects of psychotherapy and other behavioral interventions on clinically depressed older adults: a meta-analysis. Aging Ment Health 11:645–657

Raskin J, Wiltse CG, Siegal A, Sheikh J, Xu J, Dinkel JJ, Rotz BT, Mohs RC (2007) Efficacy of duloxetine on cognition, depression, and pain in elderly patients with major depressive disorder: an 8-week, double-blind, placebo-controlled trial. Am J Psychiatry 164:900–909

Rodda J, Walker Z, Carter J (2011) Depression in older adults. BMJ 343:d5219

Szegedi A, Jansen WT, van Willigenburg AP et al (2009) Early improvement in the first 2 weeks as a predictor of treatment outcome in patients with major depressive disorder: a meta-analysis including 6,562 patients. J Clin Psychiatry 70:344–353

Tess AV, Smetana GW (2009) Medical evaluation of patients undergoing electroconvulsive therapy. N Engl J Med 360:1437–1444

Sleep Disorders

Stefan Schwarz and Lutz Frölich

Implications for the Elderly, Epidemiology

Sleeping problems constitute one of the most frequently voiced complaints in the elderly. Patients commonly complain about insomnia (i.e., the problem of either falling asleep or sleeping through the night). While increased need for sleep and abnormal daytime sleepiness are frequent phenomena in older people, patients themselves rarely consider this a relevant problem. The present chapter focuses on insomnia, the most important and frequent sleep disorder in the elderly.

Epidemiological studies on the prevalence of insomnia have yielded differing results depending on study method, patient population, and the definition of insomnia (Ancoli-Israel and Cooke 2005). Overall, 30–60% of older people across industrialized nations report suffering from insomnia. Somatic and psychiatric comorbidity, frailty, low income, poor education, and loss of partner are predisposing factors (Bloom et al. 2009; Foley et al. 1999).

Among the elderly, 30–60% of all persons complain about insomnia.

S. Schwarz (✉) · L. Frölich
Central Institute of Mental Health, Medical Faculty
Mannheim/Heidelberg University, Square J 5, 68159
Mannheim, Germany
e-mail: stefan.schwarz@zi-mannheim.de;
lutz.froelich@zi-mannheim.de

The prevalence of insomnia is particularly high during inpatient hospital care. Hospitalized patients frequently receive hypnotics: On general wards, 31–41% of all patients are given hypnotics; on surgical wards, the percentage is at 33–88% (Flaherty 2008). These numbers alone point to the significance of insomnia.

In everyday practice, sleep disorders in elderly patients are either frequently not treated at all or, even more often, not adequately treated. Among the most frequent treatment mistakes are
- Long-term prescription of hypnotics
- Lack of careful assessment of patients' medical history
- Failure to properly diagnose patients' complaints.

Often, all three mistakes are committed in combination.

One reason for the lack of attention with regard to sleep disorders is the false belief that sleep disorders constitute only minor health problems. In fact, however, sleep disorders represent a complex, multifactorial geriatric syndrome (Vaz Fragoso and Gill 2007) with numerous causes that has considerable effects on the quality of life of patients as well as consequences on somatic disorders (Wolkove et al. 2007). Patients suffering from sleep disorders have a higher risk for developing high blood pressure and depression as well as cardiovascular and cerebrovascular disorders. Vice versa, these disorders predispose patients for developing sleep disorders. In addition, sleep disorders represent an important cause for reduced cognitive function.

M. Wehling (ed.), *Drug Therapy for the Elderly*,
DOI 10.1007/978-3-7091-0912-0_17, © Springer-Verlag Wien 2013

For example, patients suffering from sleep apnea will often visit their physician because of cognitive deficits instead of sleep problems.

The majority of elderly patients with insomnia are not treated adequately. Indiscriminate prescription of hypnotics is a frequent treatment mistake.

With increasing age, changes in physiological sleep structure and need for sleep may occur (Bloom et al. 2009; Vaz Fragoso and Gill 2007). While infants require 16–20 h of sleep per day, the amount of sleep required by adults amounts to only 7–8 h, that of older persons over 60 years of age to only 6.5 h. Of course, these are only average values; a person's individual need for sleep varies greatly. In addition to a shorter overall sleep duration, the proportion of deep delta-sleep cycles (stages III and IV) and REM (rapid eye movement) sleep is also reduced. Furthermore, sleep-wake-cycles also undergo changes, with older people going to bed and waking up earlier than younger adults. In the elderly, sleep is highly fragmented, which is in part due to a lower arousal threshold to external stimuli.

These physiological changes in association with advanced age explain a large portion of subjective sleep disorders in the elderly. Many patients already profit from the mere information that their subjectively perceived sleep deficit is not a sign of illness, but rather the result of naturally occurring changes in the amount of sleep needed in older age.

In the elderly, sleep disorders may be triggered by a whole host of possible causes. Within this context, it is sensible to differentiate between primary, idiopathic sleep disorders and comorbid (secondary) sleep disorders as a complication of other illnesses or as a side effect of medication. The exact cause-effect relationship, however, remains often unclear in patients with comorbidities associated with sleep disorders. The following summary as well as Table 1 show the most frequent causes of primary and comorbid sleep disorders.

Comorbidities and medication often contribute to sleep disorders in the elderly.

Overview of Frequent Sleep Disorders in the Elderly

1. Primary specific sleep disorders
   - Circadian sleep disorders
   - Sleep apnea syndrome
   - Restless legs syndrome
   - REM sleep disorders
   - Periodic leg movements during sleep.
2. Comorbidities associated with sleep disorders
   2.1. Somatic disorders
      - Pain syndromes
      - Heart disease, nocturnal angina pectoris
      - Obstructive lung disease, chronic rhinitis
      - Reflux disorder, diarrhea, obstipation
      - Nocturia, incontinence.
   2.2. Neurological-psychiatric disorders
      - Stroke
      - Parkinson's disease
      - Dementia
      - Delirious states
      - Major depression.
   2.3. Behavioral aspects
      - Inactive lifestyle
      - Afternoon nap
      - Early bedtime
      - Alcohol, coffee, black tea during evening hours
      - Heavy meals during evening hours.
   2.4. Environmental factors
      - Noise, light, unfavorable room temperature
      - Unsuitable bed or bed linens.

Therapeutically Relevant Special Features of Elderly Patients

Adequate treatment of insomnia in the elderly should include the following therapy goals:
1. Careful clarification of all causes requiring treatment,
2. Thorough patient information,
3. Improvement of sleep disturbances and, as a consequence,

Table 1 Medication and other compounds frequently associated with sleep disorders (selection)

Substance	Remark
Alcohol	Induces sleep, but shortens and fragments sleep duration
Caffeine, black tea	Should not be consumed during evening hours
Nicotine	Stimulating effect
Amphetamine	Stimulating effect, sleep disturbances, nightmares
Antidepressants (SSRI/SSNRI, bupropion)	Sleeplessness as frequent side effect
Tricyclic antidepressants, mirtazapine	Increased sleepiness
Thyroxine	Overdosing leads to sleeplessness, underdosing may cause hypersomnia
Theophylline	Increases sleeplessness
Phenytoin	May cause sleeplessness or sleepiness
Diuretics	Increased nocturia, medication should preferably be taken in the morning
Levodopa and other dopaminergic Parkinson medications	Insomnia, nightmares
Beta-blockers	Change in sleep architecture
Acetylcholine esterase inhibitors, memantine	Insomnia, nightmares
Glucocorticoids	Stimulating effect, insomnia, nightmares

SSRI selective serotonin reuptake inhibitor, *SSNRI* selective serotonin norepinephrine reuptake inhibitor.

4. Improvement of patients' quality of life and general health.

As a rule, the diagnostic and therapeutic principles do not differ from those in younger adults.

The following overview summarizes the relevant diagnostic and therapeutic procedures.

Treating Elderly Patients Suffering from Insomnia

- Sleep history
  - Determine whether patient is actually suffering from insomnia
  - Precise history of symptoms (sleep onset, duration, and course)
  - 24-h sleep pattern (wake/sleep cycles)
  - Family history of sleep disorders (e.g., sleep apnea)
  - Sleep history by significant other/sleeping partner.
- Examinations
  - Sleep diary (at least over 1 week)
  - Physical and psychiatric examination
  - Laboratory tests and technical examinations according to individual conditions.
- Diagnosis
  - Primary sleep disorder

- Comorbid sleep disorder
  - Somatic disorders
  - Psychiatric disorders
  - Behavior-related sleep disorders
  - Sleep disorders caused by external factors
  - Medication effects.
- Treatment
  - Treatment of primary causes whenever possible
  - Informing patients about their disorder
  - Measures of sleep hygiene
  - Nonpharmacological measures
  - Pharmacological treatment if absolutely necessary
  - When appropriate, referral to specialist.

In light of the extensive range of differential diagnoses, it goes without saying that the assessment and treatment of sleep disorders in the elderly is complex. A brief consultation at the general practitioner's office does not suffice when an extensive medical history and careful differential diagnosis are called for. Whenever family practitioners cannot afford to invest the time necessary for performing these steps, it is undoubtedly advisable to send older patients with insomnia to a specialist or specialized medical center instead of starting inadequate pharmacological treatment without prior careful screening due to a lack of time.

By far the most frequent mistake in the treatment of insomnia in elderly patients is the common practice to prescribe hypnotics without adequate diagnostic evaluation.

Initially, it is of particular importance to determine whether patients are indeed suffering from a sleep disorder in need of medical treatment. Many older people complain about sleeplessness; often, however, a careful analysis of sleep patterns and sleep durations reveals that these patients actually have normal sleep duration, but that their daily life offers so few activities and distractions that they subjectively perceive their sleep duration as being too short. In this large patient population, pharmacological interventions would be contraindicated. In case of comorbid sleep disorders, physicians must first attempt to treat the potentially underlying cause before additional symptomatic treatment is indicated. A summary of the most important differential diagnoses is provided in the overview on frequent causes of sleep disorders in the elderly. As case in point, the symptomatic treatment of sleep apnea syndrome with sedating hypnotic medication would in fact contribute to the deterioration of symptoms, whereas adequate treatment not only would improve the symptom of insomnia but also would alleviate a major cardiovascular risk factor.

In numerous patients, an extensive analysis of sleep and behavior patterns will reveal factors that could be directly implemented in a discussion of sleep hygiene (see summary).

Measures for Improving Sleep hygiene in Patients with Insomnia

– Beds should only be used for sleeping and sexual activities
  Patients should leave the bed whenever they cannot fall asleep and engage in other activities before returning to bed.
– No daytime naps
  Patients should not sleep or lay down to rest during the day; at night, they should refrain from going to bed too early.
– Ensure an optimal sleep environment

Low noise level, optimal and comfortable temperatures, ventilation, light sources, and bed linens, and so on should be taken into consideration.
– Avoiding activities that have a deleterious effect on sleep
  Patients should refrain from consuming alcohol, heavy meals, nicotine, or coffee during evening hours.
– Activities to promote sound sleep
  During the day, patients should be physically active and plan different measures and sleep rituals, such as a warm bath, relaxation exercises, yoga, sleep-promoting teas, or small meals rich in tryptophan (e.g., bananas) or carbohydrates.

When taking older patients' history, it often becomes apparent that many patients complaining of insomnia tend to spend their days rather inactively, maybe even lay in bed during the day, take a nap in the afternoon, or go to bed very early in the evening. Under these circumstances, it is not surprising that the duration of their nighttime sleep cannot be long. Simply by modifying these behavior patterns, patients can achieve improvement of their symptoms.

Before prescribing medication, physicians should first exhaust all nonpharmacological measures available, such as, for example, all measures and techniques for improving sleep hygiene. In some patients, specific measures such as behavior therapy or light therapy may be of use. For many patients with sleep disorders, learning relaxation techniques such as autogenic training, progressive muscle relaxation, or yoga proves to be helpful.

Improving sleep hygiene and other nonpharmacological approaches have priority over pharmacological interventions.

With regard to the pharmacological treatment of insomnia, we differentiate between acute or chronic insomnia. Typical examples for acute insomnia are grief and bereavement or inpatient hospital treatment, when unfamiliar environment and external disturbing factors such as nightly rounds or snoring roommates constitute disturbing factors. In these patients, temporary pharmacotherapy with hypnotics may indeed be useful. Generally, however, medication with hypnotics should not exceed a period of about 10 days.

With acute insomnia in association with temporarily stressful situations, the use of a hypnotic substance for a maximum of 10 days may be indicated.

Generally not useful, on the other hand, is the prescription of hypnotics in patients with chronic insomnia. Instead, physicians are called on to ward off the frequently voiced wish of patients for medication and to suggest alternative, nonpharmacological treatment approaches. Given for chronic insomnia, pharmacological substances have numerous disadvantages: Due to their centrally active sedative effect and muscle relaxant properties, benzodiazepines, and to some degree also nonbenzodiazepine hypnotic agents, reduce muscle tone and increase patients' risk of falling (see chapter "Fall Risk and Pharmacotherapy"). Many substances, particularly benzodiazepines and nonbenzodiazepine benzodiazepine receptor agonists ("Z-drugs," e.g., zolpidem), are associated with a high addiction risk, particularly if taken over longer stretches of time. Other medication groups such as antidepressants or antipsychotic drugs that are frequently employed as hypnotics are associated with a considerable potential for side effects, while the long-term efficacy and safety of newer substances, such as extended-release melatonin or melatonin receptor agonists, have not been sufficiently examined in older patients.

In patients with chronic insomnia, pharmacological interventions should generally be avoided.

Under ideal circumstances, in which both physicians and patients act in accordance with state-of-the-art medical knowledge, hypnotics would rarely be used to treat chronic insomnia. In reality, however, hypnotics are among the most frequently prescribed medication groups despite numerous side effects and an overall low efficacy profile in older patients. This is mainly for the sake of physicians' convenience, for whom handing out prescriptions is easier than getting involved in lengthy and often poorly paid consultations on sleep hygiene and behavior. Moreover, although many patients experience high psychological strain in association with their sleep disorder, unfortunately they are often not motivated or able actually to implement even simple useful rules on sleep hygiene or behavioral modifications.

It is thus not surprising that hypnotics represent the substance group that is most frequently abused by older patients. Unfortunately, neither the general public nor physicians show particular sensibility with regard to medication abuse in the elderly, so that the great majority of addiction disorders involving legal substances are not diagnosed and remain untreated. In the United States, approximately 11% of elderly citizens are thought to abuse medication, with hypnotics prescribed for the treatment of insomnia playing the most important role (Culberson and Ziska 2008). According to a large-scale study, in 2001, nearly a quarter of all patients in nursing homes were unnecessarily treated with benzodiazepines (Svarstad and Mount 2001).

Unfortunately, many physicians have been swayed by misleading marketing strategies to consider nonbenzodiazepine benzodiazepine receptor agonists to be unproblematic or "safe" concerning the development of addiction. This is a major reason why nonbenzodiazepine benzodiazepine receptor agonists are incorrectly prescribed over longer stretches of time and have replaced benzodiazepines as a hypnotic of first choice. In many countries, there is some uncertainty on the prescription of benzodiazepines as benzodiazepines like nonbenzodiazepine benzodiazepine receptor agonists are inexpensive and increasingly prescribed by way of private prescription or obtained via the Internet, thus escaping statistical recording. It has to be emphasized that in the development of medication addiction in elderly patients, in contrast to addiction disorders in young patients, physicians play the most important role. Accordingly, the prescription of these substances should be handled exceedingly restrictively, prescribing only minimal quantities and only if clearly indicated. However, many patients manage to acquire their addictive drug through "doctor shopping" by consulting different physicians as a means of securing repeat prescriptions for their drug of choice or by buying their drugs over the Internet.

Medication abuse is a frequent problem among the elderly. Due to uncritical and incorrect prescription practices, hypnotics are the most frequently used drugs of abuse.

Evidence-Based, Rationalistic Drug Therapy and Classification of Drugs According to Their Fitness for the Aged (FORTA)

Reflecting the insufficient data from adequate clinical trials on hypnotics in the elderly, there is a substantial heterogeneity between different countries or continents in the selection and use of these medications. Drugs that are commonly prescribed in some countries may not be available at all in other regions. For example, eszopiclone, one of the most commonly employed hypnotic agents in the United States, is not licensed in Europe. Trazodone, another substance frequently used in the United States to treat insomnia, is only rarely prescribed in Europe. On the other hand, in many European countries there is a tradition of off-label use of low-potency typical antipsychotics such as pipamperone or melperone to promote sleep in elderly patients, which is not a frequent practice in other countries. Scientific evidence is almost nonexistent for both trazodone and low-potency typical antipsychotics to treat insomnia in elderly patients.

Suitability of Substance Groups for Use in the Elderly

As a rule, the use of hypnotics should be avoided with sleep disorders. If at all, they should only be used in acute sleep disorders over a short treatment period. A summary of frequently prescribed hypnotics is found in Table 2.

An example for a pragmatic incremental regimen for short-term treatment with hypnotics in inpatients is shown in the overview that follows. The information provided relates only to the short-term application of hypnotics over a maximum period of 10 days in hospitalized patients. Beyond this time frame, the use of hypnotics is generally not recommended in elderly patients, although some of these substances have been licensed for use without time limitations. Whenever hypnotics must be administered for longer periods due to individual considerations (e.g., in dementia disorders, in palliative medicine, with major depression, etc.), the indication should be reassessed regularly, and a concept for possible dose reductions should be established.

Escalation Scheme for Short-Term Pharmacological Treatment of Insomnia in Elderly Patients (Example)

This scheme was developed for older patients undergoing inpatient treatment. The respective contraindications for each drug must be considered on an individual basis. As a rule, the duration of treatment should not exceed 10 days. The listing of the drugs is based on clinical experience and not on a purely scientific basis. Extended-release melatonin is not approved by the Food and Drug Administration (FDA), but freely available as a supplement in the United States. Alternatively, ramelteon may be used (8 mg).

General Rules
- Sleeping pills should be avoided.
- For the treatment of sleep disorders, benzodiazepines should only be used under particular circumstances.
- Sleep medication should generally not be administered after midnight (for exceptions, see the following discussion).

First Step: Eszopiclone
- Give an initial dose of 1 mg eszopiclone before bedtime.
- Given lack of effect, an additional dose of 1 mg should be administered after 30 min.
- Patients who had previously been given 2 mg should possibly be started on that dose.

Table 2 Pharmacological compounds frequently used for the treatment of insomnia in elderly patients

Drug	Compound group	Dosage in older patients	FORTA	Remarks
Zolpidem	Nonbenzodiazepine benzodiazepine receptor agonist	5–10 mg	C	For short-term treatment (<10 days) of acute insomnia after nonpharmacological measures have failed and treatment is absolutely necessary. Low efficacy. Risk for addiction with longer use
Zopiclone	GABA receptor agonist	3.75–7.5 mg	C	See zolpidem
Eszopiclone	GABA receptor agonist	0.5–2.0 mg	C	See zolpidem. S-enantiomer of zopiclone. Studies on prolonged use are available. However, in elderly patients, prolonged use is not recommended
Zaleplon	Nonbenzodiazepine benzodiazepine receptor agonist	5–10 mg	C	See zolpidem. Due to its short half-life particularly useful with sleep-onset disorders
Oxazepam	Benzodiazepine	10 mg	D	Poor efficacy, numerous side effects. High risk for addiction. Not recommended
Triazolam	Benzodiazepine	0.25 mg	D	Poor efficacy, numerous side effects. High risk for addiction. Not recommended
Pipamperone	Antipsychotic with sedative effect	Initially 20 mg, increase up to 80 mg/ at night[a]	C	Effect not shown, numerous side effects. Despite lack of scientific proof of efficacy suitable for short-term use with acute sleep disorder based on extensive clinical experience. Drug of second choice
Mirtazapine	Noradrenergic and serotonergic AD	15 mg, possible increase to 30 mg[a]	D[b]	Orthostatic dysregulation. Weight gain. Metabolic effects. Efficacy not shown. Not recommended for use in patients not suffering from depression
Opipramole	Tricyclic anxiolytic	50 mg[a]	D[b]	Efficacy not shown, numerous side effects. Not recommended for use in older patients
Doxepin	Tricyclic antidepressant	25–50 mg[a]	D[b]	Efficacy not shown, numerous side effects. Not recommended
Trazodone	Tricyclic antidepressant	25–100 mg[a]	D[b]	Efficacy not shown, numerous side effects. Not recommended
Diphenhydramine	Antihistamine	50 mg	D	Efficacy not shown, numerous side effects. Not recommended
Ramelteon	Melatonin receptor agonist	8 mg	C	Well tolerated. No risk for developing tolerance or withdrawal symptoms. Low risk for addiction. No extensive experience. Low efficacy. Drug of second choice for short-term treatment of acute insomnia
Melatonin (extended release)	Melatonin	2–4 mg	C	Not FDA approved. Available as a supplement in the United States. Well tolerated. No risk for developing tolerance or withdrawal symptoms. Low risk for addiction. No extensive experience. Most likely low efficacy. Drug of second choice for short-term treatment of acute insomnia

The reference substances listed are frequently used in everyday clinical practice for the treatment of insomnia in older patients. Their superiority over comparable substances not listed in this table has not been shown. FORTA classifications strictly refer to short-term use of no longer than 10 days after nonpharmacological measures have failed and when therapy is absolutely necessary.

AD antidepressant, *FDA* Food and Drug Administration, *FORTA* Fit for the Aged.

[a]Dosage recommendations based on clinical experience.

[b]Listing refers to the indication "insomnia".

- Give a maximum dose of 2 mg eszopiclone at night.
- In countries where zopiclone is available, zopiclone can be employed as an equivalent (starting dose 3.75 mg, maximum dose 7.5 mg/night).

Second Step Given Lack of Efficacy of Step 1: Extended-Release Melatonin (Not FDA Approved, Supplement in the United States)

- Give an initial dose of 2 mg extended-release melatonin.
- Given lack of effect, an additional 2 mg of extended-release melatonin may be given after 30 min.
- Patients who had previously already received the maximum dose may be started on 4 mg extended-release melatonin.
- Give a maximum dose of 4 mg extended-release melatonin per night.

Medication After Midnight

Medication should only be administered after midnight if no other sleep medication has been given during the night. As a rule, sleep medications should never be administered after 3 a.m.

- If sleep medication after midnight is unavoidable:
  - Step 1: Give 2 mg extended-release melatonin.
  - Step 2: Given lack of effect, one additional dose of 2 mg extended-release melatonin may be administered after 30 min.
- Patients who had previously failed to respond to 2 mg extended-release melatonin may immediately receive an initial one-time dose of 4 mg slow-release melatonin.
- In countries in which zaleplon (FDA approved) is available, 5 mg zaleplon can be used as an alternative to extended-release melatonin.

Treatment Approaches in Patients Who Primarily Experience Problems with Falling Asleep (No Disturbance of Sleep Continuity)

- Step 1: Give 2 mg extended-release melatonin (alternatively 5 mg zaleplon, if available).
- Step 2: Given lack of efficacy of Step 1, an additional, one-time, dose of 2 mg extended-release melatonin may be administered after 30 min.

- Given lack of effect after 30 min, proceed as described previously.

Specifically in the elderly both the efficacy and the tolerability of hypnotics have scarcely been examined. There are hardly any valid clinical trials comparing the different substances in elderly individuals.

The compounds cited in this chapter are those frequently administered to older patients in day-to-day practice. This does not imply that substances that have not been discussed within this chapter are inferior to those mentioned.

Benzodiazepines

In 1960, the first benzodiazepine was introduced to the market under the trade name Librium® (chlordiazepoxide), followed by diazepam in 1963. In 1970, flurazepam was approved, the first benzodiazepine specifically sold to treat sleep disorders. Compared with their predecessors (i.e., barbiturates and chloral hydrate), benzodiazepines quickly prevailed due to their greater efficacy and fewer adverse effects. A major advantage was the wide therapeutic spectrum of benzodiazepines, which rapidly led to a marked reduction in suicide rates due to medication overdose that had been alarmingly high in association with barbiturates. The most important problem in association with benzodiazepines (i.e., the rapid development of medication tolerance and dependency) was initially not appropriately recognized.

Today, a large number of benzodiazepines are available, differing not only with regard to their pharmacokinetic properties but also concerning their efficacy on different aspects, such as anxiety, sedation, and sleep promotion.

In young adults, the efficacy of benzodiazepines in the treatment of sleep disorders is well documented. In older patients, their usefulness for the treatment of insomnia is far less convincingly established. A meta-analysis of all available studies of sedative hypnotics (benzodiazepines and nonbenzodiazepine benzodiazepine receptor agonists) in older patients showed a significant improvement with regard to important sleep parameters, although the absolute effect size was relatively small and of questionable clinical relevance (Glass et al. 2005). The rate of undesired side effects in association with hypnotics, on the other hand, was increased, leading the authors to conclude that this relatively low benefit does not justify the risk.

A number of problems limit the use of benzodiazepines. Many substances and their active metabolites have a very long half-life and long effective duration, which will often lead to a hangover with daytime sleepiness during the following day. In the elderly, the half-life of flurazepam, for example, may exceed 100 h. This problem affects particularly older patients, whose metabolism has slowed considerably due to their advanced age, or patients with liver failure, in whom the effect of a single dose of a benzodiazepine may last for many days. For these reasons, short-acting benzodiazepines such as triazolam, with a half-life of 1.5–5 ho, were developed. Due to an increased risk of abuse and addiction, lorazepam should not be prescribed to treat sleep disorders.

In the elderly, a markedly increased risk for falls due to the centrally active sedating and muscle-relaxing effect of benzodiazepines is well documented (see chapter "Fall Risk and Pharmacotherapy").

Particularly in older patients with prior cognitive impairment, benzodiazepines will lead to the aggravation of cognitive deficits. Accordingly, benzodiazepines should be avoided in patients with dementia or mild cognitive impairment.

The half-life of benzodiazepines may be reduced within a few days, thereby increasing the risk of development of tolerance and addiction. Following prolonged use, patients will almost always develop withdrawal symptoms, which may even be life threatening. These include
- Epileptic seizures
- Autonomous nervous system dysfunction
- Agitation and anxiety
- Delirious states

After prolonged benzodiazepine consumption, withdrawal attempts should only be carried out under close outpatient supervision or, preferably, on an inpatient basis.

Under these considerations, benzodiazepines are not recommended for the treatment of sleep disorders in older patients.

Frequent side effects of benzodiazepines are risk for falls, sedation, and development of addiction. Benzodiazepines are not recommended to treat insomnia in older patients.

Nonbenzodiazepine Benzodiazepine Receptor Agonists

During the 1980s, nonbenzodiazepine benzodiazepine receptor agonists (Z-drugs) were introduced to the market. Although these substances act on the $\omega 1$ subunit of the benzodiazepine receptor, their chemical structure is not related to that of benzodiazepines. Due to their mode of action, they are associated with similar effects and side effects as benzodiazepines.

Compared with benzodiazepines, however, these substances have several advantages. They do not lead to the development of tolerance, have an overall shorter effective period, and are thus less frequently associated with daytime sleepiness and sedation the next morning. Due to these advantages nonbenzodiazepine benzodiazepine receptor agonists have replaced benzodiazepines as drugs of first choice to treat insomnia.

While initially the risk of potential abuse in association with nonbenzodiazepine benzodiazepine receptor agonists was falsely considered to be very low, these substances now take second place to benzodiazepines as the most frequent cause of medication abuse in the elderly. With prolonged use of more than 4 weeks, nonbenzodiazepine benzodiazepine receptor agonists may show an addiction potential comparable to that of benzodiazepines (Kupfer and Reynolds 1997). Moreover, their use has been linked to the development of depression (Kripke 2007).

The most commonly used nonbenzodiazepine benzodiazepine receptor agonists is zolpidem. The short-acting substance zaleplone has been taken off the market in many countries. Strictly speaking, zopiclon and eszopiclone (the S-enantiomer of zopiclone is FDA approved but not available on the European market) do not belong to the group of nonbenzodiazepine benzodiazepine receptor agonists as they do not exert their GABAergic effects via the benzodiazepine site of the GABA receptor complex. However, they are commonly listed in this group of substances, although this is not correct from a pharmacological point of view.

Overall, data on the use of nonbenzodiazepine benzodiazepine receptor agonists in older patients are sparse. Based on their meta-analysis of all research trials in older patients, Dolder et al. (2007) concluded that while only showing a modest effect on sleep quality and sleep onset latency, but not sleep duration, these drugs—unlike benzodiazepines—are generally well tolerated. Most frequently reported side effects were headaches, dizziness, and fatigue, which, however, were seen as frequently under placebo. In general, there was no relevant development of tolerance in association with nonbenzodiazepine benzodiazepine receptor agonists.

In the elderly, nonbenzodiazepine benzodiazepine receptor agonists lead to a modest improvement in sleep quality and sleep onset latency while being generally well tolerated.

In comparison with benzodiazepines, nonbenzodiazepine benzodiazepine receptor agonists have a smaller impact on patients' muscle tone and risk of falling. To date, only zolpidem has been clearly associated with an increased risk for falls, although this may be explained by the fact that this substance has been analyzed most extensively. Among the rarer but clinically relevant psychiatric complications in elderly patients are delirium, hallucinations, and delusions.

After discontinuing medication, patients may experience rebound insomnia. Overall, however, withdrawal effects are generally much less pronounced than with benzodiazepines.

To date, potential differences between individual nonbenzodiazepine benzodiazepine receptor agonists have not been examined extensively, so that clear differential recommendations cannot be offered (Dundar et al. 2004).

In most countries, zolpidem is one of the most frequently prescribed nonbenzodiazepine benzodiazepine receptor agonists. With a half-life of 2.5 h, zolpidem does not change sleep architecture or lead to the development of tolerance.

With a half-life of only 1 h, zaleplon has the shortest half-life of all nonbenzodiazepine benzodiazepine receptor agonists. Accordingly, zaleplon is particularly well suited for treating sleep onset delays. However, the substance is not marketed in all countries.

As GABA receptor agonists, zopiclone and eszopiclone have a slightly different mode of action but are commonly nonetheless listed among the group of nonbenzodiazepine benzodiazepine receptor agonists. The half-lives are 5.5 and 6.5 h, respectively. In general, zopiclone and eszopiclone exert only a minimal impact on patients' performance during the following day.

Eszopiclone is the S-enantiomer of the racemate zopiclon. Eszopiclone was introduced to the market shortly before the end of the patent protection of zopiclone. Whether the substance actually shows clinically relevant advantages over zopiclon has not been unequivocally proven (Hair et al. 2008). As a consequence, the European Medicines Agency (EMA) did not consider eszopiclone as a "new active substance," causing the manufacturer to refrain from introducing it to the European markets. Eszopiclone has a half-life of 6.5 h. Results from a meta-analysis of five trials showed good tolerability and efficacy, particularly in elderly patients (Melton et al. 2005). Eszopiclone is one of the very few substances for which studies over a longer period of time have been conducted, demonstrating good efficacy as well as tolerability and no development of tolerance over a period up to 3 months in elderly patients (Ancoli-Israel et al. 2010).

Antidepressants

Antidepressants have not been developed for the treatment of sleep disorders and not approved for this indication. Traditionally, antidepressants with sedative side effects are nevertheless frequently used off label to treat insomnia.

Typically, tricyclic antidepressants such as trazodone, opipramole (not available in the United States), and mirtazapine are given at lower doses than those necessary to treat depression. While opipramole is not an antidepressant but used against anxiety disorders, it is listed here due to its related chemical structure.

To date, we do not have sufficient evidence from clinical studies to support the use of antidepressants against insomnia. Research on the efficacy of antidepressants in sleep disorders has almost exclusively been conducted in patients with depression, in whom insomnia is often a key symptom.

Neither the effectiveness nor the optimal dose of antidepressants in the treatment of insomnia without accompanying depression have been demonstrated. The limited number of studies in primary insomnia did not yield results supporting the use of antidepressants (Erman 2005).

Aside from the fact that there are almost no data showing their efficacy, the numerous adverse side effects of the individual substances speak against the use of antidepressants in older patients.

In light of unproven efficacy and well-documented side effects, the use of antidepressants for the treatment of insomnia without accompanying depression is not recommended.

Antipsychotics

As is the case with antidepressants, antipsychotics have not been developed for the treatment of sleep disorders. In clinical practice, however, many physicians take advantage of the sedating side effect of most antipsychotics to treat sleep disorders. Particularly older, low-potency typical antipsychotics are given at low doses due to their less-pronounced antipsychotic but pronounced sedative properties.

In parallel to inconclusive clinical studies in antidepressants, there are no large systematic studies supporting the use of antipsychotics in sleep disorders. Their optimal doses for the treatment of sleep disorders are not known. At the same time, antipsychotics have a high rate of side effects, such as
- Extrapyramidal symptoms
- Negative metabolic effects
- Weight increase
- Malignant neuroleptic syndrome in rare cases
- Association with increased mortality in patients with dementia.

Despite the aforementioned lack of scientific evidence, physicians have been using antipsychotics in everyday clinical practice. From Euro-

pean experiences, pipamperone, melperone, and tiapride (not FDA approved) are well tolerated given over a limited number of days. However, this observation is not based on scientific data but rather on clinical experience.

The efficacy and tolerability of antipsychotics in the treatment of insomnia have not been sufficiently assessed.

Melatonin and Melatonin Receptor Agonists

Large randomized studies of chemically unaltered melatonin are not available, likely due to the missing commercial potential of this substance, which is produced naturally in the body and thus difficult to license. Smaller studies could demonstrate advantages with regard to sleep quality and sleep onset latency. From a theoretical viewpoint, melatonin is particularly useful in sleep onset disorders. Given short-term use, the substance is well tolerated. While melatonin is not available in some countries, the substance is freely available as a nutritional supplement in the United States and several other countries. However, nutritional supplements hardly guarantee sufficient pharmacological quality control. As their optimal dose is also unknown, the consumption of such supplement preparations must be discouraged.

Recently, an extended-release preparation of melatonin (extended-release preparations of melatonin are available as a supplement in the United States) has been approved in Europe for the treatment of sleep disorders specifically in persons older than 55 years of age. While the respective approval trials (phase III trials) showed excellent tolerability, its effect was comparably small. As there are relatively few data on the long-term use of melatonin, the substance is only approved for short-term use. The risk for the development of tolerance or addiction is presumably low. Thus far, clinical experience with retarded melatonin suggests good tolerability in older patients. Again, however, its effect is apparently comparably small. In cases of predominant sleep onset disorder, melatonin appears useful.

Recently, the selective melatonin agonist ramelteon, carrying additional effects as a serotonin reuptake inhibitor, has been introduced in the United States and several other countries. While its short-term tolerability is excellent, its effect size was small. Largely for this reason, the substance was not approved for use in Europe. The long-term tolerability has not been well investigated yet.

Antihistamines, Anticonvulsives, Phytotherapeutic Agents, and Chloral Hydrate

The very heterogeneous substances antihistamines, anticonvulsives, phytotherapeutic agents, and chloral hydrate were grouped together as neither their efficacy nor their tolerability in older patients has been sufficiently examined to allow for reliable recommendations.

In patients with pain syndromes and depression, pregabalin has been shown to have a positive influence on sleep quality and sleep duration. Whether this finding also holds for patients with insomnia has not been shown thus far. Occasionally, physicians take advantage of the sedating effect of valproic acid for the treatment of sleep disorders. Based on scientific data, this approach cannot be justified.

Diphenhydramine is a freely available, low-priced, first-generation antihistamine substance frequently used to treat insomnia. Neither its use nor possible side effects have been thoroughly examined. The few available studies on diphenhydramine have either yielded inconclusive results or were methodologically flawed (Ancoli-Israel and Cooke 2005). Its sedative effect is subject to the swift development of tolerance. In addition, diphenhydramine and other antihistamines also show anticholinergic effects rendering its use in elderly patients problematic. As a case in point, the use of diphenhydramine led to pronounced cognitive deficits in older patients who had previously shown no cognitive impairment.

Due to their anticholinergic side effects and uncertain efficacy, diphenhydramine and other antihistamines are not recommended for use in elderly patients.

To this day, the hypnotic chloral hydrate that was first introduced in 1869 is still used occasionally. There are no reliable studies of its efficacy, but a number of well-documented side effects, such as rapid induction of tolerance, prolongation of the QT interval, liver failure, and its addiction potential, speak against its use.

Numerous over-the-counter drugs, such as St. John's wort, camomile, hops, kava kava, and passion flower extracts, are marketed for the treatment of sleep disorders. For none of these substances, however, are there adequate data on efficacy and tolerability. In many countries, the sale of kava extracts is prohibited due to isolated cases of associated liver failure. Finally, the pharmaceutical quality of many of these products is not guaranteed.

Principally, considerable placebo effects can be assumed in the treatment of sleep disorders. Keeping this in mind, physicians should not actively advise against the consumption of harmless phytopharmaceuticals if they are well tolerated and patients experience subjective improvement of symptoms.

Classification of Drugs for the Prevention and Therapy of Sleep Disorders (Insomnia) According to Their Fitness for the Aged (FORTA)

(See Chapter "Critical Extrapolation of Guidelines and Study Results: Risk-Benefit Assessment for Patients with Reduced Life Expectancy and a New Classification of Drugs According to Their Fitness for the Aged")

Substance class	Compound	FORTA classification
Nonbenzodiazepine benzodiazepine receptor agonist	Zolpidem, zaleplone	C
GABA receptor agonist	Zopiclone, eszopiclone	C
Benzodiazepine	Oxazepam, triazolam	D
Antipsychotic with sedative effect	Pipamperone, melperone	C[a]
Noradrenergic and serotonergic AD	Mirtazapine	D[a]
Tricyclic anxiolytic	Opipramole	D[a]

(continued)

Tricyclic antidepressant	Doxepin, trazodone	D[a]
Antihistamine	Diphenhydramine	D
Melatonine receptor agonist	Ramelteon	C
Melatonin (extended release)	Melatonin	C[a]

[a]Not approved for the treatment of insomnia in all countries; in everyday practice, however, frequent off-label use.

References

Ancoli-Israel S, Cooke JR (2005) Prevalence and comorbidity of insomnia and effect on functioning in elderly populations. J Am Geriatr Soc 53:S264–S271

Ancoli-Israel S, Krystal AD, McCall MV et al (2010) The effect of eszopiclone 2 mg on sleep/wake function in older adults with primary and comorbid insomnia. Sleep 33:225–234

Bloom HG, Ahmed I, Alessi CA et al (2009) Evidence-based recommendations for the assessment and management of sleep disorders in older persons. J Am Geriatr Soc 57:761–789

Culberson JW, Ziska M (2008) Prescription drug misuse/abuse in the elderly. Geriatrics 63:22–31

Dolder C, Nelson M, McKinsey J (2007) Use of non-benzodiazepine hypnotics in the elderly: are all agents the same? CNS Drugs 21:389–405

Dundar Y, Dodd S, Strobl J et al (2004) Comparative efficacy of newer hypnotic drugs for the short-term management of insomnia: a systematic review and meta-analysis. Hum Psychopharmacol 19:305–322

Erman MK (2005) Therapeutic options in the treatment of insomnia. J Clin Psychiatry 66(Suppl 9):18–23

Flaherty JH (2008) Insomnia among hospitalized older persons. Clin Geriatr Med 24:51–67

Foley DJ, Monjan A, Simonsick EM et al (1999) Incidence and remission of insomnia among elderly adults: an epidemiologic study of 6,800 persons over three years. Sleep 22(Suppl 2):S366–S372

Glass J, Kl L, Herrmann N et al (2005) Sedative hypnotics in older people with insomnia: meta-analysis of risks and benefits. BMJ 331:1169

Hair PI, McCormack PL, Curran MP (2008) Eszopiclone. A review of its use in the treatment of insomnia. Drugs 68:1415–1434

Kripke DF (2007) Greater incidence of depression with hypnotic use than with placebo. BMC Psychiatry 7:42

Kupfer DJ, Reynolds CF 3rd (1997) Management of insomnia. N Engl J Med 336:341–346

Melton ST, Wood JM, Kirkwood CK (2005) Eszopiclone for insomnia. Ann Pharmacother 39:1659–1666

Svarstad BL, Mount JK (2001) Chronic benzodiazepine use in nursing homes: effects of federal guidelines, resident mix, and nurse staffing. J Am Geriatr Soc 49:1673–1678

Vaz Fragoso CA, Gill TM (2007) Sleep complaints in community-living older persons: a multifactorial geriatric syndrome. J Am Geriatr Soc 55:1853–1866

Wolkove N, Elkholy O, Baltzan M et al (2007) Sleep and aging: 1. Sleep disorders commonly found in older people. CMAJ 176:1299–1304

Treatment Decisions and Medical Treatment of Cancer in Elderly Patients

Ulrich Wedding and Stuart M. Lichtman

Relevance for Elderly Patients, Epidemiology

Introduction

The current demographic changes will result in an increasing number of older people. Aging is the single most important risk factor for the development of cancer. The incidence and mortality rates of most malignant disorders increase substantially with increase in age. Both developments combined result in an increasing number of elderly cancer patients (Smith et al. 2009).

Whether behavior of malignant cells, such as growth rate or ability to metastasize, differs between tumors developed in a young or an old organism cannot be answered generally. Tumor biology can be more favorable, indifferent, or worse in elderly patients, depending on the kind of tumor.

The population of old people is very heterogeneous. Individual resources and deficits are insufficiently described by chronological age

itself. Geriatric medicine established the comprehensive geriatric assessment (CGA) to describe these individual resources and deficits.

Recent scientific trials addressed the question of whether the integration of CGA in the care of elderly patients with cancer improves diagnostic accuracy by a better description of patient-related prognostic variables and in the consequence clinical decision making and therapeutic outcome.

Epidemiology of Cancer

Age is the major risk factor for the development of cancer. Table 1 reports the age-dependent increase of incidence and mortality rates in the U.S. population according to gender.

Current Situation of Care

Registries for primary care report that in elderly people compared to younger ones
1. Primary prevention is less often addressed and performed, and
2. Cancer screening is less often addressed and performed.

Cancer registries report that in elderly patients with cancer (Goodwin et al. 1986; Samet et al. 1986; Turner et al. 1999; Bouchardy et al. 2007),
1. The diagnosis is less often confirmed by histology,
2. The disease is more often diagnosed in advanced stage,

U. Wedding (✉)
Clinic for Internal Medicine II, Division of Palliative Care, University Clinics Jena, Erlanger Allee 101, 07740, Jena, Germany
e-mail: ulrich.wedding@med.uni-jena.de

S.M. Lichtman
65+ Clinical Geriatric Program, Memorial Sloan-Kettering Cancer Center, 650 Commack Road, Commack, NY 11725, USA
e-mail: lichtmas@mskcc.org

M. Wehling (ed.), *Drug Therapy for the Elderly*,
DOI 10.1007/978-3-7091-0912-0_18, © Springer-Verlag Wien 2013

Table 1 All cancer sites (invasive) Surveillance Epidemiology and End Result (SEER) incidence[a] and U.S. death[b] rates, age-adjusted and age-specific rates, by race and sex

	All races Total	Males	Females	Whites Total	Males	Females	Blacks Total	Males	Females
SEER incidence									
Age at diagnosis									
Age-adjusted rates, 2004–2008									
All ages	464.4	541.0	411.6	471.8	543.8	423.0	491.2	626.1	400.9
Under 65	223.8	219.1	229.6	226.4	218.9	235.4	247.2	280.6	221.3
65 and over	2,127.8	2,766.2	1,669.7	2,168.3	2,788.1	1,719.8	2,177.5	3,013.8	1,642.7
All ages (IARC world std.)[c]	315.1	355.1	285.6	320.0	356.3	293.6	339.7	426.6	277.6
Age-specific rates, 2004–2008									
<1	23.5	25.6	21.4	24.2	26.5	21.9	18.6	21.0	16.1
1–4	20.7	22.3	19.0	21.6	23.2	19.9	16.1	17.4	14.8
5–9	11.5	12.4	10.6	12.1	13.2	10.9	8.9	9.4	8.5
10–14	13.6	14.2	13.1	14.4	15.0	13.8	11.0	11.0	10.9
15–19	21.6	22.6	20.6	23.1	24.4	21.8	14.7	14.4	15.0
20–24	35.7	33.9	37.7	38.5	37.3	39.9	22.7	19.7	25.8
25–29	54.1	46.5	62.1	58.1	50.6	66.4	39.1	32.7	45.2
30–34	84.3	61.8	107.6	88.7	65.6	113.6	70.4	48.4	90.7
35–39	129.6	87.7	172.6	133.7	91.9	178.0	114.5	77.6	148.2
40–44	214.1	148.1	280.5	217.0	149.8	286.5	210.6	158.2	257.8
45–49	350.6	275.6	424.5	353.1	274.9	432.1	367.8	334.3	397.5
50–54	559.5	536.0	582.2	558.9	526.2	591.3	660.7	739.9	592.7
55–59	854.1	943.2	770.1	856.3	927.9	786.9	1,034.1	1,341.6	780.4
60–64	1,263.5	1,501.2	1,045.8	1,275.6	1,491.6	1,073.2	1,513.2	2,057.3	1,082.2
65–69	1,756.1	2,209.2	1,359.9	1,782.2	2,205.4	1,404.9	1,995.8	2,812.2	1,376.4
70–74	2,091.1	2,691.9	1,602.2	2,137.5	2,714.2	1,658.6	2,158.0	2,996.7	1,560.4
75–79	2,359.2	3,069.3	1,836.6	2,418.3	3,107.0	1,903.0	2,258.6	3,061.9	1,747.8
80–84	2,444.5	3,187.7	1,973.0	2,493.0	3,224.4	2,026.9	2,276.8	3,103.4	1,827.3
85+	2,257.2	3,136.5	1,852.4	2,275.5	3,169.6	1,868.4	2,363.5	3,307.1	2,004.5
U.S. mortality									
Age at death									
Age-adjusted rates, 2004–2008									
All ages	181.3	223.0	153.2	180.0	220.0	152.8	220.8	295.3	177.7
Under 65	58.7	63.0	54.7	56.8	60.7	53.3	82.4	94.2	73.0
65 and over	1,029.2	1,329.5	834.5	1,031.4	1,321.8	841.0	1,177.6	1,685.8	901.0
All ages (IARC world std.)[c]	108.0	128.0	93.2	106.7	125.7	92.6	136.5	174.7	111.9
Age-specific rates, 2004–2008									
<1	1.7	1.9	1.6	1.9	2.0	1.7	1.5	1.7	1.3
1–4	2.3	2.5	2.1	2.4	2.5	2.2	2.4	2.7	2.0
5–9	2.4	2.6	2.3	2.5	2.6	2.3	2.4	2.4	2.3
10–14	2.3	2.4	2.2	2.3	2.5	2.2	2.4	2.5	2.3
15–19	3.3	3.8	2.7	3.3	3.9	2.7	3.2	3.6	2.8
20–24	4.6	5.5	3.7	4.6	5.4	3.7	5.2	5.9	4.5
25–29	6.6	7.0	6.2	6.4	7.0	5.9	8.2	8.1	8.4
30–34	11.3	10.3	12.3	11.0	10.2	11.9	14.6	12.5	16.4
35–39	20.8	17.4	24.3	20.2	17.2	23.2	27.6	20.6	33.8

(continued)

Table 1 (continued)

	All races Total	Males	Females	Whites Total	Males	Females	Blacks Total	Males	Females
40–44	42.7	37.5	47.7	40.8	36.2	45.5	59.8	51.0	67.5
45–49	84.4	81.9	86.9	80.3	77.9	82.8	123.8	122.9	124.6
50–54	152.3	163.2	141.9	145.7	155.0	136.6	224.7	255.6	198.7
55–59	253.0	283.4	224.4	244.9	270.9	219.9	364.9	447.6	296.8
60–64	409.9	472.1	353.0	403.2	459.4	350.7	554.8	702.4	439.5
65–69	617.2	732.1	516.8	613.3	720.7	517.5	781.1	1,011.3	611.1
70–74	860.2	1,046.3	708.1	863.0	1,039.0	716.4	986.9	1,322.4	755.1
75–79	1,129.3	1,424.0	911.8	1,137.0	1,421.8	922.7	1,233.2	1,699.4	948.1
80–84	1,401.9	1,859.5	1,113.8	1,410.2	1,857.7	1,125.0	1,510.2	2,220.1	1,138.7
85+	1,682.8	2,455.0	1,339.8	1,680.3	2,438.4	1,341.8	1,964.5	3,282.5	1,485.0

Source: From SEER Cancer Statistics Review 1975–2008, National Cancer Institute.
ˉStatistic not shown. Rate based on less than 16 cases for the time interval.
[a]SEER 17 areas. Rates are per 100,000 and are age-adjusted to the 2000 US std. population (19 age groups—Census P25-1130), unless noted.
[b]US mortality files, National Center for Health Statistics, Centers for Disease Control and Prevention
Rates are per 100,000 and are age-adjusted to the 2000 US std. population (19 age groups—Census P25-1130), unless noted.
[c]Rates are per 100,000 and are age-adjusted to the IARC world standard population.

3. The stage is less often defined exactly,
4. The treatment is less often applied according to guidelines, and
5. That the referral to cancer centers occurs less often compared to younger ones.

One reason is the lack of valid clinical data (Trimble et al. 1994). Based on the limited data of clinical trials, data from cancer registries are a major source of information. For the United States, data from the Surveillance Epidemiology and End Result (SEER) Program are available and described in more detail when addressing different tumor entities (see following paragraphes). Many treatment decisions in elderly patients with cancer lack a high level of evidence.

Clinical Trials

Elderly patients with cancer are less often included in clinical trials (Monfardini et al. 1994; Hutchins et al. 1999; Lewis et al. 2003). Only 25% of patients included in trials of the Southwest Oncology Group (SWOG) were 65 years of age and older, compared to 63% of all cancer patients in the United States (Hutchins et al. 1999). Lewis et al. reported the recruitment of elderly patients with cancer in clinical trials of the National Cancer Institute (NCI). Of the patients recruited in 495 clinical trials, 32% were older than 65 years compared to 61% of all cancer patients in the U.S. population (Lewis et al. 2003). Especially, the recruitment of very elderly patients, those aged 80 years and older, in clinical trials is very poor. In the United Kingdom, in the MRC-AML-11 trial, for example, investigating treatment strategies in patients with acute myeloid leukemia (AML) aged 55 years and older, only 3 of 1,314 patients included were 80 years and older (Goldstone et al. 2001).

Only in a limited number of patients are the inclusion and exclusion criteria of clinical trials the major reason to exclude elderly patients (Harter et al. 2005). Most inclusion and exclusion criteria lack a high level of evidence. Even when patients fulfill the inclusion and exclusion criteria, advanced age is a major reason not to offer participation (Harter et al. 2005). If elderly patients are offered to participate in a clinical trial, their rate of participation is not different compared to younger ones (Kemeny et al. 2003).

Therapeutically Relevant Special Features of Elderly Patients

Who Is an Elderly Patient/Medically Not Fit?

Older people of the same chronological age can be very different regarding their overall health situation. Conventional history taking and physical examination tend to miss important changes of health and social situation typically occurring with advanced age. The CGA helps to describe elderly persons' health and social situation systematically and to detect resources and limitations.

CGA in General

Areas of CGA and tools to address them within a CGA are described in chapter "Heterogeneity and Vulnerability of Older Patients." The tools of CGA are validated for endpoints often looked at in geriatric medicine (Stuck et al. 1993), such as

1. Is the patient able to live in his or her own home without support?
2. Which kind of support does the patient need?
3. Is institutionalized care necessary?
4. Which resources help to improve the patient's ability for self-care?

These endpoints are different from questions that have to be addressed in care for elderly patients with cancer.

CGA in Oncology

Major questions relating to the care for elderly patients with cancer are

1. Is the newly diagnosed cancer determining the prognosis of the patient?

2. Will the newly diagnosed cancer cause symptoms and affect the patient's quality of life unfavorably?
3. Will the patient be able to tolerate cancer treatment without major adverse events?

In addition to the staging ("tumor assessment"), identifying characteristics of the tumor important for prognosis and for decision making, a CGA is recommended in elderly cancer patients ("patient assessment") to identify age-associated changes of a patient's individual resources and deficits (Extermann and Hurria 2007).

So far, it could be demonstrated, that

1. The use of CGA in elderly cancer patients identifies age-associated changes not recognized without CGA (Extermann et al. 1998; Repetto et al. 1998);
2. The recognized changes can result in a different treatment decision (Extermann et al. 2004; Girre et al. 2008);
3. Changes detected in CGA are of prognostic value regarding early termination of therapy (Frasci et al. 2000), severe toxicity (Freyer et al. 2005; Hurria et al. 2011; Extermann et al. 2012), early death (Honecker et al. 2009), and survival (Wedding et al. 2007b);
4. Elderly cancer patients receiving CGA-based care have a better quality of life and less pain than those treated with usual care (Rao et al. 2005).

As a consequence, the CGA should be part of qualified supportive care of elderly patients with cancer.

In the following, we report the value of the different categories of the CGA in oncology.

Life Expectancy

It is important to know the life expectancy of a person at birth and at a specific age, which actually can be quite different. Current figures for the United States are reported in Table 2.

Functional Status

In oncology, functional status is traditionally measured according to Eastern Cooperative Oncology Group (ECOG) Performance Status (PS), Karnofsky Performance Status (KPS), or

Table 2 Life expectancy at birth, at age 65, and at age 75 by sex for the United States in 2007

	At birth	At 65	At 70	At 75	At 80	At 85	At 90
Both sexes	77.9	18.6	15.0	11.7	8.8	6.5	4.6
Female	80.4	19.9	16.0	12.5	9.4	6.8	4.8
Male	75.4	17.2	13.7	10.6	7.9	5.8	4.1

Source: From Xu et al. 2010.

World Health Organization (WHO) PS (Karnofsky et al. 1948; Buccheri et al. 1996). These scores are validated and of prognostic information for tolerance of treatment and survival (Mor et al. 1984). The tools, established in oncology to measure performance status, correlate with tools established in geriatric medicine to measure functional status; however, they are not identical and replaceable (Extermann et al. 1998).

Cognitive Impairment

When caring for elderly patients with cancer, it is essential to know about their cognitive function for two major reasons: first to judge patients' ability to give informed consent and second to judge the ability for adherence within complex treatment protocols. Repetto et al. reported a decline of the relative frequency of patients with normal cognitive function with increasing age: According to them, 81% of those aged 65–74 years, 60% of those aged 75–84 years, and 32% of those aged 85 years and older had no cognitive impairment in the Mini-Mental Status Examination (MMSE) (Repetto et al. 1998).

Depression

A review of Massie reported the frequency of depression in cancer patients in general (Massie 2004). In CGA, 30% of elderly cancer patients were screened positive for prevalence of depression (Repetto et al. 1998). In patients with cancer of the ovary, prevalence of depression was independently associated with increased toxicity and impaired survival (Freyer et al. 2005).

Mobility

Scales to measure functional status integrate some measurement of mobility. Geriatric medicine, however, has established more detailed instruments to measure mobility. Data on the prognostic value of impaired mobility are missing for elderly cancer patients so far.

Social Situation

The assessment of social situation is part of a structured assessment of the psychosocial context. It is described that social support is associated with positive effects on physical and psychological well-being. A positive association of perceived social support and well-being was reported by different studies. Within a meta-analysis of 37 controlled trials, a positive association of psychosocial intervention on the quality of life of cancer patients was reported (Rehse and Pukrop 2003). DeBoer et al. reported that social integration and social support are positively associated with length of survival in cancer patients (De Boer et al. 1999). Special data for elderly patients with cancer are missing.

Comorbidity

The structured assessment of the comorbidities is necessary for the judgment of prognosis and of the risk of increased treatment associated side effects. The importance of comorbidity for the 1-year survival rates of cancer patients differs according to the stage of the disease (local, regional, and distant) and to the type of tumor (Read et al. 2004). More than 80% of patients with advanced non-small-cell lung cancer (NSCLC) and comorbidities of more than two in the Charlson Comorbidity Scale terminated chemotherapy prior to completion of a second cycle (Frasci et al. 2000). However, the results have to be confirmed in a larger sample of patients.

Polypharmacy

Comorbidities result in the need to take numerous drugs in addition to those described for the treatment of cancer. For detailed description, a recent review was presented by Lees and Chan (2011). Freyer at al. reported the prognostic relevance in patients aged 70 years and older with cancer of the ovary (Freyer et al. 2005).

Evidence-Based, Rationalistic Drug Therapy and Classification of Drugs According to Their Fitness for the Aged (FORTA)

Drug treatment of cancer patients covers tumor-specific drugs and drugs for supportive care. In the past, tumor-specific drugs mainly consisted of hormone or chemotherapy. In recent years, numerous other drugs have been approved, such as antibodies, tyrosine kinase inhibitors (TKIs), proteasome inhibitors, and others.

It is not possible to classify all drugs approved for oncologic care for age-associated differences in efficacy and toxicity or to recommend approaches for elderly patients with all different types of tumor. We therefore focus on the general principles of oncologic care for elderly patients with cancer and on treatment concepts for the most frequent cancer types. A more detailed approach was reported by Hurria and Balducci (2009).

The Fit for the Aged (FORTA) classification was recently recommended by Wehling (2009) and is described in detail in chapter "Critical Extrapolation of Guidelines and Study Results: Risk-Benefit Assessment for Patients with Reduced Life Expectancy and a New Classification of Drugs According to Their Fitness for the Aged" under the section "Categorization of Drugs with Regard to Their Fitness for the Aged." Application of this classification to drugs used in oncology has some limitations. Most drugs in oncology are used for a limited time, and most treatments are combination therapy. However, FORTA classification covers single agents and drugs permanently taken. We therefore differ from the concept of other parts of this book and do not provide a table listing the mentioned drugs according to their FORTA classification.

Tumor-Specific Medical Treatment

A number of former studies could not demonstrate an age-associated increase in toxicity rates when treating elderly patients with cancer (Begg and Carbone 1983; Gelman and Taylor 1984; Christman et al. 1992; Borkowski et al. 1994; Giovanazzi-Bannon et al. 1994). However, patients included in these analyses are biased, especially regarding referral and selection. In more recent, less-biased trials, different authors reported an association of increased hematological and nonhematological toxicity with increased age of the patients (Stein et al. 1995; Crivellari et al. 2000). However, these analyses insufficiently integrated age-associated changes of functional status and presence of comorbidity. Therefore, the question remains whether increased age itself or whether age-related changes are associated with increased toxicity of chemotherapy.

The reason for increased toxicity with advanced age can be related to changes in either pharmacokinetics or in pharmacodynamics, resulting in a prolonged exposure to the drug or in an increased vulnerability within prolonged regeneration (Wedding et al. 2007a).

In general, a classification of patients according to the presumed toxicity of treatment and to the non-cancer-related general health situation is recommended and exemplarily described for patients with prostate cancer (Droz et al. 2010).

Adjuvant Treatment

Adjuvant treatment implies a real burden for potential future benefit. Application of chemotherapy in elderly patients has to be discussed critically as advanced age is associated with increased real burden (toxicity), and potential future benefit might be less than in younger patients based on reduced life expectancy.

Preferably, patients should be included in clinical trials.

The major malignant disorders in which adjuvant or perioperative treatment is indicated in younger patients are breast cancer, colorectal cancer, lung cancer, and gastric cancer.

Breast Cancer

The treatment algorithms for breast cancer are nearly exceptionally based on disease characteristics, such as tumor size, node involvement, endocrine receptor status (endocrine responsive vs. nonresponsive), vascular invasion, and human epidermal growth factor receptor 2 (HER2) expression (Goldhirsch et al. 2006). Characteristics of elderly patients, such as comorbidity or functional status, are nearly ignored. Age-associated changes rarely set limitations to endocrine treatment. However, adjuvant chemotherapy has to be discussed critically based on age-associated increase in toxicity and reduced efficacy.

Schairer et al. demonstrated that only in women with localized disease breast cancer is the leading cause of death compared to other causes in women aged less than 50 years, and in women with regionalized disease, it is the leading cause only in women aged less than 60 years of life (Schairer et al. 2004). An analysis of the MA-17 trial reported the frequency of breast cancer associated and non-breast-cancer-associated causes of death after a median follow-up of 3.9 months. The trial included 5,710 women with breast cancer, median age 62 years, range 32–94 years, who had received 5 years of letrozole or placebo if they were free of recurrence 5 years after tamoxifen. Of deaths, 60% were not associated with breast cancer, 48% in those aged younger than 70 years, and 72% in those older than 70 years (Chapman et al. 2008).

Choice of optimal treatment might differ between younger and older women with breast cancer. Data for medical treatment are reported in more detail in the following section. However, the same is true for radiotherapy. Hughes et al. reported that in women aged 70 years and older with T1, node-negative, estrogen-receptor-positive breast cancer, the addition of radiotherapy to lumbectomy and tamoxifen only improved local recurrence, but not mastectomy rate for local recurrence, rates of distant metastases, and 5-year overall survival (Hughes et al. 2004).

Endocrine Therapy

Endocrine therapy can prolong disease-free and overall survival in women with endocrine-responsive breast cancer (Goldhirsch et al. 2007). Age-associated differences in efficacy of endocrine treatment have not been reported so far (Coates et al. 2007). While chemotherapy is mainly applied to decrease the incidence of early recurrence, endocrine therapy targets the prevention of early and late recurrence. The established 5 years of adjuvant tamoxifen treatment has been requestioned in three different approaches:

1. Up-front aromatase inhibitor (Arimidex, Tamoxifen, Alone or in Combination (ATAC) trial, Breast International Group (BIG)-1-98 trial),
2. Sequential therapy after 2–3 years of tamoxifen (Arimidex-Nolvadex (ARNO)-95 trial/ Austrilian Breast Cancer Study Group (ABCSG)-8 trial, Intergroup Exemestane Study (IES) trial, Intergruppo Tamoxifen Arimidex (ITA) trial),
3. Prolonged therapy after 5 years of tamoxifen (ABCSG-6a trial, MA-17 trial, National Surgical Adjuvant Breast and Bowel Project (NSABP)-B-33 trial).

For item 1, the ATAC trial could demonstrate an improvement of overall survival, the BIG-1-98 trial (Forbes et al. 2008; Regan et al. 2011).

For item 2, the ARNO-95 trial and the IES could report improved disease-free and overall survival (OS), with the IES trial reporting an improvement of relapse-free survival (Kaufmann et al. 2007; Bliss et al. 2012).

For item 3, the ABCSG-6a trial reported an improved disease-free survival (Jakesz et al. 2007), the MA-17 trial recently reported improved disease-free and overall survival (Jin et al. 2012), and the NSABP-B-33 trial reported a significant improvement of recurrence-free, but not of OS, survival (Mamounas et al. 2008).

For the BIG-1-98 trial, an analysis was performed for different age groups with respect to treatment adherence, disease-free survival, and treatment-related toxicity (Crivellari et al. 2008). Patients were attributed to three different age groups:

1. Young postmenopausal patients aged less than 65 years ($n = 3{,}127$)
2. Elderly patients aged 65–74 years ($n = 1{,}500$)
3. Old patients aged 75 years and older ($n = 295$).

The scheduled treatment duration of 5 years was completed by 76.4% of those younger than 65 years, 77.4% of those aged 65–74 years, and 61.1% of those aged 75 years and older. There was no significant difference in this rate between the tamoxifen arm (62.8%) and the letrozole arm (60.3%). Age-associated differences regarding efficacy were not reported. The incidence of adverse events increased with age. Differences between the arms existed regarding frequency of fractures; 8.5% of patients aged 75 years and older experienced fractures, 5.4% in the tamoxifen and 11.6% in the letrozole arm. Regarding cardiac adverse events, the results were not uniform.

Chemotherapy

The following issues suggest a decreased benefit and increased risk profile for adjuvant chemotherapy (Bonadonna and Valagussa 1981; Goldhirsch et al. 1990):

1. Shorter remaining life expectancy
2. Decreased effective dose
3. Differences in tumor biology.

Adjuvant chemotherapy improves disease-free survival and OS of patients with breast cancer. However, data regarding women aged 70 years and older are limited (Early Breast Cancer Trialists' Collaborative Group 2005).

The analysis of registry data could not find an improved OS in patients aged 65 years and older with endocrine-responsive disease when chemotherapy was added. However, these data confirmed the efficacy of adjuvant chemotherapy in endocrine-nonresponsive disease (Elkin et al. 2006; Giordano et al. 2006). In contrast, Muss et al. reported the results of a retrospective analysis of four trials conducted by the Cancer and Leukemia Group B (CALGB). They reported that older women and younger women derived similar reductions in breast cancer mortality and recurrence from regimens containing more intense chemotherapy. However, of 6,487 women with lymph-node-positive breast cancer, 542 (8%) patients were 65 years or older and 159 (2%) were 70 years or older (Muss et al. 2005).

A reduction of dose intensity to less than 85% is associated with reduced efficacy. Prior to the start of adjuvant chemotherapy, the decision has to be made whether the planned dose can be applied without major dose reduction. If the need for a dose reduction is very likely, the patient might benefit from a decision not to apply adjuvant chemotherapy.

Cyclophosphamid, Methotrexat, 5-Fluorouracil (CMF) is a well-established protocol. Colleoni et al. described an age-dependent increase in therapy-related mortality for patients aged 65 years and older compared to younger ones (Colleoni et al. 1999).

If an adjuvant chemotherapy is indicated, standard protocols and standard dosage should be applied. Muss et al. demonstrated that capecitabine is inferior to a standard CMF or AC (Adriamyin, Cyclophosphamid) regimen in women aged 65 years and older (Muss et al. 2009). The survival benefit was limited to patients with endocrine-nonresponsive disease.

Pinder et al. reported an increased risk of heart failure for women aged 65–70 years treated with an anthracycline-based regimen compared to younger ones (Pinder et al. 2007).

Based on preliminary data, the combination of docetaxel and carboplatin is a regimen not containing anthracyclines that might serve as an alternative regimen when anthracyclines are not indicated (Ewer and O'Shaughnessy 2007).

A recent EBCTCG (Early Breast Cancer Trialists' Collaborative Group) review addresses the question whether an anthracycline or a taxane based regime is superior to CMF (Early Breast Cancer Trialists' Collaborative Group 2012). However, data are limited to patients aged 70 years and older.

According to the FORTA classification, the CMF and the AC-/EC (Epirubicin, Cyclophosphamid) regimen are classified as group B therapy.

Immunotherapy/Targeted Therapy

As an example for immunotherapy/targeted therapy, the addition of trastuzumab to adjuvant chemotherapy in women with HER2-positive disease improves disease-free survival and OS (Slamon et al. 2011). An increased heart failure rate is the major additional toxicity. The relative frequency of patients with HER2-positive disease decreased with age. The trials evaluating the efficacy of the addition of trastuzumab did not include elderly women. The Finnish trial included only women younger than 66 years; the median age of the patients was 50.8 years. Only 16% of women in the trial reported by Romond et al. were over 60 years of age. The median age of women treated in the Herceptin Adjuvant Trial (HERA) trial was 49 years. The authors of the HERA trial reported that the age of the patients was not associated with the occurrence of heart failure (Piccart-Gebhart et al. 2005; Romond et al. 2005; Joensuu et al. 2006). A major question for future trials remains whether the addition of trastuzumab to endocrine therapy only results in similar efficacy.

According to the FORTA classification, trastuzumab as part of adjuvant chemotherapy is classified as group A therapy.

Colorectal Carcinoma

Of all recurrences of colorectal carcinoma, 80% occur within 3 years after primary treatment (Sargent et al. 2005). Data from patient registries (Ayanian et al. 2003; Edwards et al. 2005; Cronin et al. 2006) report that.

1. Elderly patients are less often treated with adjuvant chemotherapy.
2. Comorbidity is a reason not to apply adjuvant chemotherapy; however, chronological age is more important in this decision.

1,096 physicians were asked whether they would offer chemotherapy to a 55-year-old patient with no comorbidity, moderate comorbidity, or severe comorbidity or to an 80-year-old patient. The answers were yes in 99.0%, 88.6%, and 24.9%, respectively, for the younger patient compared to 92.6%, 47.2%, and 9.0%, respectively, for the older one (Keating et al. 2008). Whether the decision against adjuvant chemotherapy implies ageism cannot be judged. Data suggest that the factor of chronological age is overemphasized compared to the factor of functional status and comorbidity.

Clinical trials demonstrated that adjuvant chemotherapy improves disease-free survival and OS of patients with stage III colon carcinoma (Sargent et al. 2001; Andre et al. 2004).

Adjuvant radiochemotherapy improves disease-free survival and OS of patients with rectal carcinoma (Neugut et al. 2002).

Subgroup analyses for patients aged 70 years and older are published. Sargent et al. reported an improved disease-free overall survival and OS for patients aged 70 years and older with colon carcinoma stage III (Sargent et al. 2001). Sundarajan et al. could demonstrate the benefit in a retrospective analysis of data of the SEER program (Sundararajan et al. 2002). Disease-related mortality was of similar frequency in patients aged older and younger than 70 years; however, mortality from other causes was increased in older patients. In addition, besides a slightly increased rate of grade 3–4 neutropenia, toxicity of a regimen based on 5-fluorouracil (5-FU) was similar in older and in younger patients. The authors concluded that medically fit elderly patients should receive 5-FU-based adjuvant chemotherapy (Sargent et al. 2001). Many trials limited the participation of patients to those younger than 75 years of age (e.g., the Multicenter International Study of Oxaliplatin/5-Fluorouracil/Leucovorin in the Adjuvant Treatment of Colon Cancer (MOSAIC) trial; Andre et al. 2004; others did not give any age limits in the inclusion and exclusion criteria. However, the median age of recruited patients was well beyond that of all patients with the disease in the general population (e.g., Xeloda in Adjuvant Colon Cancer Therapy (X-Act) trial median age 62 years, range 22–82 years; Twelves et al. 2005). The selection criteria for inclusion or exclusion of a patient from that trial were not reported.

One of the three following protocols is recommended when treating elderly patients after R0 resection in stage III disease:

- 5-FU-based bolus or infusional regimens (Andre et al. 2004; Haller et al. 2005)
- Capecitabine (Twelves et al. 2005)
- FOLFOX-4 (5-Fluorouracil, Leukovorin, Oxapliplatin) (Andre et al. 2004)
- CAPOX Capecitabine, Oxaliplatin (Haller et al. 2011).

The choice is based on comorbidity, functional status, compliance and age. Only patients without major comorbidity should be treated with adjuvant chemotherapy after R0 resection of stage III colon carcinoma. In patients with good compliance, an oral regimen is a possible choice.

Recent preliminary data reported that patients aged 70 years and older do not benefit from the addition of oxaliplatin to a 5-FU-based adjuvant chemotherapy regimen in stage III colon carcinoma (McCleary et al. 2009).

Until now, the addition of immuno- or targeted therapy to adjuvant chemotherapy cannot be supported.

According to the FORTA classification, the 5-FU-based regimens and capecitabine are classified as group A therapy.

Lung Cancer

Current data from clinical trials and a meta-analysis support the use of postoperative adjuvant chemotherapy in elderly patients with lung cancer. A cisplatin-based adjuvant chemotherapy resulted in a 5% absolute increase in 5-year OS (Pignon et al. 2008). An analysis of pooled individual patient data reported that patients aged 70 years and older received a lower total dose of cisplatin and fewer cycles compared to younger ones. Toxicity rates were not higher, and OS was not different. Non-lung-cancer-related death was more common in older patients. However, only 9% of all patients analyzed were 70 years and older (Fruh et al. 2008). Thus, the treated population seemed to be highly selected. A detailed review was provided by Pallis et al. (2009).

According to the FORTA classification, the adjuvant cisplatin-based chemotherapy is classified as group B therapy.

Gastric Cancer

Perioperative chemotherapy improves progression-free survival (PFS) and OS in patients with gastric cancer or cancer of the gastroesophageal junction (Cunningham et al. 2006), with 21% of patients included in this trial 70 years and older. The median age was 62 years, the range 23–85 years. The patients were treated with three cycles of polychemotherapy, including epirubicin, cisplatin, and 5-FU (EFC regimen). Advanced age was not associated with a lower efficacy. A detailed

review was provided by Wagner and Wedding (2009).

According to the FORTA classification, the adjuvant Epirubicin, Cisplatin, 5-Fluorouracil (ECF) chemotherapy is classified as group A therapy.

Advanced Stage

Breast Cancer

The realistic aim of the treatment in advanced stage cancers is the maintenance or the improvement of health-related quality of life (HRQoL) and a limited prolongation of survival. One of the most important factors of HRQoL in elderly people is the maintenance of the ability for self-care. The treatment decision is based on

- The wishes of the patient,
- The hormone-receptor status,
- The HER-2 status,
- The number and type of metastases,
- The prior treatment,
- The time interval between primary treatment and treatment of advanced disease,
- The burden of symptoms,
- The general condition of the patient,
- And the comorbidities.

Endocrine Treatment

Endocrine therapy is the treatment of choice in patients with advanced breast cancer and endocrine-responsive disease. In the need for a fast response, a primary endocrine therapy is not indicated; then, chemotherapy is the treatment of choice. Antiestrogens and aromatase inhibitors are not cross resistant. Based on the higher rate of remission, aromatase inhibitors are recommended as the first-line treatment. Second-line endocrine therapy is possible (e.g. with the pure estrogen antagonist fulvestrant) (Bonneterre et al. 2000; Osborne et al. 2002). Chronological age is not a relevant treatment factor in the decision for endocrine therapy in advanced-stage disease.

According to the FORTA classification, the endocrine therapy of advanced-stage breast cancer is classified as group A therapy.

Chemotherapy

A number of active agents are available if chemotherapy is indicated in advanced stage breast cancer. A polychemotherapy may result in a slightly improved OS; however, it is associated with a higher rate of toxicity. In elderly patients with few symptoms and slowly progressive disease, single-agent chemotherapy is the treatment of choice in non-endocrine-responsive disease or after progression on endocrine treatment. In patients with considerable symptoms and rapidly progressive disease, so in need for a fast remission, polychemotherapy is recommended as first-line chemotherapy (Fossati et al. 1998).

An overlap between main toxicities and pre-existing comorbidities should be avoided (e.g., agents with neurotoxicity in patients with neuropathy, agents with cardiac toxicity in patients with heart failure, etc.).

According to the FORTA classification, the chemotherapy of advanced-stage breast cancer is classified as group B therapy.

Immunotherapy/Targeted Therapy

Regarding immunotherapy/targeted therapy, patients with HER2-positive breast cancer should receive trastuzumab in addition to chemotherapy (Slamon et al. 2001). Patients with progress of the disease during or shortly after the treatment with trastuzumab and chemotherapy can be treated with capecitabine and lapatinib (Cameron et al. 2008), a tyrosine kinase inhibitor of EGFR and HER2. This is superior to single-agent capecitabine and significantly improves the time to treatment failure, protects against central nervous system (CNS) recurrence, and has demonstrated a trend to improve OS (Geyer et al. 2006; Cameron et al. 2008).

According to the FORTA classification, the addition of trastuzumab to chemotherapy as first-line immunochemotherapy for advanced breast cancer and the combination of lapatinib and capecitabine as second-line therapy after progression on trastuzumab are classified as group A therapy.

Recently, the U.S. Food and Drug Administration (FDA) has withdrawn the approval of bevacizumab as a therapeutic option for the treatment of advanced breast cancer since the results of the ECIG 2100 trial could not be confirmed (Tanne 2011).

Colorectal Carcinoma

The treatment of choice for colorectal carcinoma reflects the wishes of the patient, the EGFR status, the k-ras status, the number and types of metastases, the prior treatment, the time interval between primary treatment of metastases, the burden of symptoms, the general condition of the patient, and the comorbidities (Kohne et al. 2008).

Chemotherapy

Poor performance status is more common in the population of elderly patients. Sargent et al. recently reported an analysis of nine trials, including a total of 6,286 patients and thereof 509 (8%) with poor performance status (i.e., ECOG-PS = 2). The median age of all patients was 63 years and did not differ according to PS, which seems to reflect patient selection, as young patients with poor PS were included, but old patients were not. Poor PS was associated

– With a lower remission rate (43.8% vs. 32.0%)
– With a shorter PFS (7.6 vs. 4.9 months)
– With a shorter OS (17.3 vs. 8.5 months)
– With a higher toxicity rate (see the following)
– With a higher 60-day mortality rate (2.8% vs. 12.0%).

The relative benefit of chemotherapy was independent of the PS of the patient (Sargent et al. 2009). Interestingly, only nausea (8.5% vs. 16.4%; $p < 0.001$) and vomiting (7.6% vs. 11.9%; $p = 0.006$) as grade 3 toxicities were more common in patients with poor PS compared to those with good PS, but not diarrhea (17.6 vs. 16.9), stomatitis (2.3 vs. 5.0), and neutropenia (33.7 vs. 34.5). However, the data do not reflect the situation of elderly patients.

According to the FORTA classification, chemotherapy of advanced colorectal carcinoma is classified as group B therapy.

Immunotherapy/Targeted Therapy

Regarding immunotherapy/targeted therapy, a couple of trials demonstrated that the addition of the VEGF (vascular endothelial growth factor) inhibitor bevacizumab to a first-line chemotherapy with 5-FU/LV (leucovorin) or irinotecan with 5-FU/LV or oxaliplatin with 5-FU/LV improves PFS (Hurwitz et al. 2004; Kabbinavar et al. 2005). A subgroup analysis of patients 65 years and older demonstrated that the addition of bevacizumab prolongs PFS (9.2 vs. 6.2 months) and OS (19.3 vs. 14.3 months), but not remission rate (34.4 vs. 29.0%) if compared to those not treated with bevacizumab. The rate of toxicities was not higher in patients aged 65 years and older compared to younger ones. The median age of the population was 72 years, range 65–90 years, and 12.8% of patients were 80 years and older (Kabbinavar et al. 2009).

According to the FORTA classification, the addition of bevacizumab to chemotherapy of advanced colorectal carcinoma is classified as group B therapy.

Currently, two EGFR inhibitors are approved for the treatment of advanced colorectal carcinoma (cetuximab and panitumumab). The treatment is only effective in patients with k-ras wild type (Amado et al. 2008; Lievre et al. 2008). The addition of cetuximab to a first-line FOLFIRI regimen improves the PFS (8.9 vs. 8.0 months; $p = 0.048$), but not the OS (19.9 vs. 18.6 months; $p = 0.31$). The cost is an increase in the toxicity rates:

- Skin toxicity grade 3 (19.7% vs. 0.2%; $p < 0.001$)
- Infusion-related toxicity grade 3–4 (2.5% vs. 0%; $p < 0.001$)
- Diarrhea grade 3–4 (15.7% vs. 10.5%; $p = 0.008$).

The median age of the patients was 61 years (Van Cutsem et al. 2009). The median age of patients with this disease is about 70 years in the general population.

The addition of cetuximab to a treatment with capecitabine, oxaliplatin, and bevacizumab is associated with decreased efficacy; the PFS is significantly reduced (9.4 months vs. 10.7 months; $p = 0.01$), and grade 3 and higher

toxicity is increased (81.7% vs. 73.2%; $p = 0.006$). The median age of the trial population was 62 years, range 27–83 years. In the subgroup of patients with k-ras wild-type carcinoma, the addition of cetuximab improved the remission rate (50.0% vs. 61.4%; $p = 0.06$) but not the PFS (10.6 vs. 10.5 months; $p = 0.30$) and OS (22.5 vs. 21.8 months; $p = 0.64$) (Tol et al. 2009).

Lung Cancer

Treatment of patients with advanced lung cancer aims to improve symptoms and to prolong life.

Chemotherapy

A number of effective agents are available for first-line chemotherapy. The Elderly Lung Cancer Vinorelbine Italian Study Group (ELVIS) demonstrated that patients aged 70 years and older benefitted from chemotherapy compared to best supportive care only. Chemotherapy improved symptoms and HRQoL and survival (The Elderly Lung Cancer Vinorelbine Italian Study Group 1999).

Compared to vinorelbine treatment, docetaxel seems to be associated with a greater prolongation of survival; however, this is at the cost of increased toxicity (Kudoh et al. 2006).

Until recently, single-agent chemotherapy was recommended for elderly patients. Quoix et al. recently reported a French trial comparing single-agent vinorelbine or gemcitabine mono-chemotherapy versus carboplatin and paclitaxel doublet chemotherapy in elderly patients with advanced NSCLC. Median age was 77 years. OS was 6.2 months in the single-agent arm versus 10.3 months for doublet chemotherapy, and 1-year survival rates were 24.5% versus 42.4%. However, toxic death rate and grade 3–4 toxicity were more common with doublet than with single-agent chemotherapy (Quoix et al. 2011).

Immunotherapy/Targeted Therapy

In patients with mutated epidermal growth factor (EGF) receptor, first-line therapy with erlotinib improved PFS compared to chemotherapy and reduced toxicity (Zhou et al. 2011). The inhibition of the EGF receptor with erlotinib was associated with prolonged survival in second- and third-line treatment compared to best supportive care in elderly patients. However, compared to younger patients, older patients experienced increased toxicity (Lynch et al. 2004).

Hematological Neoplasias

The incidence rates of the most frequent hematological neoplasias increased with increasing age. In the following, we report on four major hematological neoplasias for which treatment decision is difficult in elderly patients:

– Myelodysplastic syndrome (MDS)
– Acute myeloid leukemia (AML)
– Chronic lymphocytic leukemia (CLL)
– Multiple myeloma (MM).

Myelodysplastic Syndrome

MDS is a clonal disorder of hematopoetic stem cells, resulting in ineffective hematopoesis with cytopenia of peripheral blood cells. The consequences are anemia, increased risk of bleeding, and recurrent infections. The median age at diagnosis is 65–70 years. The stage distribution is based on disease characteristics, such as

– The blast count in the bone marrow,
– The degree of cytopenia, and
– The presence of cytogenetic changes.

In addition, patient characteristics are important (e.g., the presence of comorbidities) (Sperr et al. 2010).

At early stages, treatment of elderly patients aims to reduce the frequency of blood transfusions, to reduce the rate of infections, and to avoid the progression into AML. In late stage, treatment is similar to that of AML.

Recently, three agents have been approved for the treatment of MDS by the U.S. FDA: azycytidine, decitabine, and lenalidomide. The EMA only approved azycytidine so far. Azacytidine is approved for the treatment of patients with intermediate- or high-risk MDS according to the International Prognostic Scoring System (IPSS), chronic myelomonocytic leukemia (CMML) with a blast count of 10–29%, and AML with a blast count of 20–30% in the bone marrow and with

multilineage dysplasia according to WHO classification. The approval is based on the data of the AZA-001 trial. The median age of the patients was 69 years (range 42–83 years). Treatment with azacytidine was associated with a gain in survival of 9 months, 15 in the conventional therapy arm compared to 24 in the azacytidine arm (Fenaux et al. 2009a). Seymour et al. especially analyzed the results in the subgroup of patients aged 75 years and older. They concluded that azacytidine should be considered the treatment of choice in patients aged 75 years or older with good performance status and higher-risk MDS (Seymour et al. 2010).

Acute Myeloid Leukemia

The median age of patients newly diagnosed for AML is about 65 years. The treatment goal is for cure if no unfavorable prognostic factors of the leukemia or of the patient are present. The major prognostic factor of the leukemia is the presence of cytogenetic changes in the leukemic blasts. The major prognostic factor of the patient is the functional status. In elderly patients, unfavorable cytogenetic changes and impaired functional status are more common than in younger patients. Standard treatment within a curative treatment approach is the combination of an anthracycline and cytosine arabinoside; unfortunately, this treatment is associated with severe cytopenia and high early death rate. Elderly patients with poor functional status or unfavorable cytogenetic changes are candidates for a primary noncurative treatment approach, either with low-dose chemotherapy (e.g. cytosine arabinoside) or best supportive care only. In elderly patients with AML and low blast count, azacytidine improves OS (Fenaux et al. 2009b). Preliminary data reported an improved survival for this group of patients when treated with the hypomethylating agent decitabine (Thomas et al. 2011).

According to the FORTA classification, chemotherapy of AML is group A therapy.

Chronic Lymphocytic Leukemia

In elderly patients, treatment of CLL aims to prolong survival and to alleviate symptoms. Chlorambucil is a long-known, well-tolerated, and effective agent. In a recently published trial of the German CLL study group, fludarabine resulted in an improved remission rate but not improved survival compared to chlorambucil (Eichhorst et al. 2009b). Bendamustine was associated with an increased rate of toxicity despite improved remission rate and PFS (Knauf et al. 2009). Current treatment strategies for elderly patients were reported in more detail by Eichhorst et al. (2009a). The addition of rituximab, a CD-20 antibody, improved the remission rate, PFS, and OS in patients treated with fludarabine and cyclophosphamide (Hallek et al. 2010).

According to the FORTA classification, chemotherapy of CLL is group A therapy.

MM

In elderly patients, the goals of treatment of multiple myeloma are prolongation of survival and improvement of symptoms. No age-associated differences in the efficacy of the treatment are described. Treatment of choice is the combination of melphalan, thalidomide, and prednisolone in patients aged 64–74 years (Facon et al. 2007) and in patients aged 75 years or older (Hulin et al. 2009). Another effective regimen is the combination of bortezomib with melphalan and prednisolone. The median age of the patients was 71 years, and 30% were 75 years and older (San Miguel et al. 2008).

The European Myeloma Network provided current recommendations on how to personalize therapy in patients with multiple myeloma based on patient age and vulnerability (Palumbo et al. 2011).

According to the FORTA classification, the first-line chemotherapy of multiple myeloma with melphalan, thalidomide, and prednisolone or with melphalan, bortezomib, and prednisolone is classified as group A therapy.

Supportive Care

Supportive care aims to prevent or to improve symptoms of the tumor or the treatment and to improve patients' quality of life by other treatment strategies than targeting the tumor directly.

A variety of medical and nonmedical treatment options are available.

Hematological toxicity and emesis belong to the most common side effects of cancer treatment. Factors to stimulate the production of neutrophils are indicated in primary prophylaxis if the suspected rate of febrile neutropenia is over 20%. Risk factors for febrile neutropenia should be included in this decision, and age of 65 years and older is a risk factor for higher rates of febrile neutropenia following chemotherapy (Repetto et al. 2003; Aapro et al. 2006).

According to the FORTA classification, the treatment with granulocyte colony-stimulating factors (G-CSFs) is classified as group A therapy when given according to the indications supported by the guidelines.

Age is a risk factor for anemia (Endres et al. 2009). In elderly cancer patients, anemia affects quality of life more than in younger patients (Wedding et al. 2007c). The use of erythropoesis-stimulating agents (ESAs) in elderly cancer patients is as effective as in younger patients. It is essential to use these agents according to the license, which is restricted to chemotherapy-induced anemia (Bokemeyer et al. 2007; Aapro and Link 2008). In the United States, they are not approved for treatment with curative intent.

According to the FORTA classification, the treatment with ESAs is classified as group B therapy if indicated and in line with the guidelines.

The prophylactic use of antiemetic drugs is essential and independent of age. Elderly patients with functional impairment or comorbidity affected by nausea and vomiting are more prone to deterioration of their general health condition than younger patients or elderly patients without function impairment or comorbidities. Anticipatory nausea and vomiting is less common in elderly cancer patients (Watson et al. 1992).

According to the FORTA classification, the use of antiemetics is classified as group A therapy.

Definition of Aims of Treatment

A clear definition of aims of treatment is the most essential step before starting tumor therapy.

Aims of treatment include whether they

- Are curative
- Are noncurative
- Prolong survival
- Prolong time without symptoms
- Maintain quality of life
- Improve quality of life
- Improve symptoms
- Allow dying with dignity.

When considering risks and benefits of treatment, elderly patients might abstain from chemotherapy more often than younger patients as their risk of toxicity from chemotherapy is higher, as the effect on their survival is less, and as their treatment preferences might differ from younger patients. However, chronological age itself is no barrier to cancer treatment. Elderly patients can benefit in a similar way from cancer treatment as younger ones. Chronological age itself does not justify diagnostic or therapeutic nihilism. Unfortunately, the scientific base as far as high level of evidence is concerned is very limited in elderly cancer patients. The chronological age itself is not a good descriptor of an elderly patient's health situation. A CGA is much better to describe the individual deficits and resources of an elderly patient. Deficits recognized in the CGA are risk factors for toxicity and for less treatment benefit. Current data describe both under- and overtreatment of elderly cancer patients.

References

Aapro MS, Link H (2008) September 2007 update on EORTC guidelines and anemia management with erythropoiesis-stimulating agents. Oncologist 13 (Suppl 3):33–36

Aapro MS, Cameron DA, Pettengell R et al (2006) EORTC guidelines for the use of granulocyte-colony stimulating factor to reduce the incidence of chemotherapy-induced febrile neutropenia in adult patients with lymphomas and solid tumours. Eur J Cancer 42:2433–2453

Amado RG, Wolf M, Peeters M et al (2008) Wild-type KRAS is required for panitumumab efficacy in patients with metastatic colorectal cancer. J Clin Oncol 26:1626–1634

Andre T, Boni C, Mounedji-Boudiaf L et al (2004) Oxaliplatin, fluorouracil, and leucovorin as adjuvant treatment for colon cancer. N Engl J Med 350:2343–2351

Ayanian JZ, Zaslavsky AM, Fuchs CS et al (2003) Use of adjuvant chemotherapy and radiation therapy for colorectal cancer in a population-based cohort. J Clin Oncol 21:1293–1300

Begg CB, Carbone PP (1983) Clinical trials and drug toxicity in the elderly. The experience of the Eastern Cooperative Oncology Group. Cancer 52:1986–1992

Bliss JM, Kilburn LS, Coleman RE et al (2012) Disease-related outcomes with long-term follow-up: an updated analysis of the Intergroup Exemestane Study. J Clin Oncol 30(7):709–717

Bokemeyer C, Aapro MS, Courdi A et al (2007) EORTC guidelines for the use of erythropoietic proteins in anaemic patients with cancer: 2006 update. Eur J Cancer 43:258–270

Bonadonna G, Valagussa P (1981) Dose–response effect of adjuvant chemotherapy in breast cancer. N Engl J Med 304:10–15

Bonneterre J, Thurlimann B, Robertson JF et al (2000) Anastrozole versus tamoxifen as first-line therapy for advanced breast cancer in 668 postmenopausal women: results of the Tamoxifen or Arimidex Randomized Group Efficacy and Tolerability study. J Clin Oncol 18:3748–3757

Borkowski JM, Duerr M, Donehower RC et al (1994) Relation between age and clearance rate of nine investigational anticancer drugs from phase I pharmacokinetic data. Cancer Chemother Pharmacol 33:493–496

Bouchardy C, Rapiti E, Blagojevic S et al (2007) Older female cancer patients: importance, causes, and consequences of undertreatment. J Clin Oncol 25:1858–1869

Buccheri G, Ferrigno D, Tamburini M (1996) Karnofsky and ECOG performance status scoring in lung cancer: a prospective, longitudinal study of 536 patients from a single institution. Eur J Cancer 32A:1135–1141

Cameron D, Casey M, Press M et al (2008) A phase III randomized comparison of lapatinib plus capecitabine versus capecitabine alone in women with advanced breast cancer that has progressed on trastuzumab: updated efficacy and biomarker analyses. Breast Cancer Res Treat 112:533–543

Chapman JA, Meng D, Shepherd L et al (2008) Competing causes of death from a randomized trial of extended adjuvant endocrine therapy for breast cancer. J Natl Cancer Inst 100:252–260

Christman K, Muss HB, Case LD et al (1992) Chemotherapy of metastatic breast cancer in the elderly. The Piedmont Oncology Association experience. JAMA 268:57–62

Coates AS, Keshaviah A, Thurlimann B et al (2007) Five years of letrozole compared with tamoxifen as initial adjuvant therapy for postmenopausal women with endocrine-responsive early breast cancer: update of study BIG 1-98. J Clin Oncol 25:486–492

Colleoni M, Price KN, Castiglione-Gertsch M et al (1999) Mortality during adjuvant treatment of early breast cancer with cyclophosphamide, methotrexate, and fluorouracil. International Breast Cancer Study Group. Lancet 354(9173):130–131

Crivellari D, Bonetti M, Castiglione-Gertsch M et al (2000) Burdens and benefits of adjuvant cyclophosphamide, methotrexate, and fluorouracil and tamoxifen for elderly patients with breast cancer: the International Breast Cancer Study Group Trial VII. J Clin Oncol 18:1412–1422

Crivellari D, Sun Z, Coates AS et al (2008) Letrozole compared with tamoxifen for elderly patients with endocrine-responsive early breast cancer: the BIG 1-98 trial. J Clin Oncol 26:1972–1979

Cronin DP, Harlan LC, Potosky AL et al (2006) Patterns of care for adjuvant therapy in a random population-based sample of patients diagnosed with colorectal cancer. Am J Gastroenterol 101:2308–2318

Cunningham D, Allum WH, Stenning SP et al (2006) Perioperative chemotherapy versus surgery alone for resectable gastroesophageal cancer. N Engl J Med 355:11–20

De Boer MF, Ryckman RM, Pruyn JF et al (1999) Psychosocial correlates of cancer relapse and survival: a literature review. Patient Educ Couns 37:215–230

Droz JP, Balducci L, Bolla M et al (2010) Management of prostate cancer in older men: recommendations of a working group of the International Society of Geriatric Oncology. BJU Int 106:462–469

Early Breast Cancer Trialists' Collaborative Group (2012) Comparisons between different polychemotherapy regimens for early breast cancer: meta-analyses of long-term outcome among 100,000 women in 123 randomised trials. Lancet 379 (9814):432–444

Early Breast Cancer Trialists' Collaborative Group (2005) Effects of chemotherapy and hormonal therapy for early breast cancer on recurrence and 15 years survival: an overview of the randomised trials. Lancet 365 (9472): 1687–1717

Edwards BK, Brown LM, Wingo PA et al (2005) Annual report to the nation on the status of cancer, 1975–2002, featuring population-based trends in cancer treatment. J Natl Cancer Inst 97:1407–1427

Eichhorst B, Goede V, Hallek M (2009a) Treatment of elderly patients with chronic lymphocytic leukemia. Leuk Lymphoma 50:171–178

Eichhorst BF, Busch R, Stilgenbauer S et al (2009b) First-line therapy with fludarabine compared with chlorambucil does not result in a major benefit for elderly patients with advanced chronic lymphocytic leukemia. Blood 114:3382–3391

Elkin EB, Hurria A, Mitra N et al (2006) Adjuvant chemotherapy and survival in older women with hormone receptor-negative breast cancer: assessing outcome in a population-based, observational cohort. J Clin Oncol 24:2757–2764

Endres HG, Wedding U, Pittrow D et al (2009) Prevalence of anemia in elderly patients in primary care: impact on 5-year mortality risk and differences between men and women. Curr Med Res Opin 25:1143–1158

Ewer MS, O'Shaughnessy JA (2007) Cardiac toxicity of trastuzumab-related regimens in HER2-overexpressing breast cancer. Clin Breast Cancer 7:600–607

Extermann M, Hurria A (2007) Comprehensive geriatric assessment for older patients with cancer. J Clin Oncol 25:1824–1831

Extermann M, Overcash J, Lyman GH et al (1998) Comorbidity and functional status are independent in older cancer patients. J Clin Oncol 16:1582–1587

Extermann M, Meyer J, McGinnis M et al (2004) A comprehensive geriatric intervention detects multiple problems in older breast cancer patients. Crit Rev Oncol Hematol 49:69–75

Extermann M, Boler I, Reich RR et al (2012) Predicting the risk of chemotherapy toxicity in older patients: the Chemotherapy Risk Assessment Scale for High-Age Patients (CRASH) score. Cancer 118:3377–3386

Facon T, Mary JY, Hulin C et al (2007) Melphalan and prednisone plus thalidomide versus melphalan and prednisone alone or reduced-intensity autologous stem cell transplantation in elderly patients with multiple myeloma (IFM 99-06): a randomised trial. Lancet 370(9594):1209–1218

Fenaux P, Mufti GJ, Hellstrom-Lindberg E et al (2009a) Efficacy of azacitidine compared with that of conventional care regimens in the treatment of higher-risk myelodysplastic syndromes: a randomised, open-label, phase III study. Lancet Oncol 10:223–232

Fenaux P, Mufti GJ, Hellstrom-Lindberg E et al (2009b) Azacitidine prolongs overall survival compared with conventional care regimens in elderly patients with low bone marrow blast count acute myeloid leukemia. J Clin Oncol 28:562–569

Forbes JF, Cuzick J, Buzdar A et al (2008) Effect of anastrozole and tamoxifen as adjuvant treatment for early-stage breast cancer: 100-month analysis of the ATAC trial. Lancet Oncol 9:45–53

Fossati R, Confalonieri C, Torri V et al (1998) Cytotoxic and hormonal treatment for metastatic breast cancer: a systematic review of published randomized trials involving 31,510 women. J Clin Oncol 16:3439–3460

Frasci G, Lorusso V, Panza N et al (2000) Gemcitabine plus vinorelbine versus vinorelbine alone in elderly patients with advanced non-small-cell lung cancer. J Clin Oncol 18:2529–2536

Freyer G, Geay JF, Touzet S et al (2005) Comprehensive geriatric assessment predicts tolerance to chemotherapy and survival in elderly patients with advanced ovarian carcinoma: a GINECO study. Ann Oncol 16:1795–1800

Fruh M, Rolland E, Pignon JP et al (2008) Pooled analysis of the effect of age on adjuvant cisplatin-based chemotherapy for completely resected non-small-cell lung cancer. J Clin Oncol 26:3573–3581

Gelman RS, Taylor SGT (1984) Cyclophosphamide, methotrexate, and 5-fluorouracil chemotherapy in women more than 65 years old with advanced breast cancer:

the elimination of age trends in toxicity by using doses based on creatinine clearance. J Clin Oncol 2:1404–1413

Geyer CE, Forster J, Lindquist D et al (2006) Lapatinib plus capecitabine for HER2-positive advanced breast cancer. N Engl J Med 355:2733–2743

Giordano SH, Duan Z, Kuo YF et al (2006) Use and outcomes of adjuvant chemotherapy in older women with breast cancer. J Clin Oncol 24:2750–2756

Giovanazzi-Bannon S, Rademaker A, Lai G et al (1994) Treatment tolerance of elderly cancer patients entered onto phase II clinical trials: an Illinois Cancer Center study. J Clin Oncol 12:2447–2452

Girre V, Falcou MC, Gisselbrecht M et al (2008) Does a geriatric oncology consultation modify the cancer treatment plan for elderly patients? J Gerontol A Biol Sci Med Sci 63.724–730

Goldhirsch A, Castiglione M, Gelber RD (1990) Adjuvant chemo-endocrine therapy in postmenopausal women with breast cancer and axillary-node metastases. Lancet 335(8697):1099–1100

Goldhirsch A, Coates AS, Gelber RD et al (2006) First—select the target: better choice of adjuvant treatments for breast cancer patients. Ann Oncol 17:1772–1776

Goldhirsch A, Wood WC, Gelber RD et al (2007) Progress and promise: highlights of the international expert consensus on the primary therapy of early breast cancer 2007. Ann Oncol 18:1133–1144

Goldstone AH, Burnett AK, Wheatley K et al (2001) Attempts to improve treatment outcomes in acute myeloid leukemia (AML) in older patients: the results of the United Kingdom Medical Research Council AML11 trial. Blood 98:1302–1311

Goodwin JS, Samet JM, Key CR et al (1986) Stage at diagnosis of cancer varies with the age of the patient. J Am Geriatr Soc 34:20–26

Hallek M, Fischer K, Fingerle-Rowson G et al (2010) Addition of rituximab to fludarabine and cyclophosphamide in patients with chronic lymphocytic leukaemia: a randomised, open-label, phase 3 trial. Lancet 376(9747):1164–1174

Haller DG, Catalano PJ, Macdonald JS et al (2005) Phase III study of fluorouracil, leucovorin, and levamisole in high-risk stage II and III colon cancer: final report of Intergroup 0089. J Clin Oncol 23:8671–8678

Haller DG, Tabernero J, Maroun J et al (2011) Capecitabine plus oxaliplatin compared with fluorouracil and folinic acid as adjuvant therapy for stage III colon cancer. J Clin Oncol 29:1465–1471

Harter P, du Bois A, Schade-Brittinger C et al (2005) Non-enrolment of ovarian cancer patients in clinical trials: reasons and background. Ann Oncol 16:1801–1805

Honecker FU, Wedding U, Rettig K et al (2009) Use of the Comprehensive Geriatric Assessment (CGA) in elderly patients with solid tumors to predict mortality. J Clin Oncol 27(15s):9549

Hughes KS, Schnaper LA, Berry D et al (2004) Lumpectomy plus tamoxifen with or without irradiation in women 70 years of age or older with early breast cancer. N Engl J Med 351:971–977

Hulin C, Facon T, Rodon P et al (2009) Efficacy of melphalan and prednisone plus thalidomide in patients older than 75 years with newly diagnosed multiple myeloma: IFM 01/01 trial. J Clin Oncol 27:3664–3670

Hurria A, Balducci L (eds) (2009) Geriatric oncology. Springer, Heidelberg

Hurria A, Togawa K, Mohile SG et al (2011) Predicting chemotherapy toxicity in older adults with cancer: a prospective multicenter study. J Clin Oncol 29:3457–3465

Hurwitz H, Fehrenbacher L, Novotny W et al (2004) Bevacizumab plus irinotecan, fluorouracil, and leucovorin for metastatic colorectal cancer. N Engl J Med 350:2335–2342

Hutchins LF, Unger JM, Crowley JJ et al (1999) Underrepresentation of patients 65 years of age or older in cancer-treatment trials. N Engl J Med 341:2061–2067

Jakesz R, Greil R, Gnant M et al (2007) Extended adjuvant therapy with anastrozole among postmenopausal breast cancer patients: results from the randomized Austrian Breast and Colorectal Cancer Study Group Trial 6a. J Natl Cancer Inst 99:1845–1853

Jin H, Tu D, Zhao N et al (2012) Longer-term outcomes of letrozole versus placebo after 5 years of tamoxifen in the NCIC CTG MA.17 trial: analyses adjusting for treatment crossover. J Clin Oncol 30(7):718–721

Joensuu H, Kellokumpu-Lehtinen PL, Bono P et al (2006) Adjuvant docetaxel or vinorelbine with or without trastuzumab for breast cancer. N Engl J Med 354:809–820

Kabbinavar FF, Schulz J, McCleod M et al (2005) Addition of bevacizumab to bolus fluorouracil and leucovorin in first-line metastatic colorectal cancer: results of a randomized phase II trial. J Clin Oncol 23:3697–3705

Kabbinavar FF, Hurwitz HI, Yi J et al (2009) Addition of bevacizumab to fluorouracil-based first-line treatment of metastatic colorectal cancer: pooled analysis of cohorts of older patients from two randomized clinical trials. J Clin Oncol 27:199–205

Karnofsky DA, Adelmann WH, Craver FL (1948) The use of nitrogen mustard in the palliative treatment of carcinoma. Cancer 1:634–656

Kaufmann M, Jonat W, Hilfrich J et al (2007) Improved overall survival in postmenopausal women with early breast cancer after anastrozole initiated after treatment with tamoxifen compared with continued tamoxifen: the ARNO 95 Study. J Clin Oncol 25:2664–2670

Keating NL, Landrum MB, Klabunde CN et al (2008) Adjuvant chemotherapy for stage III colon cancer: do physicians agree about the importance of patient age and comorbidity? J Clin Oncol 26:2532–2537

Kemeny MM, Peterson BL, Kornblith AB et al (2003) Barriers to clinical trial participation by older women with breast cancer. J Clin Oncol 21:2268–2275

Knauf WU, Lissichkov T, Aldaoud A et al (2009) Phase III randomized study of bendamustine compared with chlorambucil in previously untreated patients with chronic lymphocytic leukemia. J Clin Oncol 27:4378–4384

Kohne CH, Folprecht G, Goldberg RM et al (2008) Chemotherapy in elderly patients with colorectal cancer. Oncologist 13:390–402

Kudoh S, Takeda K, Nakagawa K et al (2006) Phase III study of docetaxel compared with vinorelbine in elderly patients with advanced non-small-cell lung cancer: results of the West Japan Thoracic Oncology Group Trial (WJTOG 9904). J Clin Oncol 24:3657–3663

Lees J, Chan A (2011) Polypharmacy in elderly patients with cancer: clinical implications and management. Lancet Oncol 12:1249–1257

Lewis JH, Kilgore ML, Goldman DP et al (2003) Participation of patients 65 years of age or older in cancer clinical trials. J Clin Oncol 21:1383–1389

Lievre A, Bachet JB, Boige V et al (2008) KRAS mutations as an independent prognostic factor in patients with advanced colorectal cancer treated with cetuximab. J Clin Oncol 26:374–379

Lynch TJ, Bell DW, Sordella R et al (2004) Activating mutations in the epidermal growth factor receptor underlying responsiveness of non-small-cell lung cancer to gefitinib. N Engl J Med 350:2129–2139

Mamounas EP, Jeong JH, Wickerham DL et al (2008) Benefit from exemestane as extended adjuvant therapy after 5 years of adjuvant tamoxifen: intention-to-treat analysis of the National Surgical Adjuvant Breast and Bowel Project B-33 trial. J Clin Oncol 26:1965–1971

Massie MJ (2004) Prevalence of depression in patients with cancer. J Natl Cancer Inst Monogr 32:57–71

McCleary NAJ, Meyerhardt J, Green E et al (2009) Impact of older age on the efficacy of newer adjuvant therapies in >12,500 patients with stage II/III colon cancer: findings from the ACCENT Database. J Clin Oncol 27:15s (suppl; abstr 4010)

Monfardini S, Sorio R, Kaye S (1994) Should elderly cancer patients be entered in dose-escalation studies? Ann Oncol 5:964–965

Mor V, Laliberte L, Morris JN et al (1984) The Karnofsky performance status scale. An examination of its reliability and validity in a research setting. Cancer 53:2002–2007

Muss HB, Woolf S, Berry D et al (2005) Adjuvant chemotherapy in older and younger women with lymph node-positive breast cancer. JAMA 293:1073–1081

Muss HB, Berry DA, Cirrincione CT et al (2009) Adjuvant chemotherapy in older women with early-stage breast cancer. N Engl J Med 360:2055–2065

Neugut AI, Fleischauer AT, Sundararajan V et al (2002) Use of adjuvant chemotherapy and radiation therapy for rectal cancer among the elderly: a population-based study. J Clin Oncol 20:2643–2650

Osborne CK, Pippen J, Jones SE et al (2002) Double-blind, randomized trial comparing the efficacy and tolerability of fulvestrant versus anastrozole in postmenopausal women with advanced breast cancer progressing on prior endocrine therapy: results of a North American trial. J Clin Oncol 20:3386–3395

Pallis AG, Gridelli C, van Meerbeeck JP et al (2009) EORTC Elderly Task Force and Lung Cancer Group and International Society for Geriatric Oncology (SIOG) experts' opinion for the treatment of non-small-cell lung cancer in an elderly population. Ann Oncol 21:692–706

Palumbo A, Bringhen S, Ludwig H et al (2011) Personalized therapy in multiple myeloma according to patient age and vulnerability: a report of the European Myeloma Network (EMN). Blood 118:4519–4529

Piccart-Gebhart MJ, Procter M, Leyland-Jones B et al (2005) Trastuzumab after adjuvant chemotherapy in HER2-positive breast cancer. N Engl J Med 353:1659–1672

Pignon JP, Tribodet H, Scagliotti GV et al (2008) Lung adjuvant cisplatin evaluation: a pooled analysis by the LACE Collaborative Group. J Clin Oncol 26:3552–3559

Pinder MC, Duan Z, Goodwin JS et al (2007) Congestive heart failure in older women treated with adjuvant anthracycline chemotherapy for breast cancer. J Clin Oncol 25:3808–3815

Quoix E, Zalcman G, Oster JP et al (2011) Carboplatin and weekly paclitaxel doublet chemotherapy compared with monotherapy in elderly patients with advanced non-small-cell lung cancer: IFCT-0501 randomised, phase 3 trial. Lancet 378(9796):1079–1088

Rao AV, Hsieh F, Feussner JR et al (2005) Geriatric evaluation and management units in the care of the frail elderly cancer patient. J Gerontol A Biol Sci Med Sci 60:798–803

Read WL, Tierney RM, Page NC et al (2004) Differential prognostic impact of comorbidity. J Clin Oncol 22:3099–3103

Regan MM, Neven P, Giobbie-Hurder A et al (2011) Assessment of letrozole and tamoxifen alone and in sequence for postmenopausal women with steroid hormone receptor-positive breast cancer: the BIG 1-98 randomised clinical trial at 8.1 years median follow-up. Lancet Oncol 12:1101–1108

Rehse B, Pukrop R (2003) Effects of psychosocial interventions on quality of life in adult cancer patients: meta analysis of 37 published controlled outcome studies. Patient Educ Couns 50:179–186

Repetto L, Venturino A, Vercelli M et al (1998) Performance status and comorbidity in elderly cancer patients compared with young patients with neoplasia and elderly patients without neoplastic conditions. Cancer 82:760–765

Repetto L, Carreca I, Maraninchi D et al (2003) Use of growth factors in the elderly patient with cancer: a report from the Second International Society for Geriatric Oncology (SIOG) 2001 meeting. Crit Rev Oncol Hematol 45:123–128

Romond EH, Perez EA, Bryant J et al (2005) Trastuzumab plus adjuvant chemotherapy for operable HER2-positive breast cancer. N Engl J Med 353:1673–1684

Samet J, Hunt WC, Key C et al (1986) Choice of cancer therapy varies with age of patient. JAMA 255:3385–3390

San Miguel JF, Schlag R, Khuageva NK et al (2008) Bortezomib plus melphalan and prednisone for initial treatment of multiple myeloma. N Engl J Med 359:906–917

Sargent DJ, Goldberg RM, Jacobson SD et al (2001) A pooled analysis of adjuvant chemotherapy for resected colon cancer in elderly patients. N Engl J Med 345:1091–1097

Sargent DJ, Wieand HS, Haller DG et al (2005) Disease-free survival versus overall survival as a primary end point for adjuvant colon cancer studies: individual patient data from 20,898 patients on 18 randomized trials. J Clin Oncol 23:8664–8670

Sargent DJ, Kohne CH, Sanoff HK et al (2009) Pooled safety and efficacy analysis examining the effect of performance status on outcomes in nine first-line treatment trials using individual data from patients with metastatic colorectal cancer. J Clin Oncol 27:1948–1955

Schairer C, Mink PJ, Carroll L et al (2004) Probabilities of death from breast cancer and other causes among female breast cancer patients. J Natl Cancer Inst 96:1311–1321

Seymour JF, Fenaux P, Silverman LR et al (2010) Effects of azacitidine compared with conventional care regimens in elderly (≥75 years) patients with higher-risk myelodysplastic syndromes. Crit Rev Oncol Hematol 76:218–227

Slamon DJ, Leyland-Jones B, Shak S et al (2001) Use of chemotherapy plus a monoclonal antibody against HER2 for metastatic breast cancer that overexpresses HER2. N Engl J Med 344:783–792

Slamon D, Eiermann W, Robert N et al (2011) Adjuvant trastuzumab in HER2-positive breast cancer. N Engl J Med 365:1273–1283

Smith BD, Smith GL, Hurria A et al (2009) Future of cancer incidence in the United States: burdens upon an aging, changing nation. J Clin Oncol 27:2758–2765

Sperr WR, Wimazal F, Kundi M et al (2010) Comorbidity as prognostic variable in MDS: comparative evaluation of the HCT-CI and CCI in a core dataset of 419 patients of the Austrian MDS Study Group. Ann Oncol 21:114–119

Stein BN, Petrelli NJ, Douglass HO et al (1995) Age and sex are independent predictors of 5-fluorouracil toxicity. Analysis of a large scale phase III trial. Cancer 75:11–17

Stuck AE, Siu AL, Wieland GD et al (1993) Comprehensive geriatric assessment: a meta-analysis of controlled trials. Lancet 342(8878):1032–1036

Sundararajan V, Mitra N, Jacobson JS et al (2002) Survival associated with 5-fluorouracil-based adjuvant chemotherapy among elderly patients with node-positive colon cancer. Ann Intern Med 136:349–357

Tanne JH (2011) FDA cancels approval for bevacizumab in advanced breast cancer. BMJ 343:d7684

The Elderly Lung Cancer Vinorelbine Italian Study Group (1999) Effects of vinorelbine on quality of life and survival of elderly patients with advanced non-small-cell lung cancer. J Natl Cancer Inst 91:66–72

Thomas XG, Dmoszynska A, Wierzbowska A et al (2011) Results from a randomized phase III trial of decitabine versus supportive care or low-dose cytarabine for the treatment of older patients with newly diagnosed AML. J Clin Oncol 29:6509

Tol J, Koopman M, Cats A et al (2009) Chemotherapy, bevacizumab, and cetuximab in metastatic colorectal cancer. N Engl J Med 360:563–572

Trimble EL, Carter CL, Cain D et al (1994) Representation of older patients in cancer treatment trials. Cancer 74(7 Suppl):2208–2214

Turner NJ, Haward RA, Mulley GP et al (1999) Cancer in old age—is it inadequately investigated and treated? BMJ 319(7205):309–312

Twelves C, Wong A, Nowacki MP et al (2005) Capecitabine as adjuvant treatment for stage III colon cancer. N Engl J Med 352:2696–2704

Van Cutsem E, Kohne CH, Hitre E et al (2009) Cetuximab and chemotherapy as initial treatment for metastatic colorectal cancer. N Engl J Med 360:1408–1417

Wagner AD, Wedding U (2009) Advances in the pharmacological treatment of gastro-oesophageal cancer. Drugs Aging 26:627–646

Watson M, McCarron J, Law M (1992) Anticipatory nausea and emesis, and psychological morbidity: assessment of prevalence among out-patients on mild to moderate chemotherapy regimens. Br J Cancer 66:862–866

Wedding U, Honecker F, Bokemeyer C et al (2007a) Tolerance to chemotherapy in elderly patients with cancer. Cancer Control 14:44–56

Wedding U, Rohrig B, Klippstein A et al (2007b) Age, severe comorbidity and functional impairment independently contribute to poor survival in cancer patients. J Cancer Res Clin Oncol 133:945–950

Wedding U, Rohrig B, Pientka L et al (2007c) Anaemia-related impairment in quality of life in elderly cancer patients prior to chemotherapy. J Cancer Res Clin Oncol 133:279–286

Wehling M (2009) Multimorbidity and polypharmacy: how to reduce the harmful drug load and yet add needed drugs in the elderly? Proposal of a new drug classification: fit for the aged. J Am Geriatr Soc 57:560–561

Xu J, Kochanek K, Murphy SL, Tejada-Vera B (2010) Deaths: final data for 2007. National Vital Statistics Reports, 58(19). http://www.cdc.gov/NCHS/data/nvsr/nvsr58/nvsr58_19.pdf. Accessed 17 Jan 2012

Zhou C, Wu YL, Chen G et al (2011) Erlotinib versus chemotherapy as first-line treatment for patients with advanced EGFR mutation-positive non-small-cell lung cancer (OPTIMAL, CTONG-0802): a multicentre, open-label, randomised, phase 3 study. Lancet Oncol 12:735–742

Pharmacotherapy and Geriatric Syndromes

Fall Risk and Pharmacotherapy

Heinrich Burkhardt

Introduction

Maintaining postural stability in the supine position is a complex task and therefore vulnerable to disturbance by a variety of factors that may cause loss of stability and result in falls. In the elderly, as opposed to younger patients, a fall from standing or a fall while walking at low speed may end up in clinically significant incidents, namely, fractures. Typical falls in the elderly have to be distinguished from syncope, which describes a short-time loss of consciousness of sudden onset. In every fall incident, a syncope has to be ruled out as its management requires different diagnostic and therapeutic algorithms aiming at underlying cardiac diseases. Syncopes may also be provoked by drug therapy due to bradycardia, torsades, or orthostatic hypotension. In the following, we focus on typical falls in the elderly.

It is estimated that one third of all ambulatory elderly aged 65+ years will experience a fall event at least once a year. Among those aged 80+ years, this portion is estimated to rise to about 50% (Tinetti et al. 1988). This also leads to an increased risk of mortality and aggravated morbidity in the elderly (Stel et al. 2004), which is even more pronounced in elderly living in nursing homes or comparable institutions (e.g., hospitals) (Kron et al. 2003).

In the elderly, the fracture rate attributed to falls is about 5%. Most common fractures are hip and radius fractures. Mortality rates of fracture incidents are rising with advancing age. In this context, hip fractures are most significant. The 12-month mortality rate after hip fracture increases to 24% in the elderly, as revealed by a U.S. government study (U.S. Congress, Office of Technology Assessment 1994). Besides this, more than 40% of all elderly patients suffering a hip fracture were not able to return home and had to be discharged to nursing homes or similar facilities. A major reason for this increasing threat in the elderly accompanying fall incidents is the increasing prevalence of osteoporosis in this population. In addition, in the elderly changes of physiological responses may lead to less-effective compensations in case of falls (e.g., reduced protective reflexes). In this context, the most significant changes in the elderly are

- Reduced muscle mass (sarcopenia)
- Reduced visual acuity
- Changes in the nervous system
- Frequent orthostatic hypotension.

Prevalence of orthostatic hypotension may exceed 30% in elderly aged 75+ years (Gupta and Lipsitz 2007). Some of these arguments match with the criteria that define frailty (see chapter "Pharmacotherapy and the Frailty Syndrome"), thus pointing to the high inherent risk of falls in frail elderly.

H. Burkhardt (✉)
IVth Department of Medicine, Geriatrics, University Medical Centre Mannheim, Theodor-Kutzer-Ufer 1-3, Mannheim 68167, Germany
e-mail: heinrich.burkhardt@umm.de

M. Wehling (ed.), *Drug Therapy for the Elderly*,
DOI 10.1007/978-3-7091-0912-0_19, © Springer-Verlag Wien 2013

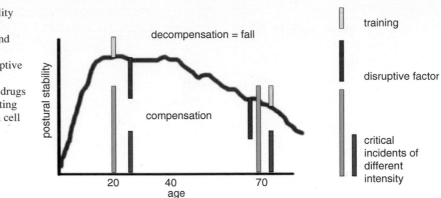

Fig. 1 Postural stability according to age and different stabilizing and destabilizing factors. Destabilizing or disruptive factors cover a wide variety, ranging from drugs to intermittent distracting events like a call on a cell phone while walking

Falls in the elderly, however, are rarely triggered by only one factor. In most cases, several factors—both internal (within the patient) and external (environmental) ones—may interact in a complex system and finally result in a fall.

In most instances, falls in elderly are triggered by multiple factors.

Among external factors, such as inappropriate lighting and terrain difficulties, drugs are regularly involved. For some fall-risk-increasing drugs (FRIDs), this unwanted property may easily be explained by the mechanism of action. Thus, all centrally acting drugs ("central nervous system [CNS] drugs") are associated with an increased risk of falls. A general model explaining the elevated risk incidence may elucidate this. The compensatory reserve in the elderly, especially in the frail elderly, decreases with advancing age; this results in the fact that irritating factors even of low intensity may impair postural stability. In this context, FRIDs may pose a much more significant burden on the stability-maintaining systems in the elderly than in younger adults (Fig. 1).

Despite this, the role of drugs as fall-risk-increasing factors is still widely underemphasized, and the detailed analysis of fall risk in the elderly is mostly missing even in the pharmacological literature (e.g., concerning anticoagulants in stroke prevention). In addition, only very few clinical studies on elderly patients measure and document falls as a significant adverse drug reaction (ADR). To estimate the fall risk, in most studies extrapolation from reports of related symptoms like dizziness, drowsiness, and confusion is necessary. For the explanation of this shortcoming, three arguments may be relevant:

– The reasons for falls are often multifactorial; therefore, the exact role of a prescribed drug may be difficult to define.

– Identifying defined drugs in epidemiologic studies or registers is often impaired by the fact that they are included in groups of similar substances and preparations, thus disabling the possibility of obtaining data for individual compounds.

– Different dosages may complicate analyses even further.

The last explains why almost no analysis could define threshold doses for increased fall risk by FRIDs. However, two main general risk factors for falls from drugs can be extracted from literature:

– Prescription of psychotropic drugs
– Polypharmacy with a simultaneous prescription of four and more drugs.

Among over 400 risk factors for an increased fall risk, some are more closely discussed with regard to pharmacotherapy, especially with a range of defined drugs. It is not possible to give a complete list of all factors, but Fig. 2 provides a simplified model and may explain interaction pathways that lead to an increased fall risk. Table 1 lists drugs for which data on the associated fall risk exist. Also, a risk stratification is given for different clinical settings (Blain et al. 2000; Campbell 1991; Cumming 1998; Leipzig 1998).

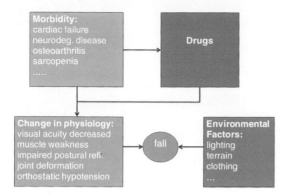

Fig. 2 Drugs in the context of the multifactorial genesis of falls in the elderly

Fall-Risk-Increasing Drugs

As mentioned, drugs that increase fall risk are summarized under the acronym FRIDs (fall-risk-increasing drugs). This may alleviate further analysis of fall risk and also help to update recommendations. Main groups of FRIDs are as follows:

- **Tranquilizers (benzodiazepines)**
- **Neuroleptics (D2 antagonists and serotonin-dopamine antagonists)**
- **Antidepressants (tricyclics, selective serotonin reuptake inhibitors [SSRIs], serotonin norepinephrine reuptake inhibitors [SNRIs] and monoamine oxidase [MAO] B inhibitors)**
- **Antihypertensives (diuretics, β-blockers, α-blockers, Ca antagonists, angiotensin-converting enzyme [ACE] inhibitors)**
- Antiarrhythmics
- Nitrates and other vasoactive substances
- Digoxin
- Opioids
- Anticholinergics
- Antihistaminics
- Antidiabetics.

Van der Velde et al. used this definition in a prospective cohort study to test whether FRIDs can be reduced or stopped without aggravating the risk for the patient. They found that in the majority of cases these medications could be reduced or stopped at no cost of deterioration,

but fall risk was impressively lowered to about 50% (Van der Velde et al. 2006). Therefore, an exact analysis of current medications and carefully reducing or simplifying drug schedules are substantial parts of any fall prevention program. These programs must be multifaceted, with drugs being a major aspect (Chang et al. 2004). The list given, however, may be seen to be too complex, and focusing on the four most important drug classes in that context may work as well. These are highlighted in the list in bold characters. In a classical review by Leipzig et al. (1999), odds ratios of fall risk were calculated for different drugs and drug classes, providing a matrix for fall risk comparison. This issue was recently reevaluated in an extensive meta-analysis. Unfortunately, only 22 of over 11,000 papers could be included in this analysis because of low quality or inappropriately addressing the problem (Woolcott et al. 2009). Nevertheless, with the methodological problems mentioned in mind, this still is only an estimate and far from precise measurements.

Fall risk is not triggered by a single brain receptor system but rather represents a network or systemic instability.

Although discussed as a major contributor to fall risk, there is only a weak association between the anticholinergic activity of a drug and the fall risk associated with it, though the total anticholinergic activity of all drugs may be a better measure and predictor of fall risk. Fall risk may not be strongly associated to a single receptor system in the brain (e.g., the serotonergic system/SSRI; see following discussion), but rather reflects the integration of network influences on a complex regulatory and multicomponent system. In the following chapters, two drug classes are outlined in more detail, and comments on some other drugs of relevance are given.

Centrally Acting Drugs (CNS Drugs)

The prescription of a centrally acting drug is widely accepted as an important risk factor for falls (Souchet et al. 2005). In this context, the kind of CNS drug involved does not seem to be

Table 1 Fall risk estimation for different drugs in the elderly

Drug	Setting Ambulatory	Nursing home	Hospital	Evidence	OR*
Tricyclic antidepressants	+	+	+	++	1.51–1.68
SSRI	+	+		+	1.68
Long-acting benzodiazepines	+	+	+	++	1.32–1.57
Short-acting benzodiazepines	+	(+)	(+)	+	1.44–1.57
Phenothiazines	(+)	(+)	(+)	(+)	(1.5–1.59[a])
Butyrophenones	(+)		+	?	
NSAIDs	(+)	+		(+)	1.16–1.21
Vasodilatory agents	(+)	(+)		(+)	1.13
Diuretics	(+)	(+)	0	(+)	1.08
Digoxin	(+)	(+)	+	0	1.22
Class I antiarrhythmics	+			+	1.59
Antihypertensives	(+)	(+)		0	1.24
ACE inhibitors	0			0	1.2

0 in studies no risk associated, (+) occasional reports found an associated risk of falls. + majority of reports described an increased risk of falls, ++ high probability for increased falls risk, * pooled OR cited from Leipzig et al. 1999 and Woolcott et al. 2009

ACE angiotensin-converting enzyme, *NSAID* nonsteroidal anti-inflammatory drug, *SSRI* selective serotonin reuptake inhibitor

[a]Neuroleptics are not divided in subclasses according to their chemical structure

of paramount importance as a large-scale analysis based on health insurance data in the United States revealed (French et al. 2006). Among CNS drugs, tricyclic antidepressants were uniformly associated with a high fall risk, and a decreased fall rate was expected to be associated with modern antidepressants (especially SSRIs) as these act much more specifically on the serotonergic system. However, in reality differences were found to be small or nil (Sleeper et al. 2000); this may again highlight that fall risk does not depend on one brain receptor system and is only weakly associated with the anticholinergic action of drugs.

A similar comparative evaluation of different antipsychotics or neuroleptics is rather challenging as this group comprises quite heterogeneous drugs. Two arguments may be considered: Phenothiazines, widely used in agitation treatment, are thought to carry an increased fall risk among neuroleptics due to their sedative component. In contrast, although providing only little sedative effect, some of the highly effective modern, so-called atypical antipsychotics may be associated with a high fall risk mainly mediated by orthostatic hypotension. This has been shown for clozapine, risperidone, and quetiapine (Haddad and Sharma 2007).

Benzodiazepines also are associated with an increased fall risk, and among those, long-acting drugs are considered to largely increase this risk; thus, short-acting benzodiazepines were recommended instead. However, epidemiologic data do not fully support this assumption. The dosage of benzodiazepines is more predictive than its duration of action. The higher the dose, the higher the risk to induce a fall in the patient. In addition, a large-scale Canadian cohort showed additional differences that seemed substance related but not explained by these two parameters. In this study, flurazepam, chlordiazepoxid, and oxazepam were associated with the highest fall risk (Tamblyn et al. 2005).

Antihypertensives

Despite the inherent risk to induce orthostatic hypotension and thereby increase the risk of falling, epidemiologic data do not support this unequivocally (Räihä et al. 1995). Increased risk is seen in the initial phase of antihypertensive treatment and mostly due to dosing errors—initial dose too high, escalation interval too short. If these pitfalls are avoided and treatment goals reflect individual restrictions by loss of Windkessel function or orthostatic instability (see chapter "Arterial Hypertension"), antihypertensive drugs rarely increase fall risk. Yet, especially vulnerable populations tending to pronounced orthostatic hypotension need to be preemptively identified: patients suffering from Parkinson's disease or multisystem atrophy (see chapter "Parkinson's Disease"). As in all patients, blood pressure should be controlled in an upright and standing position. If there is a drop of systolic blood pressure to 100 mmHg or below or by more than 20 mmHg, antihypertensive drug dosage has to be adapted.

Miscellaneous Drugs

From epidemiologic data, nonsteroidal anti-inflammatory drugs (NSAIDs) were also found to be associated with an increased fall risk. However, it is still unclear if this may result from minor central actions of these drugs or rather reflects an association with the osteoarthritis as a main indication (coincidence). Finally, diuretics, digoxin, and antiarrhythmics should be mentioned as FRIDs. Diuretics may increase fall risk by dehydration or asthenia (due to potassium loss from skeletal muscle) and have to be prescribed with caution in the elderly. Digoxin and class I antiarrhythmics (and some class III antiarrhythmics, e.g., sotalol) are both discouraged in the elderly due to the high rates of proarrhythmic effects and a narrow therapeutic range (in particular digoxin). Moreover, again epidemiologic data do not distinguish between increased fall risk as a drug ADR or reflecting a coincidence with the underlying diseases, such as cardiac failure associated with a high rate of significant arrhythmias and fall incidents/syncopes. In this context, it has to be kept in mind that in many fall incidents it remains challenging to distinguish fall from syncope.

Digoxin and class I antiarrhythmics are discouraged in the elderly due to their high ADR risk.

Drugs to Improve Fall Risk

Although drugs may represent a major risk factor for falls in the elderly, beneficial effects of pharmacotherapy on fall risk are a matter of ongoing discussions. However, as an intervention to prevent typical falls in the elderly has to act in a multifaceted manner, pharmacotherapy may only contribute in part to these efforts. Potential targets of fall risk attenuation are skeletal muscle mass and strength. As vitamin D dose dependently influences muscle performance and improves strength and function (Chapuy et al. 1992; Pfeifer et al. 2009), it may improve balance and postural control and thus mitigate the risk of fall. Vitamin D supplementation therefore has been repeatedly studied in this context. A recent meta-analysis of several double-blind, placebo-controlled clinical trials confirmed that in elderly patients regular supplementation of vitamin D with at least 700 IU/day effectively reduces fall risk in both the ambulatory and nursing home settings (Bischoff-Ferrari et al. 2009). The authors found a risk reduction of up to 38% within the first months of treatment and a persistent risk reduction of 18% up to 36 months after initial treatment. Therefore, in addition to its recommendation in osteoporosis prevention and treatment (see chapter "Osteoporosis"), vitamin D supplementation should be recommended in elderly patients with increased fall risk, especially in those with a previous fall history of more than one fall per month. There is still some debate concerning the optimal dose, and some authors recommend very high doses of up to 1,800 IU/day, which may depend on the measurement of vitamin D plasma levels. In summary, if contraindications are respected (hypercalcemia, hyperparathyroidism), a daily dose of 800 IU is safe and effective (Annweiler et al. 2010), but higher doses may be required at low vitamin D plasma levels.

Vitamin D supplementation of 800 IU/day is safe and effective to reduce fall risk in the elderly.

In addition, testosterone and dehydroepiandrosterone supplementations are discussed to improve muscle mass and performance in frail elderly (Mohr et al. 2007) at increased fall risk. However, a well-defined, but rather small, study in elderly men failed to confirm a beneficial effect of transdermal testosterone on functionality, although surrogate markers for bone turnover showed an improvement (Kenny et al. 2010a). As fall risk critically depends on functionality, an effect on fall risk is also questionable. Another small study from the same work group found an improvement of functionality in elderly women after a combined intervention, including training of muscle strength and supplementation of dehydroepiandrosterone (Kenny et al. 2010b). To date, sex hormone replacement remains controversial in this context and its risk-benefit ratio unclear. Not all elderly with an increased risk of falls show decreased levels of sex hormones, and cutoff values of these levels to guide clinical decisions for replacement therapy are widely discussed. Testosterone replacement is also considered as a therapeutic approach in the frailty and immobilization syndromes (see chapters "Immobility and Pharmacotherapy" and "Pharmacotherapy and the Frailty Syndrome"). Future developments, however, may lead to better options in this field.

Testosterone replacement to date cannot be recommended as treatment in fall prevention.

Another option of pharmacotherapy to improve fall risk is to ameliorate orthostatic hypotension. Although drugs are considered as major risk factors for orthostatic hypotension in the elderly, especially antihypertensives, elderly patients may suffer from orthostatic hypotension secondary to chronic degenerative diseases (e.g., Parkinson's disease, multisystem atrophy). In this subpopulation, drugs may help in a multifactorial treatment schedule, including physical therapy, physical activation, or support stockings. Fludrocortisone and midodrine may be recommended with caution in this context (see chapters "Immobility and Pharmacotherapy" and "Pharmacotherapy and the Frailty Syndrome"). NSAIDs are not recommended in the elderly due to their ADR spectrum.

References

Annweiler C, Montero-Odasso M, Schott AM, Berrut G, Fantino B, Beauchet O (2010) Fall prevention and vitamin D in the elderly: an overview of the key role of the non-bone effects. J Neuroeng Rehab 7:50–63

Bischoff-Ferrari HA, Dawson-Hughes B, Staehelin HB, Orav JE, Stuck AE, Theiler R, Wong JB, Egli A, Kiel DP, Henschkowski J (2009) Fall prevention with supplemental and active forms of vitamin D: a meta-analysis of randomised controlled trials. BMJ 339:b3692

Blain H, Blain A, Trechot P, Jeandel C (2000) Role des medicaments dans les chutes des sujets ages. Presse Med 29:673–680

Campbell AJ (1991) Drug treatment as a cause of falls in old age. Drugs Aging 1:289–302

Chang JT, Morton SC, Rubenstein LZ et al (2004) Interventions for the prevention of falls in older adults: systematic review and meta-analysis of randomised clinical trials. BMJ 328(7441):680–687

Chapuy MC, Arlot ME, Duboeuf F et al (1992) Vitamin D and calcium to prevent hip fractures in elderly women. N Engl J Med 327:1637–1642

U.S. Congress, Office of Technology Assessment (1994) Hip fracture outcomes in people 50 and over—background paper, OTA-BP-H120, U.S. Government Printing Office, Washington, DC

Cumming RG (1998) Epidemiology of medication-related falls and fractures in the elderly. Drugs Aging 12:43–53

French DD, Campbell R, Spehar A, Cunningham F, Bulat T, Luther SL (2006) Drugs and falls in community-dwelling older people: a national veterans study. Clin Ther 28(4):619–630

Gupta V, Lipsitz LA (2007) Orthostatic hypotension in the elderly. Am J Med 120:841–847

Haddad PM, Sharma SG (2007) Adverse effects of atypical antipsychotics: differential risk and clinical implications. CNS Drugs 21(11):911–936

Kenny AM, Boxer RS, Kleppinger A, Brindisi J, Feinn R, Burleson JA (2010a) Dehydroepiandrosterone combined with exercise improves muscle strength and physical function in frail older women. J Am Geriatr Soc 58:1707–1714

Kenny AM, Kleppinger A, Annis K, Rathier M, Browner B, Judge JO, McGee D (2010b) Effects of transdermal testosterone on bone and muscle in older men with low bioavailable testosterone levels, low bone mass, and physical frailty. J Am Geriatr Soc 58:1134–1143

Kron M, Loy S, Sturm E, Nikolaus T, Becker C (2003) Risk indicators for falls in institutionalized frail elderly. Am J Epidemiol 158:645–653

Leipzig RM (1998) Avoiding adverse drug effects in elderly patients. Cleve Clin J Med 65:479–485

Leipzig RM, Cumming RG, Tinetti ME (1999) Drugs and falls in older people: a systematic review and meta-analysis: I. Psychotropic drugs. J Am Geriatr Soc 47:30–39

Mohr BA, Bhasin S, Kupelian V et al (2007) Testosterone, sex hormone-binding globulin, and frailty in older men. J Am Geriatr Soc 55:548–555

Pfeifer M, Begerow B, Minne HW, Suppan K, Fahrleitner-Pammer A, Dobnig H (2009) Effects of a long-term vitamin D and calcium supplementation on falls and parameters of muscle function in community-dwelling older individuals. Osteoporos Int 20:315–322

Räihä I, Luutonen S, Piha J, Seppanen A, Toikka T, Sourander L (1995) Prevalence, predisposing factors, and prognostic importance of postural hypotension. Arch Intern Med 155:930–935

Sleeper R, Bond CA, Rojas-Fernandez C (2000) Psychotropic drugs and falls: new evidence pertaining to serotonin reuptake inhibitors. Pharmacotherapy 20:308–317

Souchet E, Lapeyre-Mestre M, Montastruc JL (2005) Drug related falls: a study in the French Pharmacovigilance database. Pharmacoepidemiol Drug Saf 14:11–16

Stel VS, Smit JH, Pluijm SMF, Lips P (2004) Consequences of falling in older men and women and risk factors for health service use and functional decline. Age Ageing 33:58–65

Tamblyn R, Abrahamowicz M, du Berger R, McLeod P, Bartlett G (2005) A 5-year prospective assessment of the risk associated with individual benzodiazepines and doses in new elderly users. J Am Geriatr Soc 53:233–241

Tinetti ME, Speechley M, Ginger SF (1988) Risk factors for falls among elderly persons living in the community. N Engl J Med 319:1701–1707

Van der Velde N, Stricker BH, Pols HA, Van der Cammen TJM (2006) Risk of falls after withdrawal of fall-risk increasing drugs: a prospective cohort study. Di J Clin Pharmacol 63:232–237

Woolcott JC, Richardson KJ, Wiens MO et al (2009) Meta-analysis of the impact of 9 medication classes on falls in elderly persons. Arch Intern Med 169:1952–1960

Central Nervous System (CNS) Medications and Delirium

Donna M. Fick

Delirium is a condition of acute and reversible confusion characterized by fluctuation, inattention, disorganized thinking, and an altered level of consciousness. The instrument most commonly used to assess delirium in the acute setting is the confusion assessment method or CAM. The CAM has been validated against geriatric psychiatrists' ratings using *DSM-III-R (Diagnostic and Statistical Manual of Mental Disorders, Third Edition, Revised;* American Psychiatric Association [APA] 1987) criteria and has been shown to have sensitivity between 94% and 100% and specificity between 90% and 95% (Inouye et al. 1990). It is based on *DSM-III* (APA 1980) and *DSM-IV* (APA 1994) criteria for delirium (Table 1) and assesses four features of delirium:

1. Acute and fluctuating,
2. Inattention,
3. Disorganized thinking, and
4. Altered level of consciousness.

Delirium is common in older adults, ranging from 13% to 89% depending on the care setting (Fick et al. 2002). Although delirium has many causes (see partial list in Table 2), it is often related to CNS-active medication use, which is reversible, treatable, and preventable. Certain groups are more vulnerable to drug-induced delirium, most notably older adults and persons with dementia who already have a decreased cognitive reserve (Kolanowski et al. 2010). While the mechanism for drug-induced delirium is not well understood, evidence points to the major roles of anticholinergic failure and GABAergic function (Inouye and Ferrucci 2006). Older adults also are more susceptible to delirium due to age-related changes such as a decrease in total body water and lean body mass, an increase in body fat, and a decrease in glomerular filtration rate and albumin (Cassell et al. 2003).

Drug-induced delirium may result from several different agents—these include drugs with anticholinergic properties such as antihistamines (diphenhydramine), tricyclic antidepressants (amitriptyline), narcotics, sedative-hypnotics, and antipsychotics. Benzodiazepines have been found to be associated with delirium in several studies with older adults across all care settings. Another drug category shown to sometimes cause delirium is antibiotics. Several such medications in the Beer's criteria have been found to trigger delirium (Stockl et al. 2010). **Although delirium is often caused by drug toxicity, it also may stem from drug withdrawal if not properly tapered—as in the case of benzodiazepines.**

Finally, central nervous system (CNS)-active medications, which are widely prescribed to older adults for the management of behavior problems and other chronic conditions, are sometimes inappropriately given. Older adults with

D.M. Fick (✉)
School of Nursing, The Pennsylvania State University, University Park, PA 16802, USA
e-mail: dmf21@psu.edu

M. Wehling (ed.), *Drug Therapy for the Elderly,*
DOI 10.1007/978-3-7091-0912-0_20, © Springer-Verlag Wien 2013

Table 1 *DSM-IV-TR* criteria for delirium

A. Disturbance of consciousness (i.e., reduced clarity of awareness of the environment) with reduced ability to focus, sustain, or shift attention
B. A change in cognition (such as memory, disorientation, language disturbance) or the development of a perceptual disturbance that is not better accounted for by a preexisting established or evolving dementia
C. The disturbance develops over a short period of time (minutes, hours, days, sometimes a week) and tends to change during the course of the day
D. There is evidence from the history and physical examination that the disturbance is caused as a direct physiological consequence of a general medical condition

Source: Adapted from the *Diagnostic and Statistical Manual of Mental Disorders*, fourth edition, text revision (*DSM-IV-TR;* American Psychiatric Association 2000)

Table 2 Common causes of delirium with issues to consider

Medications	Were any new medications added or changed?
	Any recent increase or decrease in dosage or in organ failure that might have an impact on toxicity?
Lack of medication or withdrawal	Is this person withdrawing from medication or alcohol?
	Is the person's pain assessed and well controlled?
Infection	Fever, urinary or respiratory symptoms?
	Are WBCs elevated? Older adult may not mount an increased WBC count or temperature
Dehydration	Has a recent BUN or creatinine clearance been checked?
Electrolyte disturbances	Sodium, potassium, glucose, thyroid
Sensory deprivation	Are glasses and or hearing aides on?
	Are they stimulated appropriately?
Intracranial	Is there evidence of focal neurological signs?
	Has there been a fall in the past days or weeks?
Cardiac/pulmonary	Have the heart rate, lung sounds, and oxygen saturation been assessed?
Urinary/fecal	When was the last bowel movement?
	Is there urinary incontinence or retention?
Environmental and activity	Has the individual experienced a recent relocation or loss? Does the person have orientation devices in his or her room? Is the person being mobilized?

Source: Adapted from Flanagan and Fick 2010; Inouye 2006
BUN blood urea nitrogen, *WBC* white blood cell

dementia who frequently experience delirium are commonly prescribed CNS-active medications.

There is conflicting evidence on whether persons with dementia are prescribed greater numbers of medications than other older individuals (Giron et al. 2001), but they do take a greater number of CNS-active medications, including antipsychotics, anxiolytics, and antidepressants. Many of these prescribed drugs have limited effectiveness in older individuals with dementia, are associated with falls and fractures (Vestergaard et al. 2006), and are known to cause delirium and further cognitive deterioration because of their potent anticholinergic properties (Boustani et al. 2007; Fick et al. 2007). Even drugs prescribed appropriately to older adults can precipitate what has been described as a "prescribing cascade." For example, cholinesterase inhibitor use has been associated with an increased risk of receiving an anticholinergic drug to manage the resulting urinary incontinence (Gill et al. 2006).

Despite increased postmarketing surveillance for drug-induced diseases, the strongest level of evidence that certain drugs cause or worsen delirium is lacking for several reasons. These include the difficulty in fully implicating drugs as the etiology of delirium, and the lack of randomized clinical trials on this topic (Applegate and Curb 1990). Like many drug-induced diseases, delirium is a multicausal problem. Therefore, identifying specific drugs' contribution to the condition of delirium is often difficult, especially in the context of delirium superimposed on dementia (Voyer et al. 2009) and chronically ill older adults. A clinical review of studies revealed that much of the research is observational in nature, although stronger evidence exists for some categories of medications, including benzodiazepines and anticholinergics, opiates (meperidine), and sedative hypnotics such as flurazepam and zolpidem (see Table 3).

As noted, several studies have strongly associated benzodiazepines with delirium. A systematic review by Clegg and Young (2011) highlighted 14 such studies and found a moderate relationship between all benzodiazepines and delirium and a higher risk with longer-acting benzodiazepines and a higher versus lower dose of benzodiazepines. Marcantonio, Lepouse and colleagues, and Pandharipande and colleagues found a moderate relationship between benzodiazepines and delirium or cognitive deterioration (Marcantonio et al. 1998; Lepousé et al. 2006; Pandharipande et al. 2006; Wright et al. 2009). Marcantonio et al. and Pandharipande et al. studied hospitalized older adults, while Wright et al.'s study included a longitudinal community population. Clegg and Young (2011) and Gaudreau and colleagues (2005) found a moderate relationship with opioid medications and delirium, although studies have shown delirium to be associated with untreated pain, so these studies should be interpreted cautiously. The side effects of opioids must be carefully balanced with the proper assessment and treatment of pain when delirium is suspected (Reid et al. 2011). Some of the newer sedative hypnotics, such as zolpidem, have been implicated in multiple case reports as causing or worsening delirium; in larger studies, they have been associated with fractures and falling (Finkle et al. 2011; Sidana et al. 2002; Toner et al. 2000). Less evidence has been found for a delirium association with corticosteroids, H2 antagonists, nonsteroidal anti-inflammatory drugs

(NSAIDs), antiparkinson drugs, and tricyclic antidepressants (Clegg and Young 2011; Kotlyar et al. 2011).

Although several drugs are being tested for the treatment of delirium (haloperidol, olanzapine, risperidone), current evidence and delirium guidelines for delirium treatment recommend using medications as a last resort if the patient is in danger of hurting him- or herself or others and other nondrug alternatives have failed. Current trials on drugs to treat delirium can be accessed at http://clinicaltrials.gov/ (accessed 19 Dec 2011).

Explorations of the potential causes of delirium should always include a look at medication, especially in studies of older adults who are more vulnerable to drug-induced delirium due to physiological changes associated with aging. The APA's (Cook 2004) practice guidelines for the treatment of patients with delirium indicate that research has not proven benzodiazepines to be an effective monotherapy for delirium except in cases of benzodiazepine or alcohol withdrawal or the need for seizure prevention. Yet, while the APA guidelines suggest that physicians avoid prescribing these drugs for patients with delirium, they continue to be widely ordered. All in all, when it comes to the problem of delirium in older adults, clinicians should consider a less-is-more approach to medication use. Delirium treatment should include a careful assessment and treatment of the causes of the delirium. Clinicians should avoid covering up the behavior with a sedating medication. Treatment of behavior problems in persons with dementia or delirium requires expert assessment of the cause of the underlying behavior and an individualized approach for understanding and treating the problem behavior.

In conclusion, increased research is needed in the area of delirium and medication use. Several studies have identified drugs that may cause or worsen delirium in older adults (see Table 1 in chapter "Pharmacotherapy and Special Aspects of Cognitive Disorders in the Elderly"). Decreasing exposure to these drugs in older adults, especially those who are more vulnerable due to older age and baseline cognitive impairment, is crucial to the prevention and management of delirium.

Table 3 Overview of studies linking medication use and delirium

Reference	Purpose, hypothesis, or research question	Study design, setting, country, sample size	Drug categories	Major findings
Moore and O'Keeffe 1999	To focus on clinically relevant cognitive impairment, in particular the major confusional syndromes: delirium and dementia, caused by drugs	Review — Ireland	Cognitive impairment in the elderly	Drugs have been reported as the cause of delirium in 11–30% of cases
			Delirium	Any drug can cause delirium, especially in a vulnerable patient
			Dementia	The relative odds of developing drug-induced confusion increased from 1.0 when 0–1 drug was used to 9.3 when 4–5 drugs were used
			Drug-induced cognitive impairment	
			Drug toxicity as a cause of delirium	
			Dementia due to drug toxicity	
			Cognitive impairment due to anticholinergic drugs	Studies have suggested that it is often the total burden of anticholinergic drugs that determines development of delirium rather than any single agent
			Cognitive impairment due to psychoactive drugs	Psychoactive drugs are the most common causes of drug-induced cognitive impairment
			Cognitive impairment due to non-psychoactive drugs	Sudden withdrawal from short-acting benzodiazepines is a common cause of delirium in hospital patients
			Prevention of drug-induced cognitive impairment	Opioids are also among the most important causes of delirium in post-operative patients
			Management of drug-induced cognitive impairment	Delirium is also a well-recognized feature of lithium toxicity
				Newer antidepressants cause decreased delirium
				Anticonvulsants can impair cognitive function (phenytoin has been most clearly linked to development of delirium and dementia)
				Nonpsychoactive drugs such as histamine H2 receptor antagonists, cardiac drugs, corticosteroids, NSAIDS, and antibiotics have been linked to cognitive impairment, but diagnosis is easily missed unless there is high suspicion

Toner et al. 2000	To report a series of cases in which patients developed delirium, nightmares, and hallucinations during zolpidem treatment and to review zolpidem's pharmacology, discuss previous reports of central nervous system side effects, examine the impact of drug interactions with concurrent use of antidepressants, and examine gender differences and side effects and explore the significance of protein binding in producing side effects	Case reports	Zolpidem	The elimination of zolpidem tends to be reduced in patients with liver cirrhosis and renal disease
		United States		Delirium and confusional behavior have been reported in multiple studies involving treatment with zolpidem, but there has only been one case report in the literature to date
				17 case reports of hallucinations caused by the use of zolpidem
				Nightmares seem to be a side effect of zolpidem that can occur at any dose, delirium and hallucinations seem to be caused by toxic levels of this medication
				Four major variables postulated to consider when prescribing zolpidem: gender (cases reported more with females), dose (hallucinations occurred with >5 mg), protein-binding affinity (drug is highly protein bound), and degree of cytochrome P450 3A4 isoenzyme inhibition by concomitantly used antidepressants
Brodeur and Stirling 2001	To report a case of an elderly woman sustaining an episode of delirium after one dose of zolpidem	Case report	Zolpidem	Other case reports discussed regarding the adverse effects of zolpidem administration Case reports included a 20-year-old

(continued)

Table 3 (continued)

Reference	Purpose, hypothesis, or research question	Study design, setting, country, sample size	Drug categories	Major findings
				woman, 34-year-old woman, 26-year-old woman, 74-year-old woman, and a 71-year-old woman
		United States		
		N = 1	**Case Summary:** 86-year-old female admitted to the hospital for blurred vision, nausea, vomiting, and increasing headache was given zolpidem 5 mg on day 3. She became very restless, would not follow commands, attempted to get out of bed, and walked with an unsteady gait. She was not oriented to place or time. She received 5 mg i.m. haloperidol and was restrained. Haloperidol was continued every 12 h for 2 days. Symptoms resolved by day 5	Zolpidem is approximately 92% bound to plasma proteins; therefore, pharmacokinetics is involved.
			Patient also had other variables that can contribute to delirium, such as hospitalization, histamine receptor blocker, and gabapentin	
Han et al. 2001	To investigate the effect of anticholinergic (ACH) medication exposure on the subsequent severity of delirium symptoms in hospitalized elderly patients diagnosed with delirium	**Prospective RCT** of either a delirium geriatric service or in an **observational cohort study** of outcomes of delirium (prognosis study	Anticholinergics	The clinician-rated ACH score was statistically significant correlate of delirium severity on the following day, when adjusted for the number of non-ACH medications, and this effect remained statistically significant when adjusting for the total number of medications
			Delirium index Medication(DI) exposures	
			1. Summers drug risk number (DRN)	
			2. Clinician-rated ACH score	

Study	Objectives/Hypotheses	Setting	Country	N	Drug	Results
		University-affiliated primary acute hospital			3. Number of ACH medications	The effect of increasing the number of non-ACH medications was also statistically significant, but the effect of ACH medications was almost 5 times stronger
					4. Number of non-ACH medications	
					5. Total number of medications	The effect of ACH medications remained significant after adjusting for sex, serum urea nitrogen-creatinine ratio, and alcohol/drug abuse
	Hypotheses: Current exposure to ACH medications is independently associated with increased severity of delirium symptoms, and the effect of ACH medication exposure on delirium severity may depend on dementia status, with demented patients being more sensitive to ACH medications than those without dementia		United States	N = 278		
				N = 95, trial, intervention		
				N = 96, trial, control		
				N = 87; prognosis study		
Sidana et al. 2002	To report a rare side effect in the form of zolpidem-induced delirium, which is not mentioned in the literature	Letter to the editor			Zolpidem	The day after taking zolpidem 10 mg p.o. h.s, the patient displayed symptoms of irrelevant talk, suspicious attitude, hearing of voices. Acute psychosis diagnosis was made, and patient was admitted. The patient continued to display delirious symptoms and his diagnosis was changed to acute delirium
		Psychiatry outpatient department (OPD) of government medical college hospital				

(continued)

Table 3 (continued)

Reference	Purpose, hypothesis, or research question	Study design, setting, country, sample size	Drug categories	Major findings
		India		
		N = 1		
Alagiakrishnan and Wiens 2004	To provide an approach for clinicians to prevent, recognize, and manage drug-induced delirium. To review the mechanisms for this condition and discuss the age-related changes that may contribute to altered pharmacological effects	Review article	Clinical recognition of drug-induced delirium	Causative drugs for delirium include narcotics, benzodiazepines, and anticholinergics (observational studies).
		Canada	Medications associated with delirium	Both hyperactive and mixed delirium is commonly seen in cholinergic toxicity, alcohol intoxication, and certain illicit drug intoxication, serotonin syndrome, and alcohol and benzodiazepine withdrawal. Hypoactive delirium is often due to benzodiazepine, narcotic overdose, or sedative hypnotic or alcohol intoxication
			Mechanisms of drugs causing delirium	
			Factors that may have a role in the susceptibility of an individual to drug-induced delirium	
			Investigations	Benzodiazepines are lipid soluble, which causes a prolonged half-life in the elderly because of the accumulation of lipid tissue
			Management	Of the SSRIs, paroxetine has the greatest affinity for muscarinic receptors
				Lithium can cause delirium at therapeutic levels
				Demerol is avoided due to decreased renal function
				Alternative medicine products such as henbane, jimson weed, and

Author/Year	Hypothesis	Design	Method	Setting/Sample	Exposure	Results
						mandrake can contribute to delirium
						Evidence supports a major role for cholinergic failure in delirium
						In stroke and dementia, there is an impaired integrity of the blood–brain barrier
						Haloperidol is the drug of choice to manage symptoms of delirium
Gaudreau et al. 2005	Hypothesis: Exposure to certain psychoactive medications, including anticholinergics, benzodiazepines, corticosteroids, or opioids, increases the risk for delirium in hospitalized patients	Prospective cohort	Patients with a histologic diagnosis of cancer were followed up with the Nursing Delirium Screening Scale (developed by the group) for up to 4 weeks, and exposure to psychoactive medications was documented daily	Hemato-oncology/internal medicine unit; Canada; N = 261	Exposure to psychoactive medications	43 (16.5%) of the 261 patients became delirious during the 4-week follow-up
						Clinical variables associated with increased risk of delirium included history of delirium and liver metastases
						Patients exposed to higher than 2 mg of daily benzodiazepines were at twice the risk of developing delirium
						Patients exposed to daily corticosteroid doses higher than 15 mg had a 2.7-fold increase in the risk of delirium
						Patients exposed to opioids higher than 90 mg were 2.1 times more at risk of developing delirium
						No association was found between anticholinergics and delirium occurrence in this study

(continued)

Table 3 (continued)

Reference	Purpose, hypothesis, or research question	Study design, setting, country, sample size	Drug categories	Major findings
Rudolph et al. 2008	To validate the Anticholinergic Risk Scale (ARS) score against clinical symptoms of anticholinergic toxic reactions in a retrospective geriatric evaluation and management (GEM) cohort also in a prospective older primary care population	Retrospective cohort and Prospective cohort	Anticholinergic risk scale	Among both cohorts, the prevalence and numbers of anticholinergic adverse effects were statistically significantly increased with higher ARS scores
		Retrospective: GEM clinics at the Veterans Affairs Boston Health Care System	The 500 most prescribed medications within the Veterans Affairs Boston Healthcare System were reviewed by a geriatrician and 2 geropharmacists to identify medications with potential to cause anticholinergic adverse effects. Medications were ranked from 0 to 3, with 3 being very strong. Statistically significant agreement was found among the reviewers and in the agreement among the ARS medication rankings	Higher ARS scores statistically significantly increased the risk of anticholinergic adverse effects in both cohorts
		N = 132		
	Hypothesis: The ARS score would be positively associated with the risk of anticholinergic symptoms, central adverse effects would be more prevalent among the GEM cohort than among the primary care cohort, and the GEM and primary care cohorts would be equally susceptible to peripheral adverse effects, and the ARS would identify increased risk of peripheral adverse effects similarly in both cohorts	Prospective: Primary care clinics at the Veterans Affairs Boston		
		Healthcare System		
		N = 117 male	Anticholinergic adverse effects	

Voyer et al. 2009	To identify the predisposing factors associated with delirium among demented long-term care (LTC) residents	Cross sectional	Participants recruited from three LTC facilities and one LTC unit of a large regional hospital		Age, severity of dementia, level of functional autonomy, number of medications, pain, behavioral symptoms, dehydration, brachial perimeter, and geriatric fever were all significantly associated with delirium at the .05 level	Age, severity of dementia, level of functional autonomy, number of medications, pain, behavioral symptoms, dehydration, brachial perimeter, and geriatric fever were all significantly associated with delirium at the .05 level
	To assess if the number of predisposing factors present for a given resident were linked to the likelihood of the resident having delirium	Canada		Age and severity of dementia were the most associated factors of delirium	Age and severity of dementia were the most associated factors of delirium	
		N = 155		Delirium (definite and probable) measured with the onfusion sessment ethod (CAM)		
				Dementia status was indicated by the presence of a medical diagnosis of dementia		
				Hierarchic Dementia scale rated dementia severity		
				Pain rated using the DOLOPLUS-II		
				Cornell Depression Scale		
				Charlson Comorbidity Index		
				Functional Autonomy Measurement System		
				Insomnia Severity Index		
				Visual and hearing impairment measured using the two items from the SMAF		
				Oxygen saturation, geriatric fever, hydration, weight loss, number of medications		

(continued)

Table 3 (continued)

Reference	Purpose, hypothesis, or research question	Study design, setting, country, sample size	Drug categories	Major findings
Wright et al. 2009	To evaluate the combined effect of CNS medication use on cognitive decline and incident cognitive impairment in older community-dwelling adults	Longitudinal cohort	CNS medication (benzodiazepine, opioid receptor agonists, antipsychotics, antidepressants) at baseline (1 year), 3, and 5 years	At baseline (1 year), 13.9% of subjects used at least one CNS active medication. At years 3 and 5, the prevalence increased to 15.3% and 17.1%, respectively
				Antidepressants were more commonly used than any other CNS medication class. SSRIs were the most commonly used type of antidepressant
	Hypothesis: Older adults using CNS medications would have a higher risk of decline in cognitive function than those who did not use any CNS medication	Adults ages 65 and older enrolled in the Health, Aging, and Body Composition study without baseline cognitive impairment		By year 5, 7.7% of baseline participants had 3MS scores that dropped below 80 (cognitive impairment). One quarter of participants demonstrated cognitive decline by year 5
		United States		
		N = 2,737		
Levin et al. 2010	To present a complex case of delirium that was determined to be caused by a CYP3A4 interaction between fentanyl and diltiazem	Case report	Three days after the initiation of diltiazem, the patient once again became delirious (hypoactive delirium). Concomitantly this patient was receiving a fentanyl drip at 25 μg/h	Delirium was diagnosed secondary to narcotic toxicity due to the interaction between diltiazem and fentanyl. Once fentanyl was discontinued, delirium symptoms started to resolve
		Cancer center		
		United States		Diltiazem is a CYP3A4 inhibitor, and fentanyl is metabolized by CYP3A4
		N = 1		

Reference	Study design / Country	Aim and Hypothesis	Study population	Medication groups (N)	Outcomes measured	Results
Stockl et al. 2010	Retrospective Cohort Study United States	To evaluate the risk of selected adverse events and healthcare costs for elderly patients receiving specific Beers high severity (BHS) potentially inappropriate medication versus comparable elderly patients not receiving potentially inappropriate medications Hypothesis: The use of specific Beers high-severity (BHS) medications designated as "always avoid" or "rarely appropriate" in the elderly would result in increased adverse events and health care costs.	Patients aged 65 and older who started 1 of 23 potentially inappropriate medications (PIMs) matched with control subjects who were not receiving PIMs	BHS anticholinergics N = 37,358 BHS narcotics N = 395 Trimetho-benzamide hydrochloride BHS sedative hypnotics N = 13,542	Primary: risk of having the adverse event of interest during a post period of up to 360 days for exposed patients versus controls Adverse events of interest: delirium or hallucinations for the BHS anticholinergics; delirium, or hallucinations for the BHS narcotics; extrapyramidal effects for timethobenzamide; and falls or fractures for the BHS sedative hypnotics Annual health care costs	BHS sedative hypnotic-receiving patients were significantly more likely to have a fall or fracture than controls BHS anticholinergic receiving patients did not have higher risk of delirium or hallucinations than controls Annual adjusted medical and total healthcare costs were significantly higher for patients exposed to PIMs than for controls

(continued)

Table 3 (continued)

Reference	Purpose, hypothesis, or research question	Study design, setting, country, sample size	Drug categories	Major findings
Clegg and Young 2011	To identify prospective studies that investigated the association between medications and risk of delirium	Systematic literature review	Medication classes (neuroleptics, opioid, benzodiazepines, antihistamine H1 antagonists, histamine H2 antagonists, dihydropyridines, antimuscarinics, tricyclic antidepressants, antiparkinson, digoxin, steroids, and NSAIDS)	The risk of delirium was increased with opioids, benzodiazepines, dihydropyridines, and possibly antihistamines
		RCTs, prospective cohort studies, and case–control studies that reported on medications and delirium in hospital patients or long-term care residents		No increased risk with neuroleptics, or digoxin
				Uncertainty regarding H2 antagonists, tricyclic antidepressants, antiparkinson medications, steroids, NSAIDS, and antimuscarinics
		United Kingdom		
		N = 14 studies included in final analysis		
Devanand and Schultz 2011	To report findings related to the Clinical Antipsychotic Trials Intervention Effectiveness-Alzheimer's Disease (CATIE-AD) study	Editorial	Antipsychotics	Lower cognitive performance in dementia patients who received atypical antipsychotic medications compared with placebo
		Community-dwelling patients with a mean Mini-Mental State Examination (MMSE) score of 15.2		The CATIE-AD design allowed for comparison of olanzapine, quetiapine, and risperidone to detect individual drug effects.
		More than 400 participants		Elderly females were at increased risk of a decline in executive functioning—although mechanism not clear

Ancelin et al. 2012	To evaluate the effects of anti-inflammatories on cognitive function	n = 7234 community-dwelling older adults	Anti-inflammatories	
		Longitudinal design		
Finkle et al. 2011	To determine whether zolpidem is a safer alternative to the benzodiazepines	Retrospective cohort	Nonvertebral fracture and hip fractures	The rate ratios (the ratio of the fracture rate after the initial prescription to the fracture rate in the interval 3 years to 1 year before the initial prescription) for the 90-day posttreatment interval relative to the pretreatment interval were statistically significant for zolpidem, lorazepam, and diazepam, but not for alprazolam
		Community based	Zolpidem and benzodiazepine prescription	
		United States		Excess risks for nonvertebral fractures were observed after an initial prescription for zolpidem, lorazepam, and diazepam, but not alprazolam
		Health maintenance organization members with an initial prescription for		There was excess risk for zolpidem relative to alprazolam and possibly relative to lorazepam, but risks for zolpidem and diazepam appeared similar
		Zolpidem		
		N = 43,343		
		Alprazolam		Recommendations: The findings suggest that zolpidem is unlikely to be a safer alternative to benzodiazepines in older adults, and that it may convey greater risk than alprazolam
		N = 103,790		
		Lorazepam		
		N = 150,858		
		Diazepam		
		N = 93,618		

(continued)

Table 3 (continued)

Reference	Purpose, hypothesis, or research question	Study design, setting, country, sample size	Drug categories	Major findings
Hughes and Pandharipande 2011	To detail the effects of perioperative and intensive care unit sedation on the development of delirium and cognitive impairment and provide an evidence-based approach toward analgesia and sedation paradigms to improve patient outcomes	Review article	Sedative and analgesic medications and acute and chronic brain dysfunction	Large prospective study evaluated for emergence delirium in the postanesthesia care unit found a 4.7% incidence and demonstrated an almost twofold increase in the odds of developing delirium if benzodiazepines were administered preoperatively. Also, the second study displayed the incidence delirium to be 5% and that of hypoactive to be 8%. Significant risk factors were benzodiazepines and etomidate induction, and longer anesthetic duration was a risk factor for hypoactive
		United States	Depth of sedation and outcomes	The MENDS study displayed that dexmedetomidine vs. lorazepam decreased the duration of brain organ dysfunction with less likelihood of delirium development
			Changing intensive care unit (ICU) sedation paradigms to improve patient outcomes	
			Delirium and cognitive dysfunction prevention	SEDCOM study demonstrated that dexmedetomidine vs. midazolam displayed reduction in delirium prevalence
			Delirium management	
Kotlyar et al. 2011	To address three major types of psychiatric manifestations in older people commonly related to medications: cognitive impairment, insomnia, and depression	Book chapter	Psychiatric manifestations of drugs (see findings) were addressed in this review	

Anticholinergics: age-related decreases in cholinergic function implemented. Many medications with anticholinergic effects such as TCAs, antipsychotics, first-generation antihistamines, and urinary antimuscarinic agents are prescribed. Second-generation antihistamines are preferred for the elderly. Lower doses of oxybutynin may not impair cognition in those with baseline cognitive impairment. Increased blood-brain barrier permeability. Other medications such as histamine 2 receptors, furosemide, and digoxin have serum activity

Benzodiazepines: increased risk for adverse effects because of age-related changes and inadvertent sudden withdrawal of short-acting can cause delirium

Antidepressants: TCA's are the most likely of this class to cause impaired cognition

Opioid analgesics: Demerol has been associated with an increased risk of delirium when compared to other opioids

Antiepileptics: dose-related adverse effects

Antihypertensives: much antihypertensive evidence stems from case reports and observational studies

Histamine-2 receptor antagonists–

CYP cytochrome P, *NSAID* nonsteroidal anti-inflammatory drug, *RCT* randomized controlled trial, *SSRI* selective serotonin reuptake inhibitor, *TCA* tricyclic antidepressant, *MENDS* Maximizing Efficacy of Targeted Sedation and Reducing Neurological Dysfunction, *SEDCOM* Safety and Efficacy of Dexmedetomidine compared with Midazolam

In many cases, the use of CNS-active medications could be avoided by substituting a safer nondrug alternative to handle behavior or sleep issues. Although such studies have been limited, there is increasing evidence of the beneficial effects of music therapy, physical and cognitive activity therapies, and nondrug sleep interventions (Agostini et al. 2001; Kolanowski et al. 2011).

Future studies should include larger sample sizes and more rigorous study designs to better assess for drug-induced delirium. Future research should also address the testing of nondrug interventions for behavior and sleep problems—conditions for which CNS-active drugs are frequently prescribed.

References

Agostini JV, Leo-Summers LS, Inouye SK (2001) Cognitive and other adverse effects of diphenhydramine use in hospitalized older patients. Arch Intern Med 161:2091–2097

Alagiakrishnan K, Wiens CA (2004) An approach to drug induced delirium in the elderly. Postgrad Med J 80:388–393

American Psychiatric Association (1980) Diagnostic and statistical manual of mental disorders, 3rd edn. American Psychiatric Association, Washington, DC

American Psychiatric Association (1987) Diagnostic and statistical manual of mental disorders, 3rd edn. American Psychiatric Association, Washington, DC, rev

American Psychiatric Association (1994) Diagnostic and statistical manual of mental disorders, 4th edn. American Psychiatric Association, Washington, DC

American Psychiatric Association (2000) Diagnostic and statistical manual of mental disorders, 4th edn. American Psychiatric Association, Washington, DC, text revn

Ancelin ML, Carrière I, Helmer C et al (2012) Steroid and nonsteroid anti-inflammatory drugs, cognitive decline, and dementia. Neurobiol Aging 33:2082–2090

Applegate WB, Curb JD (1990) Designing and executing randomized clinical trials involving elderly persons. J Am Geriatr Soc 38:943–950

Boustani M, Hall KS, Lane KA et al (2007) The association between cognition and histamine-2 receptor antagonists in African Americans. J Am Geriatr Soc 55:1248–1253

Brodeur MR, Stirling AL (2001) Delirium associated with zolpidem. Ann Pharmacother 35:1562–1564

Cassell CK, Leipzig RM, Cohen HJ et al (2003) Geriatric medicine: an evidence-base approach, 4th edn. Springer, New York

Clegg A, Young JB (2011) Which medications to avoid in people at risk of delirium: a systematic review. Age Ageing 40:23–29

Cook I (2004) Guideline Watch: Practice Guideline for the Treatment of Patients with Delirium, American Psychiatric Association. Psychiatry online 1–4. Acessed June 30, 2012

Devanand DP, Schultz SK (2011) Consequences of antipsychotic medications for the dementia patient. Am J Psychiatry 168:767–769

Fick D, Kolanowski A, Waller J (2007) High prevalence of central nervous system medications in community–dwelling older adults with dementia over a three year period. Aging Ment Health 11(5):588–595

Fick DM, Agostini JV, Inouye SK (2002) Delirium superimposed on dementia: a systematic review. J Am Geriatr Soc 50:1723–1732

Finkle WD, Der JS, Greenland S et al (2011) Risk of fractures requiring hospitalization after an initial prescription for zolpidem, alprazolam, lorazepam, or diazepam in older adults. J Am Geriatr Soc 59:1883–1890

Flanagan NM, Fick DM (2010) Delirium superimposed on dementia. Assessment and intervention. J Gerontol Nurs 36:19–23

Gaudreau JD, Gagnon P, Harel F, Tremblay A (2005) Psychoactive medications and risk of delirium in hospitalized cancer patients. J Clin Oncol 23:6712–6718

Gill SS, Bronskill SE, Normand SL et al (2006) Antipsychotic drug use and mortality in older adults with dementia. Ann Intern Med 146:775–786

Giron MS, Forsell Y, Bernsten C, Thorslund M, Winblad B, Fastborn J (2001) Psychotropic drug use in elderly people with and without dementia. Int J Geriatr Psychiatry 16:900–906

Han L, McCusker J, Cole M et al (2001) Use of medications with anticholinergic effect predicts clinical severity of delirium symptoms in older medical inpatients. Arch Intern Med 161:1099–1105

Hughes CG, Pandharipande PP (2011) The effects of perioperative and intensive care unit sedation on brain organ dysfunction. Anesth Analg 112:1212–1217

Inouye SK (2006) Delirium in older persons. N Engl J Med 354:1157–1165

Inouye SK, Ferrucci L (2006) Elucidating the pathophysiology of delirium and the interrelationship of delirium and dementia. J Gerontol A Biol Sci Med Sci 61:1277–1280

Inouye SK, van Dyck CH, Alessi CA, Balkin S, Siegal AP, Horwitz RI (1990) Clarifying confusion: the confusion assessment method. A new method for detection of delirium. Ann Intern Med 113:941–948

Kolanowski AM, Fick DM, Clare L, Therrien B, Gill D (2010) An intervention for delirium superimposed on dementia based on cognitive reserve theory. Aging Ment Health 14:232–242

Kolanowski AM, Fick DM, Litaker MS, Clare L, Leslie D, Boustani M (2011) Study protocol for the recreational stimulation for elders as a vehicle to resolve delirium superimposed on dementia (reserve for DSD) trial. Trials 12:119

Kotlyar M, Gray SL, Maher RL, Hanlon JT (2011) Psychiatric manifestations of medications in the elderly. In: Agronin MA, Maletta GJ (eds) Principles and practice of geriatric psychiatry. LWW, Baltimore

Lepousé C, Lautner CA, Liu L, Gomis P, Leon A (2006) Emergence delirium in adults in the post-anaesthesia care unit. Br J Anaesth 96:747–753

Levin TT, Bakr MH, Nikolova T (2010) Case report: delirium due to a diltiazem-fentanyl CYP3A4 drug interaction. Gen Hosp Psychiatr 32:648

Marcantonio ER, Goldman L, Orav EJ, Cook EF, Lee TH (1998) The association of intraoperative factors with the development of postoperative delirium. Am J Med 105:380–384

Moore AR, O'Keeffe ST (1999) Drug-induced cognitive impairment in the elderly. Drugs Aging 15:15–28

Pandharipande P, Shintani A, Peterson J et al (2006) Lorazepam is an independent risk factor for transitioning to delirium in intensive care unit patients. Anesthesiology 104:21–26

Reid MC, Bennett DA, Chen WG et al (2011) Improving the pharmacologic management of pain in older adults: identifying the research gaps and methods to address them. Pain Med 12:1336–1357

Rudolph JL, Salow MJ, Angelini MC, McGlinchey RE (2008) The anticholinergic risk scale and anticholinergic adverse effects in older persons. Arch Intern Med 168:508–513

Sidana A, Singh GP, Sharma RP (2002) Zolpidem induced delirium (letter to the editor). Indian J Psychiatr 44:398

Stockl KM, Le L, Zhang S, Harada AS (2010) Clinical and economic outcomes associated with potentially inappropriate prescribing in the elderly. Am J Manag Care 16(1):e1–e10

Toner LC, Tsambiras BM, Catalano G, Catalano MC, Cooper DS (2000) Central nervous system side effects associated with zolpidem treatment. Clin Neuropharmacol 23:54–58

Vestergaard P, Rejnmark L, Mosekilde L (2006) Anxiolytics, sedatives, antidepressants, neuroleptics and the risk of fracture. Osteoporos Int 17:807–816

Voyer P, Richard S, Doucet L, Carmichael PH (2009) Predisposing factors associated with delirium among demented long-term care residents. Clin Nurs Res 18:153–171

Wright RM, Roumani YF, Boudreau R et al (2009) Effect of central nervous system medication use on decline in cognition in community-dwelling older adults: findings from the Health, Aging and Body Composition Study. J Am Geriatr Soc 57:243–250

Pharmacotherapy and Special Aspects of Cognitive Disorders in the Elderly

Heinrich Burkhardt

Introduction

Cognitive impairment significantly influences pharmacotherapy as a major barrier for successful adherence. This is outlined in more detail in chapter "Adherence to Pharmacotherapy in the Elderly." Cognitive function compromises not only adherence and management of pharmacotherapy but also cognitive function itself, which is an important target for pharmacotherapy to slow further deterioration in case of dementia or delirium (see chapters "Dementia" and "Central Nervous System (CNS) Medications and Delirium"). Unfortunately, drugs may also cause harm by inducing unintended cerebral symptoms such as disorientation, delusion and hallucination (delirium), dizziness, adynamia, and forgetfulness. These adverse drug reactions are often missed or misinterpreted and hereby represent a main factor of inadequate prescribing cascades (Fig. 1).

Drugs as Trigger of Cognitive Disorders

A major risk in treating frail elderly or elderly with dementia is delirium. As outlined in chapter "Central Nervous System (CNS) Medications and Delirium," delirium is triggered by more than one factor in most cases. Among those, drugs are often involved. From a clinical point of view, two pitfalls have to be mentioned in this context. First, delirium often presents with a hypoactive pattern lacking agitation and apparent vegetative signs (Lewis et al. 1995). In that case, immediate and correct diagnosis is often missing. Assessment according to the *DSM-IV* (*Diagnostic and Statistical Manual of Mental Disorders, Fourth Edition*; American Psychiatric Association 1994) criteria in clinical routine and applying standardized screening tools (confusion assessment method [CAM], delirium index) are essential and helpful to improve unacceptably high frequencies of misdiagnosis (Inouye et al. 1990; McCusker et al. 1998).

Hypoactive delirium is often missed or misinterpreted.

A second pitfall is the correct separation of delirium from dementia. This may frequently be challenging, and careful history taking is demanding. Cognitive malfunction in the elderly may be mistaken as dementia when the patient's history is not well known. This carries the risk of missing serious underlying disorders that cause delirium (e.g., pneumonia, electrolyte disorders, thyroid disorders). In addition, delirium caused by adverse drug reactions (ADRs) may be missed this way.

Sudden onset of change in cognition in the elderly is frequently caused by an underlying physiological disorder (infection, electrolyte imbalance, organ failure).

H. Burkhardt (✉)
IVth Department of Medicine, Geriatrics, University Medical Centre Mannheim, Theodor-Kutzer-Ufer 1-3, Mannheim 68167, Germany
e-mail: heinrich.burkhardt@umm.de

M. Wehling (ed.), *Drug Therapy for the Elderly*,
DOI 10.1007/978-3-7091-0912-0_21, © Springer-Verlag Wien 2013

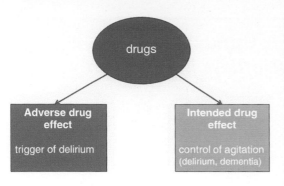

Fig. 1 Drugs may represent both trigger factors and treatment in delirium

A thorough examination therefore is essential to rule out any underlying disorder that may be cured or attenuated (Rummans et al. 1995; Cole 2004). Figure 2 highlights the multiple factors that may precipitate delirium. In addition, delirium always indicates a complex disease course and is a significant factor of both remaining disability and mortality.

As already outlined in chapter "Central Nervous System (CNS) Medications and Delirium," drugs providing anticholinergic activity are associated with the highest risk of inducing cognitive disorders and should be avoided in the elderly, especially in elderly with preexisting cerebral disorders. Therefore, they are discouraged in patients with dementia. Delirium risk is associated with the total anticholinergic burden posed by medication. In case of polypharmacy, this is an important issue, and drugs with anticholinergic properties should be rigorously avoided or at least limited in that circumstance as delirium risk is increasing according to the total anticholinergic burden to which several drugs may additively contribute (Han et al. 2001).

Risk of delirium increases with total anticholinergic drug burden.

It is noteworthy that not only central nervous system (CNS) drugs provide anticholinergic activity. Frequently, even drugs not primarily prescribed to control for CNS-related problems like digoxin and theophylline carry that risk (Tune et al. 1992). An overview and risk estimation are given in Table 1 However, due to methodological

problems such as correct drug classification and missing appropriate assessment instruments, evaluation of cohorts concerning frequency, cause, and treatment of delirium is difficult, and risk estimation is mainly not based on large case-control cohorts. For more detail, see chapter "Central Nervous System (CNS) Medications and Delirium."

As already mentioned in chapter "Central Nervous System (CNS) Medications and Delirium," drug therapy for delirium should not routinely be given, but only if agitation and hallucination are otherwise poorly controlled, and should never be used to substitute for or displace nonpharmacological measures like avoidance of further disturbing factors (e.g., noisy and crowded surroundings, lack of day-night triggers, surplus of involved staff members). These measures are the same to prevent delirium in elderly with risk factors, especially those with preexisting dementia.

Some rules to prevent and treat delirium are given here:

– Try nonpharmacologic treatment first
– Avoid any unnecessary irritation of the patient
– Check if there is any connection with newly prescribed medication
– Discontinue anticholinergic medication if possible
– In case of prescribed benzodiazepines:
  Discontinue if taken for less than 1 week
  Taper dose slowly if taken for more than 1 week
– Check pharmacokinetic aspects (renal function)
– If necessary (agitation, hallucination) control symptoms with antipsychotics
– Avoid polypharmacy

Besides the acute onset of cognitive dysfunction or delirium, drugs also may influence cognitive function in the long term. A significant association of cognitive decline and long-term benzodiazepine treatment was found by Stewart (2005). In particular, a decline in visuospatial cognition has been discussed. These changes may not be fully reversible after discontinuation of benzodiazepines. In general, benzodiazepines are unfavorable drugs in long-term treatment as

Fig. 2 Significant triggers of delirium in the elderly

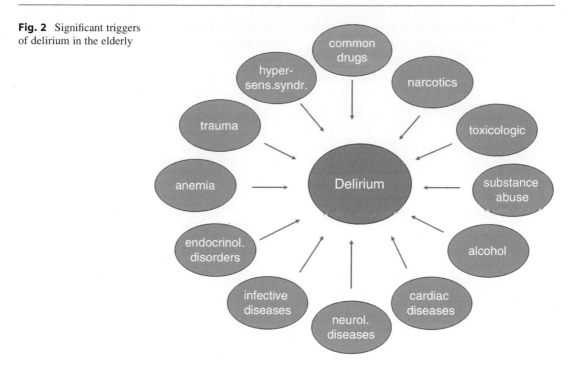

Table 1 Delirium risk associated with defined drugs

Drug class	Drug	Risk evaluation
Anticholinergics	Atropine, scopolamine	High risk especially in dementia
Antidepressants		Significant risk, especially amitriptyline
Antipsychotics		Significant risk with phenothiazines, low risk with atypical antipsychotics (e.g., olanzapine)
Lithium		High risk, in elderly even in case of normal plasma level
Benzodiazepines		Medium risk, no different risk according to different benzodiazepines
Antiparkinson drugs	Levodopa, dopamine agonists, MAO-B inhibitors	Medium risk for all of them, sometimes already occurring at low dose
Anticonvulsants	Phenobarbital, phenytoin, valproic acid	Low risk
Antihistaminics		High risk, especially cimetidine
Antiarrhythmics	Chinidine, lidocaine, disopyramide	High risk with disopyramide, low risk for the remaining
Calcium antagonists	Verapamil, nifedipine	Low risk
β-Blocker	Propanolol	Low risk
Diuretics	Thiazide diuretics	Low risk
Digoxin		Medium risk, in elderly already at normal serum levels
Antibiotics	β-Lactam antibiotics, chinolones	Medium risk, conflicting data due to methodology
Corticosteroids		Risk with high doses
Analgesics	Opioids and NSAIDs	High risk with opioids, medium risk with NSAIDs, aspirin at high doses, low risk with acetaminophen
Theophylline		Medium risk, pronounced dose-dependent effect

MAO monoamine oxidase, *NSAID* nonsteroidal anti-inflammatory drug

drug dependency, increased fall risk, and unintended sedation are significant disadvantages (Madhusoodanan and Bogunovic 2004). Benzodiazepines are clearly inappropriate in long-term treatment, and prescription should be limited to a maximum of 2 weeks.

Avoid benzodiazepines in long-term treatment.

Pharmacotherapeutic Strategies to Control Symptoms in Delirium

The primary aim of pharmacotherapy in the context of delirium is to control hyperactive symptoms like agitation, hallucination, and overactivity of the vegetative nervous system. Besides this, additional measures also involving pharmacotherapy have to be mentioned, such as the prophylaxis of thromboembolism.

The most commonly used first-line drugs to control for hyperactive CNS symptoms are antipsychotics. Haloperidol and melperone (not approved by the Food and Drug Administration [FDA]) are recommended. However, in the presence of Parkinson's disease or intercurrent motor dysfunctions resembling the Parkinson syndrome, these have to be avoided or discontinued, and so-called atypical antipsychotics like clozapine or risperidone are to be prescribed instead. Alternatively, clomethiazole (not FDA approved) may be prescribed. If delirium is caused by withdrawal of alcohol or benzodiazepines, an additional prescription of low-dose benzodiazepines is recommended. Table 2 provides an overview and outlines pharmacodynamic aspects of different drugs. Although not fully understood, antipsychotic effects in delirium are thought to be precipitated by a D2 antagonism in the dopaminergic system, whereas sedation is due to antagonism at the H1 receptor site of the histaminic system, and anxiolytic effects are provided by antagonism at the 5-HT2A receptor of the GABAergic system. Besides motor function disorders resembling parkinsonism, there are several more ADRs associated with typical antipsychotics like haloperidol. In long-term treatment, the risk to develop tardive dyskinesia increases in elderly patients, a motor function disturbance not fully reversible and difficult to control (Caligiuri et al. 1997).

The more recently developed and established atypical antipsychotics are associated with a lower rate of both acute extrapyramidal motor symptoms and tardive dyskinesia in long-term treatment. However, there is an ongoing debate whether this advantage may be offset by a different pattern of significant ADRs. Furthermore, it still is not clear whether a different risk-benefit ratio exists especially in patients with dementia and the frail elderly. Surprisingly, the efficacy of antipsychotics—regardless whether conventional or atypical—to control for agitation or aggressive behavior is not well addressed in controlled studies; as elsewhere in geriatric pharmacotherapy, it thus remains challenging to balance benefit versus risk. It is noteworthy that in several studies addressing pharmacotherapeutic control of agitation and aggressive behavior in dementia, a remarkable placebo effect was found (up to 30 %) (Schneider et al. 2006).

Postural hypotension and falls are additional ADRs with increasing clinical significance in the elderly. They are more frequently described for atypical antipsychotics (e.g., clozapine), and careful dosing, especially of atypical antipsychotics, is therefore mandated (Kindermann et al. 2002). Finally, there are data pointing to an increased risk of cerebrovascular mortality, cardiovascular mortality, and overall mortality associated with all antipsychotics, and a further increase of this added risk with advancing age is discussed. These incidences were initially reported for atypical antipsychotics, but subsequent studies failed to show a significant difference between conventional and atypical antipsychotics concerning these issues (Gill et al. 2005; Ray et al. 2009). Unfortunately, there is still a paucity of data calculating cardio- and cerebrovascular risk associated with short- and long-term antipsychotic treatment, and it remains unclear whether these ADRs represent a true class effect or are limited to defined drugs (Burke and Tariot 2009).

If delirium occurs in dementia patients and total anticholinergic burden or ADRs have already been ruled out as plausible cause, drug treatment with inhibitors of acetylcholinesterase has been discussed as a treatment option (Wengel et al. 1999). However, there is only sparse data concerning this approach, and a recent Cochrane review failed to show any significant benefit

Table 2 Drugs used in delirium treatment

Drug	ADR pattern	Comment
Haloperidol (strong D2 antagonist)	Extrapyramidal motor symptoms about 10 %, risk of tardive dyskinesia in long-term treatment up to 40 %, orthostatic hypotension about 1 %	Not recommended for long-term treatment in elderly, only to control acute agitation in delirium
Clozapine (stronger anticholinergic, antihistaminergic H1 and antiserotonergic 5-HT2 action)	Severe idiosyncratic ADR (aplastic anemia <1 %), orthostatic hypotension 1–10 %, mild leukopenia 1–10 % extrapyramidal motor symptoms <10 %	Significant indication in Parkinson's disease, frequent orthostatic hypotension, risk of severe hematologic ADR requires special monitoring
Tiapridex (weaker action at D2 receptor site, weaker sedative effect)	Extrapyramidal-motor symptoms <10 %, tardive dyskinesia rare, orthostatic hypotension rare	More favorable ADR pattern compared to haloperidol
Olanzapine (stronger anticholinergic and antihistaminergic H1 effect)	Extrapyramidal motor symptoms 10 % and over	Careful dosing as elimination rate may be decreased in the elderly
Risperidone (stronger antiserotonergic 5-HT2 effect)		Orthostatic hypotension may be significant
Melperon (not approved by FDA) (weaker effect at D2 receptor site, strong antiserotonergic action 5-HT2)		Frequently used in the elderly to control agitation, stronger sedative effect, frequently longer delay of treatment response
Clomethiazole (GABA modulator)	Bronchial hypersecretion	Second-line drug, contraindicated in case of sleep apnea and severe respiratory disorders

ADR adverse drug reaction, *FDA* Food and Drug Administration

(Overshott et al. 2008). At present, acetylcholinesterase inhibitors are therefore not recommended for delirium treatment, and further studies of this topic are needed. In delirium, inhibitors of acetylcholinesterase may be prescribed in dementia patients only based on an individual clinical assessment.

References

American Psychiatric Association (1994) Diagnostic and statistical manual of mental disorders, 4th edn. American Psychiatric Association, Washington, DC

Burke AD, Tariot PN (2009) Atypical antipsychotics in the elderly: a review of therapeutic trends and clinical outcomes. Expert Opin Pharmacother 10:2407–2414

Caligiuri MP, Lacro JP, Rockwell E, McAdams LA, Jeste DV (1997) Incidence and risk factors for severe tardive dyskinesia in older patients. Br J Psychiatry 171:148–153

Cole MG (2004) Delirium in elderly patients. Am J Geriatr Psychiatry 12:7–21

Gill SS, Rochon PA, Herrmann N et al (2005) Atypical antipsychotic drugs and risk of ischaemic stroke: population based retrospective cohort study. BMJ 330 (7489):445

Han L, McCusker J, Cole M, Abrahamowicz M, Primeau F, Elie M (2001) Use of medications with anticholinergic effect predicts clinical severity of delirium symptoms in older medical inpatients. Arch Intern Med 161:1099–1105

Inouye SK, van Dyck CH, Alessi CA, Balkin S, Siegal AP, Horwitz RI (1990) Clarifying confusion: the confusion assessment method. A new method for detection of delirium. Ann Intern Med 113:941–948

Kindermann SS, Dolder CR, Bailey A, Katz IR, Jeste DV (2002) Pharmacological treatment of psychosis and agitation in elderly patients with dementia: four decades of experience. Drugs Aging 19:257–276

Lewis LM, Miller DK, Morley JE, Nork MJ, Lasater LC (1995) Unrecognized delirium in geriatric patients. Am J Emerg Med 13:142–145

Madhusoodanan S, Bogunovic OJ (2004) Safety of benzodiazepines in the geriatric population. Expert Opin Drug Saf 3:485–493

McCusker J, Cole M, Bellavance F, Primeau F (1998) Reliability and validity of a new measure of severity of delirium. Int Psychogeriatr 10:421–433

Overshott R, Karim S, Burns A (2008) Cholinesterase inhibitors for delirium. Cochrane Database Syst Rev (1):CD005317

Ray WA, Chung CP, Murray KT, Hall K, Stein CM (2009) Atypical antipsychotic drugs and the risk of sudden cardiac death. N Engl J Med 360:225–235

Rummans TA, Evans JM, Krahn LE, Fleming KC (1995) Delirium in elderly patients: evaluation and management. Mayo Clin Proc 70:989–998

Schneider LS, Dagerman K, Insel PS (2006) Efficacy and adverse effects of atypical antipsychotics for dementia: meta-analysis of randomized, placebo-controlled trials. Am J Geriat Psychiatry 14:191–210

Stewart SA (2005) The effects of benzodiazepines on cognition. J Clin Psychiatry 66(Suppl 2):9–13

Tune L, Carr S, Hoag E, Cooper T (1992) Anticholinergic effects of drugs commonly prescribed for the elderly: potential means for assessing risk of delirium. Am J Psychiatry 149:1393–1394

Wengel SP, Burke WJ, Roccaforte WH (1999) Donepezil for postoperative delirium associated with Alzheimer's disease. J Am Geriatr Soc 47:379–380

Pharmacotherapy and Incontinence

Heinrich Burkhardt and John Mark Ruscin

Introduction

It is estimated that up to 50 million people in the developed world are affected by urinary incontinence. Incontinence includes a variety of different bladder or anorectal dysfunctions. As control of excretion of urine and feces is dependent on very complex regulation of neurologic and pelvic structures, a large number of influencing factors may lead to loss or impaired control of bowel and bladder. Both fecal and urinary incontinence are classified into different categories that share common pathogenic aspects. As therapeutic strategies vary widely between different categories of incontinence, an exact diagnosis prior to therapeutic interventions is essential for successful treatment.

Epidemiology and Etiology of Incontinence

Although incontinence is not a problem limited to the elderly population, it is more common and significant in this population. Incontinence is a common cause of loss of independence and contributes significantly to functional impairment (Coll-Planas et al. 2008). It is important to note that incontinence is not a normal consequence of aging, but a symptom with many underlying causes. Epidemiologic studies reported a prevalence rate for urinary incontinence of up to 30 % for adults aged 65 and over, with a rate approaching 70 % for those living in long-term care facilities (Ouslander 1990). The prevalence of fecal incontinence is lower than that of urinary incontinence, but it still affects up to half of those living in nursing home settings (Wald 2007). In the nursing home population in particular, there is a lack of studies investigating methods to achieve or maintain continence (Roe et al. 2011). Fecal incontinence is also known to increase with advancing age (Nelson 2004). Incontinence tends to affect women disproportionately, but this varies depending on the type of incontinence and the age of the population.

Both urinary and fecal incontinence are commonly overlooked by health care providers and underreported by patients. Many patients mistakenly consider incontinence as a burden of old age and fail to seek professional assistance. As a consequence, the opportunity for early diagnosis and treatment is often missed. In a survey, only 5 % of women affected by urinary incontinence consulted a physician for diagnosis and treatment (Minaire and Jacquetin 1992). At the same time, most patients describe incontinence as a severe health burden that reduces quality of life (Hayder and Schnepp 2008).

H. Burkhardt (✉)
IVth Department of Medicine, Geriatrics, University Medical Centre Mannheim, Theodor-Kutzer-Ufer 1-3, Mannheim 68167, Germany
e-mail: heinrich.burkhardt@umm.de

J.M. Ruscin
Department of Internal Medicine, SIU School of Medicine, 701 N. 1st Street, Springfield, IL 62702, USA
e-mail: mruscin@siumed.edu

M. Wehling (ed.), *Drug Therapy for the Elderly*,
DOI 10.1007/978-3-7091-0912-0_22, © Springer-Verlag Wien 2013

Table 1 Factors alleviating urinary incontinence in the elderly

Urological and gynecological factors	Urinary tract infection
	Bladder stone
	Bladder tumor
	Detrusor instability
	Prostate hypertrophy
	Urinary fistula
	Pelvic floor weakness
	Urogenital atrophy
	Postgynecological surgery
	Detrusor adynamia
Diseases	Severe acute diseases (functional incontinence)
	Delirium
	Impaired mobility
	Immobilization
	Drugs
	Chronic constipation
	Dementia
	Depression
	Alcohol
	Diabetes
	Obesity
Neurologic disorders	Paresis
	Brain injuries
	Brain tumor
	Stroke and poststroke residual
	Parkinson's disease
	Hydrocephalus
	Multiple sclerosis
	Polyneuropathy
	Spinal injury and tumor
Environmental factors	Inadequate toilet height
	Large distance to toilet
	Inappropriate lighting
	Missing labeling (e.g., hospital)
	Inappropriate clothing

Source: Adapted from Fonda 1995

Both urinary and fecal incontinence are often overlooked and underemphasized in elderly patients.

In the aging patient, incontinence is most often a multifactorial problem resulting from urologic, neurologic, psychiatric, and pharmacologic etiologies (Table 1). Among the more common chronic neurologic diseases associated with incontinence (fecal and urinary) are dementia and residual impairments subsequent to stroke. Other neurologic issues that can contribute to both types of incontinence symptoms include multiple sclerosis, Parkinson's disease, diabetes-related nerve damage, brain tumors, and spinal cord injuries. Also, age-associated decline in muscle mass and mobility (frailty syndrome) may unmask problems with continence control (Huang et al. 2007). Newly diagnosed incontinence in an elderly patient may also point to an accelerated frailty syndrome (Miles et al. 2001).

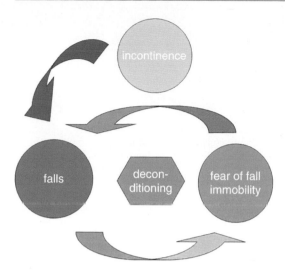

Fig. 1 Interaction between incontinence, falls, and immobility

Chronic disease is frequently associated with incontinence.

Various pharmacologic agents can produce or unmask incontinence symptoms, and patients with new-onset symptoms should have their medications reviewed to determine if drug therapy may be contributing to symptoms. Urinary tract infections and fecal impaction can also be related to urinary symptoms and should be investigated in patients with new onset symptoms. Finally, incontinence can lead to additional problems, resulting in a negative cascade of events (Fig. 1), such as embarrassment and isolation, depression, deconditioning, polypharmacy, falls, fear of falling, and further functional impairment (Brown et al. 2000). Another important issue among older adults with incontinence is reduction in fluid intake. Many patients suffering from incontinence try to compensate by restricting fluids rather than seeking professional help. This practice can lead to additional problems, such as dehydration, electrolyte imbalance, delirium, and falls.

The Significance of Drug Therapy with Regard to Incontinence Treatment

Table 2 provides an overview of the different categories of incontinence and therapeutic approaches and highlights pharmacotherapeutic strategies. The therapeutic approach depends greatly on the type of incontinence and may include pharmacologic, behavioral, or surgical interventions. In many cases, a multimodal approach is encouraged to achieve an optimized treatment result. It is important to understand that pharmacologic treatment approaches alone may be of limited value in resolving symptoms, particularly in patients with dementia or limited mobility (Ouslander 1990). The success of pharmacologic therapy can be enhanced greatly when combined with behavioral interventions (Burgio et al. 2000).

Drug Therapy in Overactive Bladder Syndrome

Overactive bladder (OAB) is the most common type of urinary symptom in adults. OAB is characterized by urinary urgency, frequency (eight or more micturitions in a 24-h period), and nocturia, with or without urinary incontinence. OAB that includes incontinence symptoms is often referred to as OAB wet, whereas OAB that does not include incontinence symptoms is referred to as OAB dry. Nocturia can be associated with sleep disruption and significant negative impact on quality of life (DuBeau et al. 1999).

To improve symptoms related to OAB and detrusor hyperactivity, antimuscarinic drugs are most commonly used. Calcium antagonists and potassium channel acting agents are less effective (Diokno et al. 2004). Older anticholinergic agents, such as atropine or propantheline bromide, are no longer recommended because of their higher potential for adverse drug effects. The risk-benefit ratio of using antimuscarinic agents in the elderly remains controversial, primarily due to the frequency of anticholinergic side effects (confusion, dry mouth, dizziness, and sedation).

Among the available drugs, tertiary amines (oxybutynin, tolterodine, fesoterodine, solifenacin, darifenacin) and quaternary amines (trospium chloride) are most frequently used (Ouslander 2004). Oxybutynin also possesses muscle-relaxing/local anesthetic properties. In general, treatment with antimuscarinic therapies

Table 2 Pharmacotherapy of incontinence

Category	Pathophysiology	Therapy	Drug therapy	Comment
Fecal incontinence				
	Anatomical or irritation (after trauma or surgery, inflammation, tumor, rectal prolapse)	Treat underlying problem (e.g., surgery, anti-inflammatory treatment)	No primary option	
	Chronic diarrhea	Treat underlying cause, otherwise symptomatic treatment	Stool-regulating drugs (psyllium, kaopectin, gum agar); loperamide, alosetron	Amitriptyline or other antimuscarinic medications not recommended in the elderly
	Chronic constipation	Treat underlying cause, otherwise symptomatic treatment	Stool-regulating drugs, psyllium, laxatives	Saline laxatives are not recommended in the elderly
	Primarily impaired sphincter function	Biofeedback	No primary option	
Urinary incontinence				
Urge incontinence	Overactive bladder (OAB) syndrome	Treat local causes (infection), primarily drug therapy, continence training	Antimuscarinc agents (tertiary and quaternary amines)	Anticholinergic adverse effects can limit utility for some patients (dry mouth, constipation, confusion, blurred vision)
Stress incontinence	Dysfunction of pelvic floor and urethral sphincter	Physiotherapy, surgery, (drug therapy)	Local application of estrogen with atrophic vaginitis, α-adrenergics, duloxetine	Drug therapy only in mild forms
Overflow incontinence	Outflow obstruction (BPH), detrusor adynamia (spinal dysfunction)	Surgery (obstruction), catheter insertion (detrusor adynamia)	Alpha-1 antagonists, 5-alpha reductase inhibitors, combination of the two	Onset of activity much more rapid with alpha-1 antagonists than with 5-alpha reductase inhibitors
Functional incontinence	May occur in patients with severe diseases or dementia	Voiding training, assisted voiding, environmental interventions	Not indicated	May consider discontinuing or decreasing if medications may be contributing to incontinence (iatrogenic)

BPH benign prostatic hypertrophy

has been shown to decrease frequency by approximately 20 % and incontinence episodes by approximately 50 %. No specific agent has been shown to be superior to another in terms of efficacy, although tolerability can differ among the agents. There have been numerous studies to test the effectiveness of antimuscarinic drugs in OAB; however, few studies have included significant numbers of elderly patients, particularly more frail older adults. An extensive recent review identified only 8 of 33 studies with ade-quate quality and a sufficient number of elderly to enter a meta-analysis (Paquette et al. 2011). These eight studies analyzed oxybutynin, solife-nacin, darifenacin, tolterodine, and trospium. A small study evaluating the effect of oxybutynin on urge incontinence in women aged 70 and over with frailty syndrome disclosed a significant improvement of incontinence. However, in up to 90 % of patients treated, there were also significant signs of anticholinergic side effects (dry mouth), and 50 % of patients experienced constipation (Szonyi et al. 1995). More recently, there has been a great deal of attention focusing on central nervous system (CNS) adverse effects such as confusion, cognitive decline, and dizziness. In the meta-analysis from Paquette et al. (2011), rather low prevalence rates were found (about 5 %). Unfortunately, few studies provided detailed information regarding CNS effects. This is due primarily to inadequate reporting and monitoring for these problems (Paquette et al. 2011). Tolterodine and oxybutynin have been associated with cognitive decline (Donnellan et al. 1997; Katz et al. 1998; Womack and Heilman 2003). However, it is important to note that all tertiary amines, to varying degrees, have the ability to cross the blood-brain barrier. The concurrent treatments for dementia and OAB create a therapeutic dilemma as many of the dementia treatments involve use of cholinesterase inhibitors, while OAB treatments are anticholinergic.

There are five know subtypes of muscarinic receptors, M1 through M5 (Morrison et al. 2002). The M1 subtype predominates in the CNS, and the M3 receptor appears to be more clinically relevant in the bladder. Most of the muscarinic medications are nonselective muscarinic antagonists. Darifenacin and solfenacin are considered to be M3-selective agents, which suggests increased selectivity for bladder tissue and lower CNS adverse effects (Simpson and Wagstaff 2005). There are studies to suggest that darifenacin is not associated with cognitive side effects (Lipton et al. 2005; Kay 2004). This has similarly been suggested for solifenacin, however, mainly in younger adults. In one study, only 6.7 % of included subjects were older than 75 years (Chapple et al. 2005). Similarly, these studies have only included cognitively normal adults. The effects of these medications on cognition in patients with cognitive impairment at baseline are not known.

Trospium chloride is a quaternary amine (polar). Therefore, from a theoretical point of view, it has a reduced ability to cross the blood-brain barrier. This has been demonstrated in an experimental setting, where no effect on cognitive function and no detectability in the CNS were found (Staskin et al. 2010). However, to date there are not enough data to show this advantage in clinical practice by a lowered adverse drug reaction (ADR) frequency (Staskin 2005; Paquette et al. 2011). Table 3 summarizes important aspects for these drugs.

Drug Therapy in Stress Incontinence

In stress incontinence, drug therapy may help in a multimodal approach, but usually is not the most significant part of treatment. Stress incontinence mainly affects middle-aged and elderly women and is rare in males. The primary causes are changes in anatomy and structure of the pelvic floor. In males, stress incontinence may occur after trauma or surgery. Stress incontinence is usually reported by patients as loss of urine with coughing, sneezing, laughing, bending over to pick up objects, or anything that increases intra-abdominal pressure (Rogers 2008).

The first-line treatment for stress incontinence should include pelvic floor exercises (Kegel exercises), which have been shown to improve symptoms (Bo 2003). For obese individuals, weight loss may improve symptoms of incontinence. The use of pessaries, intravaginal devices that provide urethral support, can also be helpful for stress incontinence, but must be fit professionally to optimize comfort and symptom relief.

Local application of estrogen has been recommended to influence atrophy of vaginal and urethral epithelium (Cardozo et al. 2004). Systemic drug therapy with α-adrenergic agents (midodrine, pseudoephedrine, clonidine) may also be considered in stress incontinence as an adjunct to pelvic floor exercises. However, the use of these agents is not supported by rigorous clinical studies. In addition, with α-adrenergic agents, there is a risk of blood pressure increases and cardiac arrhythmias. Therefore, in older patients, these agents should only be considered when benefit exceeds the risk and close cardiac monitoring can be performed. Antidepressants have been considered as agents effective to control stress incontinence by influencing presynaptic neurons in the sacral plexus (Jost et al. 2004). Duloxetine has been studied for the treatment of stress

Table 3 Pharmacotherapy in overactive bladder syndrome

Drug	Mechanism of action	ADR	Comment	FORTA
Oxybutinin	Antimuscarinic action; antispasmodic properties	Anticholinergic: dry mouth, dizziness, constipation, delirium/confusion	Anticholinergic side effects much more common with immediate-release oral dosage forms; controlled-release dosage forms and transdermal dosage forms tolerated better	C
Tolterodine	Antimuscarinic action	Anticholinergic: dry mouth, dizziness, constipation, delirium/confusion	Metabolized in the liver via cytochrome P450 2D6 to an active (5-OH methyl tolterodine) metabolite; genetically poor metabolizers of 2D6 may not respond as well	C
Fesoterodine	Antimuscarinic action	Anticholinergic: dry mouth, dizziness, constipation, delirium/confusion	Also metabolized to 5-OH metabolite but via nonspecific esterases, rather than 2D6	C
Trospium chloride	Antimuscarinic action	Anticholinergic: dry mouth, constipation; possibly less dizziness, delirium/confusion	Quaternary ammonium compound; from kinetics, may be less likely to cause central adverse effects	B
Solifenacin	Antimuscarinic action; highly uroselective (M3)	Anticholinergic: dry mouth, constipation; possibly less dizziness, delirium/confusion	From pharmacodynamic selectivity, expect less central adverse effects	C
Darifenacin	Antimuscarinic action; highly uroselective (M3)	Anticholinergic: dry mouth, constipation; possibly less dizziness, delirium/confusion	From pharmacodynamic selectivity, expect less central adverse effects	C

ADR adverse drug reaction, *FORTA* Fit for the Aged

incontinence and has been shown to reduce incontinence frequency and severity and to improve quality of life. (Millard et al. 2004; Mariappan et al. 2007; Norton et al. 2002). However, duloxetine is not approved to treat incontinence in all countries. To date, there are limited studies focusing on the elderly, and antidepressants can be troublesome in the elderly due to their ADR potential (nausea, blood pressure increase, falls, and central adverse effects).

Drug Therapy in Incontinence Caused by Urinary Retention (Overflow Incontinence)

Incontinence may occur together with urinary retention. Two forms have to be distinguished. First, obstruction of the lower urinary tract in men, commonly as a result of prostate hypertrophy, may cause incontinence. In older men, benign prostatic hyperplasia (BPH) is the main cause of lower urinary tract symptoms. In women overflow incontinence is rare and sometimes occurs in meatus stenosis. Second, bladder adynamia (e.g., after spinal cord injury, nerve damage from long-standing diabetes) may also cause incontinence. If obstruction is significant, surgical intervention may be required. With bladder adynamia, long-term placement of an indwelling catheter may be necessary. Overflow incontinence can also be caused by fecal impaction, so it is important to investigate bowel habits or perform a rectal exam in older patients (Wald 2007).

In milder forms of obstruction due to prostatic enlargement, or when surgical intervention is not possible or is unacceptable to the patient, drug therapy may be helpful. Two classes of drugs are commonly used in men with prostatic obstructive symptoms, alpha-1 antagonists and 5-alpha reductase inhibitors (Lepor et al. 1996; Kirby et al. 2003). The alpha-1 antagonists (see Table 3) have a much more rapid onset, usually within a few days to a week, and are often used initially in patients who have bothersome symptoms. The alpha-1 antagonists are all similarly effective in improving symptoms but differ in their selectivity for the bladder/prostate and side-effect profiles. The nonselective agents prazosin, terazosin, and doxazosin can lower blood pressure and are associated with dizziness and orthostasis and therefore should be titrated to patient response. The selective agents, such as tamsulosin and alfuzosin, do not commonly cause dizziness and orthostasis. The 5-alpha reductase inhibitors finasteride and dutasteride can reduce the size of the prostate gland but have a much slower onset of 3–6 months. Finasteride and dutasteride appear to be most effective in men who have significantly enlarged prostates (Gormley et al. 1992; Roehrborn et al. 2002). The alpha-1 antagonists and 5-alpha reductase inhibitors can be used in combination, and combination therapy has been shown to reduce long-term complications (urinary retention, incontinence) associated with BPH (McConnell et al. 2003).

The use of parasympathomimetics (bethanechol) in bladder adynamia is discouraged because ADR risk is unfavorably high. Alpha-1 blocking agents may be prescribed in bladder adynamia to lower outlet resistance and thereby alleviate micturition. As mentioned, these agents are associated with tachycardia and orthostatic dysregulation and an increased risk of falls. In spastic paresis, bladder dysfunction and incontinence may be treated with spasmolytic agents (e.g., baclofen). However, adverse effects with spasmolytics are common, and effectiveness has not been well established.

Drug Therapy in Fecal Incontinence

Drug therapy may be targeted for constipation or diarrhea, depending on the cause of fecal incontinence. To help identify the underlying cause of fecal incontinence, perianal inspection, digital rectal examination, and examination of the perineum is necessary (Cheung and Wald 2004). The management of symptoms should be tailored to the underlying cause, which may include modification of stool consistency, behavioral interventions, and surgical procedures to correct underlying problems (Wald 2007). Treatment of constipation with stool softeners, high fiber or psyllium, or osmotic laxatives such as lactulose, sorbitol, or polyethylene glycol may be helpful.

In some instances, fecal impaction with paradoxical diarrhea can occur (Chassagne et al. 2000). The passed feces may be soft or fluid; however, the impaction is associated with hard, difficult-to-pass, feces. In this case, stool regulation may be achieved with use of lactulose or psyllium (Bliss et al. 2001). It is important to point out that use of psyllium requires adequate fluid intake. Therefore, for patients who are fluid restricted, use of psyllium may make constipation worse. Saline laxatives should be used with caution in the elderly, and for only short periods of time, as electrolyte imbalance and dehydration are frequent.

Avoid saline laxatives in the elderly.

If the cause of incontinence is chronic diarrhea without impaction, psyllium or fiber intake may also be beneficial. If an antidiarrheal agent is necessary, loperamide may be used (Scarlett 2004; Wald 2007). It is not associated with CNS adverse effects and has been shown to be more effective than diphenoxylate-atropine in patients with fecal incontinence (Palmer et al. 1980). Irritable bowel associated with diarrhea can be treated with tricyclic antidepressants, but the anticholinergic side effects likely limit utility in older adults. Although not specifically tested in patients with fecal incontinence, 5-hydroxytryptamine type 3 antagonists (alosetron) are used to treat diarrhea associated with irritable bowel disease (Cremonini et al. 2003). This agent is costly and has been associated with ischemic colitis, making it a consideration only after other antidiarrheals have failed.

Functional Incontinence

Functional incontinence is defined as incontinence in the context of severe acute or chronic disease. In this context, incontinence is not due to any underlying disorder with the urethra, bladder, or the bladder's ability to store urine, but rather is explained as loss of self-management capacity (e.g., dementia) or mobility problems (e.g., rheumatoid arthritis). With this type of incontinence, specific drug therapy is not indicated, and functional improvement in the course of the underlying disease may resolve the incontinence problem. In dementia, there are mixed incontinence syndromes triggered by both loss of self-management capacity and primary neural changes. An exact diagnosis may be challenging. If there is evidence for a nonfunctional component of incontinence, drug treatment may be considered. In a study evaluating urodynamic measures, 41 % of patients with dementia had normal bladder function (Yu et al. 1990). Pure functional incontinence should not be treated with drug therapy, but rather by measures optimizing patients' self-management capacity through orientation therapy, assisted toileting, or other behavioral interventions (Hägglund 2010).

Iatrogenic Incontinence

Many medications can trigger urinary incontinence symptoms (Resnick 1996). Drug-induced incontinence should be considered in any patient who has new-onset symptoms or for whom symptoms become acutely worse (Fig. 2). Medications that are commonly implicated in iatrogenic incontinence include diuretics; anticholinergics (detrusor muscle relaxation); alpha-1 agonists (obstruction, overflow in males); alpha-1 antagonists (stress in females); and dihydropyridine calcium antagonists (fluid retention, nocturia). Sedative hypnotics and other centrally acting medications can also produce

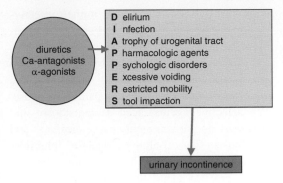

Fig. 2 Factors that may cause or alleviate incontinence and may also be influenced by therapeutic measures

functional-type incontinence as patients may not be able to pay as close attention or respond appropriately to normal bladder cues. Diuretics can be particularly problematic for older adults.

Ideally, diuretics should not be prescribed in the afternoon or evening to prevent nocturia and nighttime falls, particularly in frail patients or those who have impairment of locomotion.

If diuretics must be prescribed, agents with a longer duration of action are preferred. If potent, short-acting diuretics or high doses are unavoidable (e.g., in the case of heart failure), monitoring and safety measures should taken to prevent falls and delirium.

Fecal incontinence may also be triggered by a variety of drugs, and different pathways may lead to incontinence (Table 4). For example, antibiotic treatments may influence gut flora, and motility treatment may cause diarrhea and subsequently

Table 4 Drugs frequently affecting intestinal mobility (not exhaustive)

Constipation	Diarrhea
Opioids	Antibiotics
Anticholinergics	Digoxin
Nifedipine	NSAIDs
Diltiazem	Colchicine
Diuretics	Antidiabetics (metformin)
Phenytoin	Magnesium-containing products
Selegiline	Levothyroxine
Simvastatin	Levodopa
Verapamil	Cholinesterase inhibitors
Calcium- or aluminum-containing products	Metoclopramide

NSAID nonsteroidal anti-inflammatory drug

fecal incontinence. On the other hand, opioids and anticholinergic medications may cause constipation and fecal impaction (Ratnaike and Jones 1998).

References

Bliss DZ, Jung HJ, Savik K et al (2001) Supplementation with dietary fiber improves fecal incontinence. Nurs Res 50:203–213

Bo K (2003) Pelvic floor muscle strength and response to pelvic floor muscle training for stress urinary incontinence. Neurourol Urodyn 22:654–658

Brown JS, Vittinghoff E, Wyman JF et al (2000) Urinary incontinence: does it increase risk for falls and fractures? Study of Osteoporotic Fractures Research Group. J Am Geriatr Soc 48:721–725

Burgio KL, Locher JL, Goode PS (2000) Combined behavioral and drug therapy for urge incontinence on older women. J Am Geriatr Soc 48:370–374

Cardozo L, Lose G, McClish D, Versi E (2004) A systematic review of the effects of estrogens for symptoms suggestive of overactive bladder. Acta Obstet Gynecol Scand 83:892–897

Chapple CR, Martinez-Garcia R, Selvaggi L et al (2005) A comparison of the efficacy and tolerability of solifenacin succinate and extended release tolterodine at treating overactive bladder syndrome: results of the STAR trial. Eur Urol 48:464–470

Chassagne P, Jego A, Gloc P et al (2000) Does treatment of constipation improve faecal incontinence in institutionalized elderly patients? Age Ageing 29:159–164

Cheung O, Wald A (2004) The management of pelvic floor disorders. Aliment Pharmacol Ther 19:481–495

Coll-Planas L, Denkinger MD, Nikolaus T (2008) Relationship of urinary incontinence and late-life disability: implications for clinical work and research in geriatrics. Z Gerontol Geriatr 41:283–290

Cremonini F, Delgado-Aros S, Camilleri M (2003) Efficacy of alosetron in irritable bowel syndrome: a meta-analysis of randomized controlled trials. Neurogastroenterol Motil 15:79–86

Diokno AC (2004) Medical management of urinary incontinence. Gastroenterology 126(1 Suppl 1):S77–S81

Diokno AC, Estanol MV, Mallett V (2004) Epidemiology of lower urinary tract dysfunction. Clin Obstet Gynecol 47:36–43

Donnellan CA, Fook L, McDonald P, Playfer JR (1997) Oxybutynin and cognitive dysfunction. BMJ 315:1363–1364

DuBeau CE, Kiely DK, Resnick NM (1999) Quality of life impact of urge incontinence in older persons: a new measure and conceptual structure. J Am Geriatr Soc 47:989–994

Fonda D (1995) Management of the incontinent older patient. Internationale Continence Survey Medicom Europe, Bussom

Gormley GJ, Stoner E, Bruskewitz RC et al (1992) The effect of finasteride in men with benign prostatic hyperplasia. N Engl J Med 327:1185–1191

Hägglund D (2010) A systematic literature review of incontinence care for persons with dementia: the research evidence. J Clin Nurs 19:303–312

Hayder D, Schnepp W (2008) Urinary incontinence—the family caregivers' perspective. Z Gerontol Geriatr 41:261–266

Huang AJ, Brown JS, Thom DH, Fink HA, Yaffe K, Study of Osteoporotic Fractures Research Group (2007) Urinary incontinence in older community-dwelling women: the role of cognitive and physical function decline. Obstet Gynecol 109:909–916

Jost WH, Marsalek P, Manning M, Jünemann KP (2004) Pharmaceutical treatment of stress incontinence. New approaches via a direct effect of duloxetine on Onuf's nucleus. Urologe A 43:1249–1253, in German

Katz IR, Sands LP, Bilker W, DiFilippo S, Boyce A, D'Angelo K (1998) Identification of medications that cause cognitive impairment in older people: the case of oxybutynin chloride. J Am Geriatr Soc 46:8–13

Kay G (2004) The M3 selective receptor antagonist darifenacin has no clinically relevant effect on cognition and cardiac function. Prog Urol 14(suppl 3):22, A65

Kirby RS, Roehrborn C, Boyle P et al (2003) Efficacy and tolerability of doxazosin and finasteride, alone or in combination, in treatment of symptomatic benign prostatic hyperplasia: the Prospective European Doxazosin and Combination Therapy (PREDICT) trial. Urology 61:119–126

Lepor H, Williford WO, Barry MJ et al (1996) The efficacy of terazosin, finasteride, or both in benign prostatic hyperplasia. N Engl J Med 335:533–539

Lipton RB, Kolodner K, Wesnes K (2005) Assessment of cognitive function of the elderly population: effects of darifenacin. J Urol 173:493–498

Mariappan P, Alhasso A, Ballantye Z, Grant A, N'Dow J (2007) Duloxetine, a serotonin and noradrenaline reuptake inhibitor (SNRI) for the treatment of stress urinary incontinence: a systematic review. Eur Urol 51:67–74

McConnell JD, Roehrborn CG, Bautista OM et al (2003) The long-term effect of doxazosin, finasteride, and combination therapy on the clinical progression of benign prostatic hyperplasia. N Engl J Med 349:2387–2398

Miles TP, Palmer RF, Espino DV, Mouton CP, Lichtenstein MJ, Markides KS (2001) New-onset incontinence and markers of frailty: data from the Hispanic Established Populations for Epidemiologic Studies of the Elderly. J Gerontol A Biol Sci Med Sci 56: M19–M24

Millard RJ, Moore K, Rencken R, Yalcin I, Bump RC, Duloxetine UI Study Group (2004) Duloxetine vs placebo in the treatment of stress urinary incontinence: a four-continent randomized clinical trial. BJU Int 93:311–318

Minaire P, Jacquetin B (1992) The prevalence of female urinary incontinence in general practice. J Gynecol Obstet Biol Reprod (Paris) 21:731–738

Morrison J, Steers WD, Brading AF et al (2002) Neurophysiology and neuropharmacology. In: Abrams P, Cardoza L, Khoury S, Wein A (eds) Incontinence, 2nd edn. Health Publications, Plymouth, pp 86–163

Nelson RL (2004) Epidemiology of fecal incontinence. Gastroenterology 126(1 Suppl 1):S3–S7

Norton PA, Zinner NR, Yalcin I, Bump RC (2002) Duloxetine versus placebo in the treatment of stress urinary incontinence. Am J Obstet Gynecol 187:40–48

Ouslander JG (1990) Urinary incontinence in nursing homes. J Am Geriatr Soc 38:289–291

Ouslander JG (2004) Management of overactive bladder. N Engl J Med 350:786–799

Palmer KR, Corbett CL, Holdsworth CD (1980) Double-blind cross-over study comparing loperamide, codeine, and diphenoxylate in the treatment of chronic diarrhea. Gastroenterology 79:1272–1275

Paquette A, Gou P, Tannenbaum C (2011) Systematic review and meta-analysis: do clinical trials testing antimuscarinic agents for overactive bladder adequately measure central nervous system adverse events? J Am Geriatr Soc 59:1332–1339

Ratnaike RN, Jones TE (1998) Mechanisms of drug-induced diarrhoea in the elderly. Drugs Aging 13:245–253

Resnick NM (1996) Geriatric incontinence. Urol Clin North Am 23:55–74

Roe B, Flanagan L, Jack B, Barrett J, Chung A, Shaw C, Williams K (2011) Systematic review of the management of incontinence and promotion of continence in older people in care homes: descriptive studies with urinary incontinence as primary focus. J Adv Nurs 67:228–250

Roehrborn CG, Boyle P, Nickel JC, Hoefher K, Andriole G (2002) Efficacy and safety of a dual inhibitor of 5-alpha-reductase types 1 and 2 (dutasteride) in men with benign prostatic hyperplasia. Urology 60:434–441

Rogers RG (2008) Urinary stress incontinence in women. N Engl J Med 358:1029–1036

Scarlett Y (2004) Medical management of fecal incontinence. Gastroenterology 126(1 Suppl 1):S55–S63

Simpson D, Wagstaff AJ (2005) Solifenacin in overactive bladder syndrome. Drugs Aging 22:1061–1069

Staskin DR (2005) Overactive bladder in the elderly: a guide to pharmacological management. Drugs Aging 22:1013–1028

Staskin D, Kay G, Tannenbaum C et al (2010) Trospium chloride has no effect on memory testing and is assay undetectable in the central nervous system of older patients with overactive bladder. Int J Clin Pract 64:1294–1300

Szonyi G, Collas DM, Ding YY, Malone-Lee JG (1995) Oxybutynin with bladder retraining for detrusor instability in elderly people: a randomized controlled trial. Age Ageing 24:287–291

Wald A (2007) Fecal incontinence in adults. N Engl J Med 356:1648–1655

Womack KB, Heilman KM (2003) Tolterodine and memory: dry but forgetful. Arch Neurol 60:771–773

Yu LC, Rohner TJ, Kaltreider DL, Hu TW, Igou JF, Dennis PJ (1990) Profile of urinary incontinent elderly in long-term care institutions. J Am Geriatr Soc 38:433–439

Immobility and Pharmacotherapy

Heinrich Burkhardt

Clinical Significance of Immobilization

Immobility is a frequent and significant geriatric syndrome. It is associated with an often severe loss of independence and self-management capacity. Furthermore, immobility leads to changes in physiology that are irreversible or at least difficult to revert. Long-standing or chronic immobility in this context should be distinguished from acute immobilization, with the latter showing a wide overlap with what is termed *deconditioning* in the geriatric field (Killewich 2006). The underlying pathophysiological mechanisms are not completely identical but show common features. The most significant of these are functional and structural changes in skeletal muscles, especially of leg extensors and trunk muscles, which are most important to maintain independent locomotion.

Deconditioning along with acute disease may lead to a significant loss of muscle mass within a few days. This clinical process may be detrimental for the recovery of patients, cause loss of functional independence, and finally result in prolonged morbidity and mortality (Creditor 1993). In elderly patients with preexistent reduction of muscle mass, bed rest and deconditioning

frequently represent a massive threat for adverse outcomes, even when acute disease is not primarily complicated by sepsis, delirium, or organ failure.

Due to deconditioning, elderly are at special risk for loss of independence after acute diseases.

For illustration, a few facts concerning muscle function resources in the elderly may be summarized here: 50 % of all women older than 70 years and 15 % of all elderly older than 70 years are not capable of climbing a 30-cm step due to loss of muscle strength. In an experimental setting, muscle loss during a 28-day period of bed rest was found at 0.5 kg, and even rose to 1.5 kg if the hypothalamic-pituitary-adrenal (HPA) axis was stimulated (Paddon-Jones et al. 2006).

The cascade of deconditioning is described in Fig. 1. Its most important triggers are

- Preexisting limitation in locomotion
- Activated HPA axis
- Malnutrition
- Neurologic and cognitive limitations.

The prevalence of some of these clinical features is clearly elevated in the elderly, qualifying this entire population to be at risk. However, as methodological difficulties exist and the exact criteria of deconditioning are still under debate, clear prevalence data are hard to obtain. In addition, data on changes in functionality in the context of defined acute diseases are still rare. With these shortcomings in mind, an estimate derived from Medicare data in the United States showed that 20 % of all elderly patients hospitalized with

H. Burkhardt (✉)
IVth Department of Medicine, Geriatrics, University Medical Centre Mannheim, Theodor-Kutzer-Ufer 1-3, Mannheim 68167, Germany
e-mail: heinrich.burkhardt@umm.de

M. Wehling (ed.), *Drug Therapy for the Elderly*,
DOI 10.1007/978-3-7091-0912-0_23, © Springer-Verlag Wien 2013

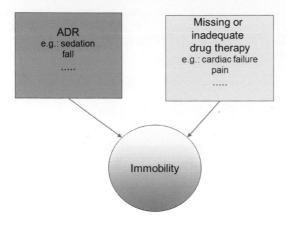

Fig. 1 The cascade of deconditioning

an acute disease experienced significant deconditioning (Kortebein 2009). In this clinical context, there are three independent risk factors for deconditioning:
– Age above 70 years
– Bed rest along with acute disease
– Surgery.

The most important clinical consequences thus are to avoid prolonged bed rest in the elderly whenever possible and to start rehabilitative measures as early as possible to recover a patient's functionality.

Bed rest affects not only muscle mass, although this is clearly the main contributor to functionality loss with bed rest. Several other changes influencing morbidity and mortality are summarized here as consequences of prolonged bed rest:
– Loss of muscle mass
– Osteoporosis
– Constipation
– Decreased effective plasma volume
– Apathy and depression
– Pressure ulcers.

Pressure ulcers, apathy, and depression may also be seen in hypoactive delirium, and care of patients at risk has to include prophylactic measures to avoid confusion and anxiety.

Patients at risk for deconditioning or already experiencing deconditioning require multimodal treatment emphasizing not only rehabilitative measures but also prophylactic aspects to avoid

further deterioration. A treatment schedule thus should cover at least:
– Preventive care (turning the patient at least every 2 h) to avoid pressure ulcers
– Physiotherapy to prevent further decline of muscle mass and function
– Nutritional care to avoid further catabolism, including supportive treatment with nutritional agents
– Personal care to avoid deprivation and depression.

If immobilization already occurred and rehabilitative treatment is no longer an option, any preventive measure to maintain remaining life quality has still to be employed, including all aspects mentioned. This particularly applies to bedridden patients with long-standing immobilization, who are prone to certain complications and hazards, such as pneumonia, urinary system infection, and venous thromboembolism, leading to increased morbidity and mortality. Care for the immobilized elderly is a challenge with many critical aspects that can only be sufficiently managed if qualified caregivers have enough time to address them.

Pharmacotherapy in the Context of Immobilization

As specified, care for immobilized patients always requires a multimodal approach. One facet is pharmacotherapy, which may contribute to success along with physiotherapy, nursing, and nutritional therapy. In particular, pharmacotherapy may prevent further complications or slow the deconditioning cascade. The following aspects may be addressed by pharmacotherapy:
– Prophylaxis of thromboembolism
– Prophylaxis of osteoporosis
– Prophylaxis and treatment of constipation
– Treatment of depression
– Treatment of confusional state.

Two of those aspects are detailed further in this chapter: prophylaxis of thromboembolism and osteoporosis. Antidepressant treatment mainly follows the recommendations given in chapter "Depression." Pharmacotherapy of delirium is outlined in chapter "special aspects of cognitive disorders" and treatment of constipation in chapter "Pharmacotherapy and Incontinence." Saline laxatives are discouraged in the elderly due to their risk of inducing electrolyte imbalances'; psyllium seed husks and lactulose are preferable.

Prophylaxis of Thromboembolism in the Immobilized Elderly Patient

The prophylaxis of thromboembolism by anticoagulants is undoubtedly effective in patients being immobilized to undergo surgery or treatment of acute disease (e.g., pneumonia). This intervention largely reduces disease-associated or perioperative morbidity and mortality. Advancing age is an independent risk factor for the occurrence of thromboembolism. Estimates from epidemiologic data show a doubling of thromboembolic risk with each decade above age 40 years (Anderson et al. 1991). In elderly aged 80+ years, Di Minno and Tufano (2004) found the 1-year incidence of clinically significant thromboembolic events to be 450–600 incidents per 100,000 persons. Furthermore, after such an incident overall mortality in the elderly is increased by 39 % compared to less than 10 % in adults younger than 40 years (Anderson et al. 1991).

The highest risk of thromboembolism is associated with orthopedic surgery, especially joint replacement and related surgery in the lower extremity.

Without any drug treatment to prevent thromboembolism, thromboembolism rate would exceed 80 %, as calculations from Geerts et al. (2001) showed. All immobilizing surgical procedures thus require pharmacotherapeutic thromboembolism prophylaxis. This beneficial effect of thromboembolism prophylaxis is not limited to bed rest along with surgery but is also found for immobilization due to acute internal (e.g., cardiac failure) and neurologic (e.g., stroke) diseases. Therefore, it is common practice to include this prophylaxis routinely in schedules of acute care treatment. In elderly patients hospitalized for nonsurgical

reasons, Oger et al. (2002) found deep vein thrombosis in screening diagnostics in 18 % of cases, although these were clinically unapparent in these patients. Although evidence in the nonsurgical field is less well established than for joint surgery, the clinical relevance and significance of this measure in nonsurgical acute diseases is without doubt.

However, evidence for the categorization of mobility limitations and initiation of thromboembolic prophylaxis is limited. This evidence cannot be extracted from available data as mobility has rarely been measured or categorized in clinical trials. Table 1 is based on an extensive analysis on thromboembolism in the United States (Kniffin et al. 1994) and provides summary comments on the risk in different clinical situations. Among nonsurgical/traumatologic risk factors, cardiac failure and cancer are carrying the highest risk. However, even in this analysis no quantitative measure of immobilization is given, such as a time score to assess the duration of immobilization. Second, these data are mainly descriptive, not allowing for an independent analysis of the identified risk factors. Despite this, prophylaxis of thromboembolism should be strictly encouraged from a clinical point of view in nonsurgical/traumatologic acute illness.

Although a wide consensus to encourage thromboembolism prophylaxis exists, the duration of prophylactic treatment is still under debate. A prolonged treatment after discharge from acute care—up to 6 weeks—showed a significant additional prophylactic effect in patients after hip surgery (Eriksson et al. 2003; Kolb et al. 2003; Comp et al. 2001). The situation concerning nonsurgical/traumatologic patients is less clear. In addition, it is unknown if patients may be identified who will benefit most from prolonged prophylactic treatment. Finally, it is also unclear if analysis of locomotion function after acute care will be useful in this context.

Conversely, chronically bedridden patients do not benefit from thromboembolic prophylaxis if acute illness is absent. Gatt et al. (2004) compared bedridden elderly with those with preserved locomotion functionality and found no difference in the incidence of thromboembolism in a 10-year follow-up interval. All patients

Table 1 Prevalence of risk factors for thromboembolism in the elderly

Risk factor	Prevalence in thromboembolism (%)	Comment
Cardiac failure	26	Prevalence is significantly higher compared to the elderly population in general (about 10 % in the United States), pointing to a significant risk
Hospitalization within last month	23	Identifies risk according to rehabilitation/reconvalescence
Surgery within last month	22	Prevalence despite pharmacotherapeutic thromboembolic prophylaxis
Cancer diagnosis within last 6 months	17	Elevated prevalence compared to elderly in general (see cardiac failure)
Living in a nursing home	8	No risk factor for thromboembolism
Stroke within last 6 months	8	In the acute phase cerebrovascular disease may be a risk factor due to immobilization; no ongoing risk (as opposed to cancer)
Myocardial infarction within last 6 months	8	In acute phase cardiovascular disease is a risk factor for thromboembolism, mechanism not well understood
Hip fracture within last 6 months	6	Like stroke, no ongoing risk factor, risk increased only in acute phase, functionality is most significant

included in this study lived in nursing homes. To date, data do not support a lifelong thromboembolism prophylaxis in bedridden patients. In summary, however, some uncertainty still exists regarding the choice of elderly patients to receive pharmacotherapeutic prophylaxis of thromboembolism and the duration of treatment. Risk models and decision algorithms integrating those aspects of morbidity, the extent of immobilization, and other patient- and situation-related factors are still missing (Lacut et al. 2008). Therefore, treatment decisions have to be based on individual evaluations of the clinical situation.

Pharmacotherapeutic prophylaxis of thromboembolism in immobilized elderly is not generally recommended if acute disease is absent.

In addition, the risk profile of prophylactic anticoagulant treatment has to be considered. Drugs of choice for thromboembolism prophylaxis during the course of an acute disease are low molecular weight heparins. Oral anticoagulants such as warfarin are not commonly used as they are associated with a higher risk of bleeding. However, in the elderly low molecular weight heparins also carry an increased risk of bleeding. This is due to

– General increase of bleeding risk with advancing age

– Reduced glomerular filtration rate and related drug accumulation (see chapter "Atrial Fibrillation").

An estimate of the actual glomerular filtration rate is mandatory to avoid these adverse drug reactions (ADRs). If glomerular filtration rate is found to be below 30 ml/min, a dose reduction to the equivalent of 30 mg enoxaparine/day is necessary (Haas and Spyropoulos 2008). A rare ADR of all heparins is thrombocytopenia; therefore, regular monitoring of platelet counts is indispensable. Newly developed anticoagulants (selective factor Xa inhibitors and thrombin antagonists) may expose a more favorable risk-benefit ratio and are also easier to handle (e.g., oral treatment). However, some of these drugs also may accumulate with reduced renal function.

Prophylaxis of Osteoporosis in the Immobilized Elderly Patient

Unlike the prophylaxis of thromboembolism, prophylaxis of osteoporosis should not be triggered by acute disease or surgery. Development of osteoporosis in immobilized patients is mainly caused by the reduction of mechanical stress on skeletal compartments, although the mechanisms are yet not fully understood. Osteoporosis is predominantly seen in spine and lower extremities, and loss of bone mass may reach up to 4 % per month after immobilization (Matkovic et al. 1990). However, a majority of studies done in this field included younger immobilized patients (e.g., after spine trauma and paralysis) or volunteers with prolonged voluntary bed rest, but not bedridden elderly (Berg et al. 2007). A well-designed study in twins nicely demonstrated the effect of chronic immobilization on bone mass of lower extremities and lumbar spine (Bauman et al. 1999). They compared monozygotic twins in whom one sibling had been chronically immobilized due to spinal trauma. A strong correlation between the duration of immobilization and loss of bone mass was found.

In immobilized patients, the oral supplementation of calcium (1 g/day) and vitamin D (1,000 IU/day) is recommended to lower loss of bone mass.

This recommendation has been validated in an extensive meta-analysis and is in concordance with the pharmacotherapeutic approach in osteoporosis—basic prevention strategy (Tang et al. 2007). However, this meta-analysis aimed mainly at osteoporosis prevention and included only a minor number of chronically immobilized patients. Therefore, the evidence for immobilized patients is still weak. As differential approaches in different forms of osteoporosis are not favored by existing evidence and thus a common basic prevention strategy may be recommended independent of primary cause of osteoporosis, the same recommendations may also be given for immobilized patients. Another argument supporting this nondifferentiated approach is the fact that the majority of elderly bedridden patients are underexposed to sunlight and therefore develop significant vitamin D deficiency, which requires common supplementation.

If osteoporosis is already present, it should be treated in the immobilized elderly according to general treatment recommendations for osteoporosis treatment (Baum and Peters 2008; Group Health Cooperative 2011). Bisphosphonates are the drugs of choice (see more detail in chapter "Osteoporosis").

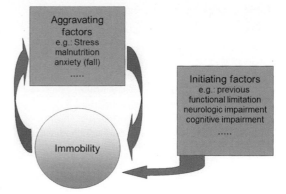

Fig. 2 Pharmacotherapy-related conditions aggravating immobility

It is a matter of debate whether in a patient without osteoporosis or increased osteoporosis risk a basic preventive strategy including calcium and vitamin D supplementation should start at the beginning of immobilization. From a clinical point of view, it might reasonable to start this therapy a soon as possible, but in clinical practice, this is rarely followed. Studies analyzing an early preventive therapy in immobilization are missing.

Drug Therapy to Improve Immobility

If immobility is not due to long-standing and permanent conditions (e.g., paralysis) but rather results from a short-term loss of muscle strength and mass, drug therapy may help to regain functionality, at least from a theoretical point of view. Nevertheless, this may not represent the first choice of therapy and—as in all rehabilitative situations—multifaceted programs may work best to regain mobility. Among these facets, the most significant ones are physical exercise (i.e., resistance training) and nutritional interventions (i.e., supplementation of protein). Both intervention areas have proven beneficial to revert deconditioning. To date, a significant benefit of drug therapy has not been established in this context. There is some debate if and to what extent testosterone supplementation may be useful. Preliminary studies on this topic are not encouraging, and the risk-benefit ratio seems to be unacceptable (for hormone replacement in sarcopenia and fall

Table 2 Drugs to improve orthostatic hypotension

Drug	ADR profile	Comment
Ibuprofen, diclofenac	Gastrointestinal bleeding, renal failure, elevated blood pressure	Utilizes fluid retention, in elderly discouraged, if applied use only in short-term course
Fludrocortisone	Edema, aggravated cardiac failure, hypertension, delirium	Drug of first choice in the elderly, cardiac failure has to be respected as a contraindication
Midodrine	Hypertension, delirium	Slow starting dose and close monitoring of blood pressure mandatory, in elderly not encouraged
Desmopressin	Aggravated cardiac failure, edema, chest pain, hyponatremia, water intoxication	Increased risk in the elderly for hyponatremia and heart failure due to increased water retention, close monitoring of fluid balance mandatory
Ergot-like drugs	Claudication, coronary ischemia, decreased cerebral perfusion	Generally discouraged in the elderly

ADR adverse drug reaction

risk mitigation, see chapters "Epidemiologic Aspects"and "Fall Risk and Pharmacotherapy").

Drugs as Risk Factors for Immobility

Drugs affecting muscle performance or central nervous system (CNS) function may decrease locomotion capabilities. In the elderly with reduced resources, these effects may precipitate falls or necessitate bed rest. Although not solitary culprits, those drugs represent at least unfavorable, but also modifiable, cofactors. Most significant drugs in this regard are CNS drugs, especially those with a marked sedative effect. The major drug groups are neuroleptics, benzodiazepines, and certain antidepressants. This list resembles the FRID (fall-risk-increasing drug; see chapter "Fall Risk and Pharmacotherapy") list. Oppositely, an insufficient or absent drug therapy also favors locomotion deficits (e.g., undertreated cardiac failure with increasing dyspnea, ineffective pain control). In the elderly with frailty syndrome and impaired locomotion abilities, a thorough analysis of the drug schedule considering these aspects should always be performed (Fig. 2).

Drugs Against Locomotion Deficits in Early Rehabilitation

If deconditioning has occurred, rehabilitative measures should be implemented as early as possible.

In this initial phase of rehabilitation, clinical problems may necessitate a pharmacotherapeutic approach. Antidepressant therapy to improve adynamy (see chapter "Depression") and treatment of orthostatic hypotension have to be mentioned here.

Orthostatic hypotension is frequently seen in the early phase of rehabilitation after bed rest and deconditioning. Hypotension results in an increased risk for falls and trauma that has even been seen in younger adults after 3 weeks of bed rest. The underlying mechanism is decreased vascular reactivity, which normally counteracts the postural blood shift into the lower extremities. In the elderly, those homeostatic mechanisms are often already primarily impaired due to age-related changes in physiology; in normal physiology, they are mainly characterized by peripheral vasoconstriction and increase in heart rate after sudden change from supine to upright position (Luutonen et al. 1995). It is not surprising that in frail elderly the prevalence of orthostatic hypotension rises to 50 % even without deconditioning in acute disease (Gupta and Lipsitz 2007). In this situation, antihypotensive drug therapy along with measures of physical therapy may be considered. Table 2 provides an overview of drugs that may be useful in this context. Furthermore, ongoing drug therapy that negatively influences postural stability has to be stopped if possible (e.g., tricyclic antidepressants, excessive antihypertensive treatment).

However, the evidence for these recommendations is weak as controlled studies are absent. In particular, there are no studies to compare drug efficacy. Therefore, the comments given in Table 2 mainly reflect the expected ADR profile. Nonsteroidal anti-inflammatory drugs (NSAIDs) are generally discouraged in the elderly, in particular for indications other than relief of acute pain. Desmopressin may be indicated in severe cases and carries the risk of aggravated heart failure. Ergot-like drugs are generally discouraged in the elderly. From a geriatric point of view, fludrocortisone may be the first choice here. Although this drug has not been studied in the early rehabilitation phase, at least some data exist for elderly with an increased fall risk. Despite short-term benefit, long-term treatment was frequently not tolerated due to increased blood pressure and aggravated cardiac failure (Hussain et al. 1996).

If drug therapy as an additional measure is chosen to improve orthostatic hypotension, prescription should be limited to the shortest period possible.

References

Anderson FA Jr, Wheeler HB, Goldberg RJ et al (1991) A population-based perspective of the hospital incidence and case fatality rates of deep vein thrombosis and pulmonary embolism. The Worcester DVT Study. Arch Intern Med 151:933–938

Baum E, Peters KM (2008) The diagnosis and treatment of primary osteoporosis according to current guidelines. Dtsch Arztebl Int 105:573–582

Bauman WA, Spungen AM, Wang J, Pierson RN Jr, Schwartz E (1999) Continuous loss of bone during chronic immobilization: a monozygotic twin study. Osteoporos Int 10:123–127

Berg HE, Eiken O, Miklavcic L, Mekjavic IB (2007) Hip, thigh and calf muscle atrophy and bone loss after 5-week bedrest inactivity. Eur J Appl Physiol 99:283–289

Comp PC, Spiro TE, Friedman RJ et al (2001) Prolonged enoxaparin therapy to prevent venous thromboembolism after primary hip or knee replacement. Enoxaparin Clinical Trial Group. J Bone Joint Surg Am 83-A:336–345

Creditor MC (1993) Hazards of hospitalization of the elderly. Ann Intern Med 118:219–223

Di Minno G, Tufano A (2004) Challenges in the prevention of venous thromboembolism in the elderly. J Thromb Haemost 2:1292–1298

Eriksson BI, Lassen MR, PENTasaccharide in HIp-FRActure Surgery Plus Investigators (2003) Duration of prophylaxis against venous thromboembolism with fondaparinux after hip fracture surgery: a multicenter, randomized, placebo-controlled, double-blind study. Arch Intern Med 163:1337–1342

Gatt ME, Paltiel O, Bursztyn M (2004) Is prolonged immobilization a risk factor for symptomatic venous thromboembolism in elderly bedridden patients? Results of a historical cohort study. Thromb Haemost 91:538–543

Geerts WH, Heit JA, Clagett GP et al (2001) Prevention of venous thromboembolism. Chest 119:132S–175S

Group Health Cooperative (2011) Osteoporosis prevention, screening, and treatment guideline copyright © 1998–2011. http://www.ghc.org/all-sites/guidelines/osteoporosis.pdf. Accessed 4 Sept 2011

Gupta V, Lipsitz LA (2007) Orthostatic hypotension in the elderly: diagnosis and treatment. Am J Med 120:841–847

Haas S, Spyropoulos AC (2008) Primary prevention of venous thromboembolism in long-term care: identifying and managing the risk. Clin Appl Thromb Hemost 14:149–158

Hussain RM, McIntosh SJ, Lawson J, Kenny RA (1996) Fludrocortisone in the treatment of hypotensive disorders in the elderly. Heart 76:507–509

Killewich LA (2006) Strategies to minimize postoperative deconditioning in elderly surgical patients. J Am Coll Surg 203:735–745

Kniffin WD Jr, Baron JA, Barrett J, Birkmeyer JD, Anderson FA Jr (1994) The epidemiology of diagnosed pulmonary embolism and deep venous thrombosis in the elderly. Arch Intern Med 154:861–866

Kolb G, Bodamer I, Galster H et al (2003) Reduction of venous thromboembolism following prolonged prophylaxis with the low molecular weight heparin Certoparin after endoprothetic joint replacement or osteosynthesis of the lower limb in elderly patients. Thromb Haemost 90:1100–1105

Kortebein P (2009) Rehabilitation for hospital-associated deconditioning. Am J Phys Med Rehabil 88:66–77

Lacut K, Le Gal G, Mottier D (2008) Primary prevention of venous thromboembolism in elderly medical patients. Clin Interv Aging 3:399–411

Luutonen S, Antila K, Erkko M, Raiha I, Rajala T, Sourander L (1995) Haemodynamic response to head-up tilt in elderly hypertensives and diabetics. Age Ageing 24:315–320

Matkovic V, Jackson RD, Mysiw WJ, Whitten R, Dekanic D (1990) Osteoporosis. In: Kottke FJ, Lehmann JF (eds) Handbook of physical medicine and rehabilitation. Saunders, Philadelphia, pp 1169–1208

Oger E, Bressollette L, Nonent M et al (2002) High prevalence of asymptomatic deep vein thrombosis on admission in a medical unit among elderly patients. Thromb Haemost 88:592–597

Paddon-Jones D, Sheffield-Moore M, Cree MG et al (2006) Atrophy and impaired muscle protein synthesis during prolonged inactivity and stress. J Clin Endocrinol Metab 91:4836–4841

Tang BM, Eslick GD, Nowson C, Smith C, Bensoussan A (2007) Use of calcium or calcium in combination with vitamin D supplementation to prevent fractures and bone loss in people aged 50 years and older: a meta-analysis. Lancet 370(9588):657–666

Pharmacotherapy and the Frailty Syndrome

Heinrich Burkhardt

Introduction

As outlined in chapter "Heterogeneity and Vulnerability of Older Patients," the frailty syndrome is a major feature to categorize elderly persons according to their vulnerability, prognosis, and risk-benefit ratio under the particular aspect of diagnostic and therapeutic interventions. Therefore, it also serves as one of the most important patient characteristics to guide differential pharmacotherapy in the elderly. The frailty syndrome describes a frequent phenotype at advanced age and refers to pathophysiologic cascades attributable to the aging process. Frailty identifies elderly persons with both reduced resources and altered body composition, factors most significant for changes in pharmacokinetics and pharmacodynamics.

Definition of the Frailty Syndrome and Underlying Mechanisms

A major characteristics of the apparent heterogeneity of the elderly is the wide range of physical fitness levels. Elderly with apparently impaired fitness and evident vulnerability are denominated as frail. In the field of geriatrics, the frailty

syndrome was defined to identify elderly at risk for advanced aging processes and increased mortality and morbidity. The frailty syndrome describes

- Increased vulnerability to different stressors
- Decreased functionality, especially regarding locomotion
- Impaired compensatory resources.

Although this phenotype is seemingly well known and described from a clinical point of view, a precise identification and classification is difficult due to missing or ill-defined arguments. In 2001 Fried et al. proposed five major aspects for the identification of the frail under clinical conditions:

- Unintentional weight loss
- Low grip strength
- Exhaustion
- Slow walking speed
- Reduced physical activity.

Frailty is a reduction of physiological capacities not restricted to a defined organ system, but rather includes multiple physiologic systems and is not based on a unique pathogenetic process (Woodhouse and O'Mahony 1997).

In this context, Rockwood et al. (1994) proposed a dynamic framework of frailty relying on the balance between health- and resource-maintaining factors on the one hand and disease- and disability-promoting factors on the other hand. A dysbalance within this framework forcing the system toward disability leads to an increased vulnerability of the patient for external stressors (Campbell and Buchner 1997). In this framework,

H. Burkhardt (✉)
IVth Department of Medicine, Geriatrics, University Medical Centre Mannheim, Theodor-Kutzer-Ufer 1-3, Mannheim 68167, Germany
e-mail: heinrich.burkhardt@umm.de

M. Wehling (ed.), *Drug Therapy for the Elderly*,
DOI 10.1007/978-3-7091-0912-0_24, © Springer-Verlag Wien 2013

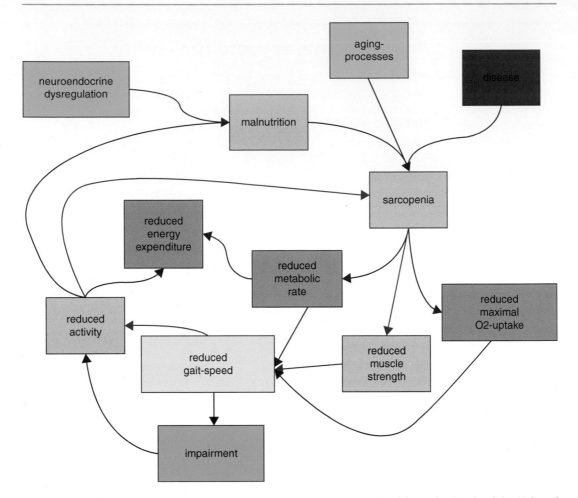

Fig. 1 The frailty cascade, including sarcopenia, reduced metabolic rate, malnutrition and reduced activity (Adapted from Fried et al. 2001)

multiple clinical and social problems may be addressed, and a close relation to the functionality of the patient is given. In 2004, the American Geriatric Society defined frailty as a physiological syndrome that is defined by reduced resources and a lower resilience against different stressors (Walston et al. 2006). This syndrome may result from the cumulative effect of decreased resources in different physiologic systems (Ferrucci et al. 2004) and is therefore also related to the concept of multimorbidity that has been frequently and alternatively used to define vulnerable elderly.

In contrast to multimorbidity, however, the frailty concept includes pathogenetic aspects of the aging process itself. In this framework, thus,

a central feature is the loss of muscle mass at advancing age. A progressive loss of muscle mass is defined as sarcopenia and is distinguished from loss of muscle mass in other clinical conditions, such as inflammation, cancer (cachexia), or starvation. Sarcopenia, which is frequent in elderly patients, may explain reduced muscle strength, early exhaustion, reduced walking speed, and reduced physical activity and thus major aspects of frailty. Different pathogenetic pathways are discussed to explain sarcopenia (Abate et al. 2007). Among these are genetic aspects, comorbidity, environmental factors, and life events. Besides this, pure aging processes are involved (Bortz 2002). Fried et al. (2001)

proposed a scheme of the frailty process as a cascade (Fig. 1), including sarcopenia, malnutrition, and reduced physical activity.

Reduced physical activity is the main contributor to sarcopenia and frailty. More closely related to the aging process itself are changes in the endocrine system (e.g., decline in sex hormone levels) and metabolism (e.g., reduction in resting metabolic rate) that also activate the frailty cascade. Finally, changes in the immune system (e.g., subclinical activation of cytokine activity) commonly described by the concept of immunoaging also contribute to this cascade. An overview provided by Morley et al. (2005) indicated that the most important markers involved are

- Sex hormones
- DHEAs (dehydroepiandrosterones)
- IGF (insulin-like growth factor) 1.

The list is incomplete, and other markers and systems may be involved as well. Clearly, physical activity, muscle metabolism, and nutrition are key factors; cognitive decline and other age-related changes in the organism contribute as well. Other features from the actual aging theory regarding cell aging research may also be represented by this concept:

- Oxidative stress
- Mitochondrial dysfunction
- Genetic and epigenetic DNA changes.

Age-related processes are not the only constituents of these changes; chronic diseases and the related frailty concept may integrate the aspect of multimorbidity as well to identify the vulnerable elderly. Years before Fried postulated the five criteria mentioned for frailty, Buchner and Wagner (1992) proposed a different approach to frailty and named three major aspects of their concept:

- Neurological impairment
- Musculoskeletal impairment
- Dysbalance of energy metabolism.

This approach is more distant to pathophysiological mechanisms than the one proposed by Fried and focuses on muscle metabolism from a general and clinical perspective. These aspects compose a dynamic framework and also allow for interventions to slow the frailty cascade (Marcell 2003; Roubenoff 2003).

The multidimensionality of the framework creates methodological difficulties to define a consented diagnostic measure integrating the most important aspects. In this context, Fried's criteria are most frequently used but were also challenged (Hubbard et al. 2009). Important aspects that are missing in Fried's criteria are balance and cognition. Alternative indices often include aspects of functionality like activities of daily living (ADLs). As Fried et al. (2001) only published quintiles from two large cohorts of elderly in the United States rather than clear absolute cutoff limits, important parameters are still not clearly defined; tendencies are detectable in the scientific discussion to leave the muscle performance-based definition and shift back to aspects of self-management (ADL/IADL [instrumental activities of daily living] concept). However, this will mix up sarcopenia and self-management capacity—two aspects that are clearly correlated (Janssen et al. 2002) but still separated by a major distinction: organ dysfunction versus impairment of the person as a whole. Another trend to define the major contributors to frailty more clearly is the direct measurement of muscle mass via, for example, DEXA (dual-emission x-ray absorptiometry) or BIA (body impedance analysis) and add this measure to Fried's criteria.

Epidemiology and Clinical Significance

The discussion of the criteria defining frailty described explains the fact that different data on epidemiologic aspects critically depend on the diagnostic criteria utilized. However, all studies consistently showed an increase of sarcopenia and the frailty syndrome with advancing age, and this was independent of the utilized diagnostic criteria. Mitnitski et al. (2005) showed this in an extensive review of cohort studies and found an almost-linear increase of prevalence with advancing age. Prevalence data are given in more detail in chapter "Epidemiologic Aspects." In general, one fourth of all persons 70 years and older fulfill frailty criteria.

The prognostic significance of frailty was shown repeatedly in longitudinal cohorts. In a meta-analysis, Stuck et al. (1999) found evidence for morbidity effects of frailty. They analyzed predictors of functional loss in the elderly. The most significant predictors were loss of muscle strength and malnutrition. Janssen (2006) analyzed sarcopenia-related aspects derived from body impedance analysis in a large U.S. cohort (5,000 men and women over 65 years) and found clear prognostic evidence for sarcopenia-related aspects on morbidity within an 8-year interval.

Data from the Zutphen study (Zutphen Elderly Study) identified reduced physical activity as a significant risk factor for increased mortality (Bijnen et al. 1999). This study included 427 elderly men in the Netherlands. Another commonly used biomarker—strength of the hand grip—was also shown to be an independent predictor of increased mortality in the elderly (Metter et al. 2004). Other studies not using singular markers of sarcopenia but rather realizing a more integrative approach to the frailty syndrome also confirmed the prognostic significance of this condition in a longitudinal setting.

Muscle force as measured by hand grip strength is an independent predictor of mortality in the elderly.

In their seminal work, Fried et al. (2001) also described the prognostic value of the frailty syndrome as defined by at least three positive factors out of the five criteria mentioned with regard to mortality. The observation time of this cohort was 72 months. The predictive impact of frailty is independent from chronological age (Schuurmans et al. 2004) and may also cover psychosocial and behavioral aspects (Schulz and Williamson 1993; Tennstedt et al. 1990).

Significance of the Frailty Syndrome for Pharmacotherapy

The concept of the frailty syndrome may be the best tool to identify a general geriatric vulnerability of the patient, linking the highly vulnerable subpopulation to an increased ADR risk. A closer relation of frailty to special aspects of ADR

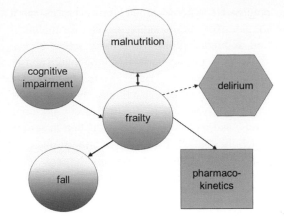

Fig. 2 Significant determinants and consequences of frailty

risk, in particular falls, can be found as frailty equals low muscle mass and force, as well as loss of compensatory resources to maintain postural stability (see chapter "Fall Risk and Pharmacotherapy"). Special concerns arise if FRIDs (fall-risk-increasing drugs) are prescribed to frail elderly. Unfortunately, FRIDs are often continued in the elderly even when evidence for a positive risk-benefit ratio no longer exists. Van der Velde et al. (2006) analyzed the impact of discontinuation or dose reduction of FRIDs on the course of the underlying disease and fall risk. Discontinuation or dose reduction of these drugs did not cause harm in many elderly patients and is thus encouraged. Another link between frailty and pharmacotherapy is described by the fact that low muscle mass often leads to an overestimation of renal function if only based on serum creatinine. This is a significant issue when drugs with a narrow therapeutic range are prescribed (e.g., digoxin). Furthermore, this relation may explain a confusional state or cognitive impairment in some cases. Some of these pathways are given in Fig. 2.

Cognitive decline is missing in the Fried criteria but is discussed among the so-called prefrailty aspects. Prefrailty aspects are features identifying elderly persons at risk as they promote the frailty syndrome by reduced activity and locomotion. Relations exist between cognitive abilities and locomotion, as shown in recent

Table 1 Drugs potentially affecting muscle strength

Drug	Kind of myopathy induced by drug	ADR frequency (%)
Amiodarone	Painful vacuolar myopathy	1–10
Chloroquine	Painful vacuolar myopathy	<1
Colchicine	Painful vacuolar myopathy	<1
Cyclosporin	Painful mitochondrial myopathy	1–10
Diuretics	Hypokalemia	Unknown
D-Penicillamine	Inflammatory myopathy	<1
Neuroleptics	Malignant neuroleptic syndrome	>0,5
Statins	Rhabdomyolyis	5
Steroids	Chronic form with atrophic myopathy, acute form with elevation of creatinin kinase	Unknown
Valproic acid	Carnitin-associated myopathy	10–20
Zidovudine	Mitochondrial myopathy	<1

ADR adverse drug reaction

interventional studies (Schwenk et al. 2010). Unfortunately, so far these aspects possibly resulting in a changed risk-benefit ratio have not been implemented in clinical trials.

Drugs That May Contribute to the Frailty Syndrome

By different mechanisms, drugs may contribute to the cascade of frailty. First, all drugs aggravating risk of fall and fear of fall contribute to the frailty cascade. They result in a reduced physical activity and thereby promote further loss of muscle mass and muscle strength. These FRIDs are described in chapter "Fall Risk and Pharmacotherapy"; they are mainly centrally acting agents.

Another pathway through which drugs may contribute to the frailty cascade are direct effects on skeletal muscle. Drugs with a direct effect on muscle strength are given in Table 1. Most significant in this context are corticosteroids, which may cause myopathy in high-dose long-term treatment (Mitsui et al. 2002). Whether elderly are more receptive to this risk remains unclear, as well as the safe threshold of dose to avoid this ADR, which may be lower in the elderly. In general, the critical threshold for long-term corticosteroid therapy is assumed to be 7.5 mg/day equivalent of prednisolone. Table 2 gives an overview of thresholds for

Table 2 Critical threshold of commonly prescribed corticosteroids to induce long-term ADR ("Cushing" syndrome)

Drug	Threshold dose (mg/day)
Cortisone	40
Dexamethasone	1.5
Hydrocortisone	30
Methylprednisolone	6
Prednisolone	7.5
Prednisone	7.5

ADR adverse drug reaction

commonly used corticosteroids. Elevated daily doses above these values are critical in long-term treatment; daily doses above 30 mg prednisolone equivalent are not recommended except for short-term treatment (Williams 2006).

As elderly with frailty syndrome may lack compensatory mechanisms and even lower stressor levels may exert negative influences on muscle strength in analogy to the model for fall risk given in chapter "Fall Risk and Pharmacotherapy," negative effects on functionality may be common in association with drug therapy. However, data are sparse in this regard. The lack of data on myopathy resulting from statin therapy or loss of muscle strength due to prescription of neuroleptics in frail elderly is remarkable. Figure 3 summarizes possible influences on muscle strength in this context. This covers not only drugs but also frequent and

Fig. 3 Significant determinants of muscle strength in the elderly. *Immunosensc* immunosenescence

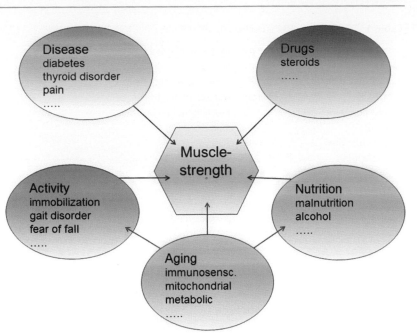

significant chronic diseases. Besides this, immobilization interacts with the frailty syndrome and is outlined in more detail in chapter "Immobility and Pharmacotherapy."

Pharmacotherapeutic Strategies to Improve the Frailty Syndrome

To date, there are no recommended pharmacotherapeutic approaches to improve the frailty syndrome, although some approaches have been proposed (Lynch 2008). Interventions to improve the course of the frailty syndrome are based on a multifaceted concept. This includes physical exercise, especially resistance training to improve muscle strength in the trunk and lower extremities, and nutritional intervention (especially protein supplementation) to stop muscle catabolism. In the case of an accelerated hypogonadism with advancing age as determined by comparison with percentiles of age-adjusted normal values, testosterone supplementation in men is discussed. However, the significance of the effect remains unclear in a clinical setting (Srinivas-Shankar and Wu 2009). An intervention study in elderly men failed to show a clear benefit from testosterone supplementation to improve frailty aspects (Kenny et al. 2010).

However, studies of this topic were small, and serious concerns about dosage and long-term adverse effects exist for sex hormone supplementation. Selective modulators of the androgen receptor (SARMs) have also been discussed (Segal et al. 2006), but to date no favorable benefit-risk ratio could be shown. For long-term treatment or long-term prevention, general recommendations cannot be given, although a limited potential of pharmacotherapy is seen that certainly remains secondary to core interventions like resistance training or nutritional supplementation of protein (Waters et al. 2010). Finally, in this context the overlap with antiaging medicine is an issue of ethical and sociocultural dimensions.

References

Abate M, Di Iorio A, Di Renzo D, Paganelli R, Saggini R, Abate G (2007) Frailty in the elderly: the physical dimension. Eura Medicophys 43:407–415

Bijnen FC, Feskens EJ, Caspersen CJ, Nagelkerke N, Mosterd WL, Kromhout D (1999) Baseline and previous physical activity in relation to mortality in elderly men: the Zutphen Elderly Study. Am J Epidemiol 150:1289–1296

Bortz WM 2nd (2002) A conceptual framework of frailty: a review. J Gerontol A Biol Sci Med Sci 57: M283–M288

Buchner DM, Wagner EH (1992) Preventing frail health. Clin Geriatr Med 8:1–17

Campbell AJ, Buchner DM (1997) Unstable disability and the fluctuations of frailty. Age Ageing 26:315–318

Ferrucci L, Guralnik JM, Studenski S, Fried LP, Cutler GB Jr, Walston JD, Interventions on Frailty Working Group (2004) Designing randomized, controlled trials aimed at preventing or delaying functional decline and disability in frail, older persons: a consensus report. J Am Geriatr Soc 52:625–634

Fried LP, Tangen CM, Walston J et al (2001) Frailty in older adults: evidence for a phenotype. J Gerontol A Biol Sci Med Sci 56:M146–M156

Hubbard RE, O'Mahony MS, Woodhouse KW (2009) Characterising frailty in the clinical setting—a comparison of different approaches. Age Ageing 38:115–119

Janssen I (2006) Influence of sarcopenia on the development of physical disability: the Cardiovascular Health Study. J Am Geriatr Soc 54:56–62

Janssen I, Heymsfield SB, Ross R (2002) Low relative skeletal muscle mass (sarcopenia) in older persons is associated with functional impairment and physical disability. J Am Geriatr Soc 50:889–896

Kenny AM, Kleppinger A, Annis K et al (2010) Effects of transdermal testosterone on bone and muscle in older men with low bioavailable testosterone levels, low bone mass, and physical frailty. J Am Geriatr Soc 58:1134–1143

Lynch GS (2008) Update on emerging drugs for sarcopenia—age-related muscle wasting. Expert Opin Emerg Drugs 13:655–673

Marcell TJ (2003) Sarcopenia: causes, consequences, and preventions. J Gerontol A Biol Sci Med Sci 58: M911–M916

Metter EJ, Talbot LA, Schrager M, Conwit RA (2004) Arm-cranking muscle power and arm isometric muscle strength are independent predictors of all-cause mortality in men. J Appl Physiol 96:814–821

Mitnitski A, Song X, Skoog I, Broe GA, Cox JL, Grunfeld E, Rockwood K (2005) Relative fitness and frailty of elderly men and women in developed countries and their relationship with mortality. J Am Geriatr Soc 53:2184–2189

Mitsui T, Azuma H, Nagasawa M, Iuchi T, Akaike M, Odomi M, Matsumoto T (2002) Chronic corticosteroid administration causes mitochondrial dysfunction in skeletal muscle. J Neurol 249:1004–1009

Morley JE, Kim MJ, Haren MT (2005) Frailty and hormones. Rev Endocr Metab Disord 6:101–108

Rockwood K, Fox RA, Stolee P, Robertson D, Beattie BL (1994) Frailty in elderly people: an evolving concept. CMAJ 150:489–495

Roubenoff R (2003) Sarcopenia: effects on body composition and function. J Gerontol A Biol Sci Med Sci 58:1012–1017

Schulz R, Williamson GM (1993) Psychosocial and behavioral dimensions of physical frailty. J Gerontol 48(Spec No):39–43

Schuurmans H, Steverink N, Lindenberg S, Frieswijk N, Slaets JP (2004) Old or frail: what tells us more? J Gerontol A Biol Sci Med Sci 59:M962–M965

Schwenk M, Zieschang T, Oster P, Hauer K (2010) Dual-task performances can be improved in patients with dementia: a randomized controlled trial. Neurology 74:1961–1968

Segal S, Narayanan R, Dalton JT (2006) Therapeutic potential of the SARMs: revisiting the androgen receptor for drug discovery. Expert Opin Investig Drugs 15:377–387

Srinivas-Shankar U, Wu FC (2009) Frailty and muscle function: role for testosterone? Front Horm Res 37:133–149

Stuck AE, Walthert JM, Nikolaus T, Bula CJ, Hohmann C, Beck JC (1999) Risk factors for functional status decline in community-living elderly people: a systematic literature review. Soc Sci Med 48:445–469

Tennstedt SL, Sullivan LM, McKinlay JB, D'Agostino RB (1990) How important is functional status as a predictor of service use by older people? J Aging Health 2:439–461

Van der Velde N, Stricker BH, Pols HA, Van der Cammen TJM (2006) Risk of falls after withdrawal of fall-risk-increasing drugs: a prospective cohort study. Br J Clin Pharmacol 63:232–237

Walston J, Hadley EC, Ferrucci L et al (2006) Research agenda for frailty in older adults: toward a better understanding of physiology and etiology: summary from the American Geriatrics Society/National Institute on Aging Research Conference on frailty in older adults. J Am Geriatr Soc 54:991–1001

Waters DL, Baumgartner RN, Garry PJ, Vellas B (2010) Advantages of dietary, exercise-related, and therapeutic interventions to prevent and treat sarcopenia in adult patients: an update. Clin Interv Aging 5:259–270

Williams O (2006) Drug induced and toxic myopathies. In: Brust JCM (ed) Current diagnosis and treatment in neurology. McGraw Hill, New York, pp 370–373

Woodhouse KW, O'Mahony MS (1997) Frailty and ageing. Age Ageing 26:245–246

Further Problem Areas in Gerontopharmacotherapy and Pragmatic Recommendations

Adherence to Pharmacotherapy in the Elderly

Heinrich Burkhardt

General Aspects of Adherence

Adherence is defined as accordance between prescribed therapy and patient behavior (Haynes 1979). This term covers not only pharmacotherapy but also other health-related advice from professional health workers. Despite the prominent significance of adherence for treatment, prevention, and rehabilitation success, rather little scientific work is done on this topic. This may be due in part to methodological problems such as how exactly to measure adherence. Second, although different categories of nonadherence are defined, their delineation seems to be rather arbitrary (e.g., intended vs. unintended nonadherence). Therefore, prevalence data of nonadherence are difficult to obtain even in well-controlled scientific studies (e.g., randomized controlled trials [RCTs]) (Kruse 1995; Spilker 1991). This explains why conflicting data concerning nonadherence exist in the literature, with prevalence rates for nonadherence ranging from 15% to 93%. For example, nonadherence to prescribed medications may be reported to be as high as 50% in arterial hypertension; in general, it will be higher in asymptomatic (such as arterial hypertension) than symptomatic diseases. Despite these large ranges concerning

prevalence data, there is evidence for a consistently increasing rate of nonadherence with increasing number of drugs prescribed (Spagnoli et al. 1989). Simultaneous prescription of five and more drugs is considered critical in this context (McElnay and McCallion 1998).

Nonadherence increases with an increasing number of simultaneously prescribed drugs.

As multimorbidity and polypharmacy are more frequent in the elderly, this population is commonly thought to show an increased rate of nonadherence compared to younger adults. However, this could not be confirmed in most studies done on this topic (Fincham 1988; Balkrishnan 1998). Hughes (2004) provided an overview of studies concerning adherence especially in the elderly. In one of those studies, Mallion et al. (1998) showed that neither age nor gender proved as strong predictors of nonadherence in antihypertensive treatment.

Nonadherence is influenced by several factors that represent not only aspects of the therapeutic schedule (e.g., complexity) but also

- Patient-related aspects (e.g., personality)
- Patient-physician interaction (e.g., shared decision making)
- Sociocultural aspects (e.g., education, access to health system)
- The patient's health belief.

A systematic overview of these factors was given in the review by Hughes (2004). Their influence may differ for different age classes and change with time in the same individual. The negative impact of some factors on adherence

H. Burkhardt (✉)
IVth Department of Medicine, Geriatrics, University Medical Centre Mannheim, Theodor-Kutzer-Ufer 1-3, Mannheim 68167, Germany
e-mail: heinrich.burkhardt@umm.de

M. Wehling (ed.), *Drug Therapy for the Elderly*,
DOI 10.1007/978-3-7091-0912-0_25, © Springer-Verlag Wien 2013

Table 1 Overview of significant factors influencing adherence to drug therapy

Domain	Factor	Comment
Drug and therapy associated	Complexity of therapeutic schedule and application route (subcutaneous versus oral), high requirements with regard to patient self-management abilities	Functionality is most significant
	Discontinuity of therapy	Impedes a stable adherence
	Number of drugs	Repeatedly proven as significant factor (critical threshold >5)
	Risk of ADR associated with therapy	Overall prevalence estimated in previous brown-bag study about 8 %; many patients are not sufficiently informed at the start of medication
	Medication package/container	Frequently overlooked as barrier
Disease associated	Chronicity of disease	Most significant in case of prophylactic treatment
	Poor prognosis	Adherence improves along with severity of disease
	Missing of symptoms	Increasingly asymptomatic presentation in the elderly may impede adherence
Patient associated	Physiological changes	May represent prerequisites for impaired functionality (e.g., visual acuity)
	Multimorbidity	Leads to polypharmacy (see there)
	Cognition	Reduced cognition is significant in the elderly as prevalence is increasing beyond age 70; besides this, 70 % of patients do not have adequate information about prescribed medication
	Health beliefs	Controversially discussed, in the elderly more stable health beliefs may even improve adherence compared to younger adults
	Psychosocial aspects	Not well analyzed
Miscellaneous	Patient-doctor relation	Controversially discussed, no general recommendations for interaction style
	Access to medication	May also depend on functionality even if health system allows general access
	Social support	May act differently in different age categories
	Poverty	Depends on health insurance system

ADR adverse drug reaction.

may decrease with advancing age; for others, it may increase. Table 1 provides an overview and comments on different contributors to adherence. The complexity of these influences easily explains methodological difficulties and clearly outlines that nonadherence in many cases depends on a complex interplay of several of these factors.

Adherence and Functionality

In the elderly, impaired functionality is obviously a more significant factor concerning adherence

than in younger adults. This is especially significant in complex therapeutic schedules that demand a large amount of self-management capacities to follow prescription and recommendations. More complex treatment schedules are associated with a greater prevalence of nonadherence (Dolce et al. 1991). This was nicely shown with special reference to geriatric patients in a study by Nikolaus et al. (1996). In geriatric patients discharged from an acute geriatric ward, they found 40% unable to adhere to recommended prescription schedules during follow-up. This was mainly due to a so-far-unrecognized

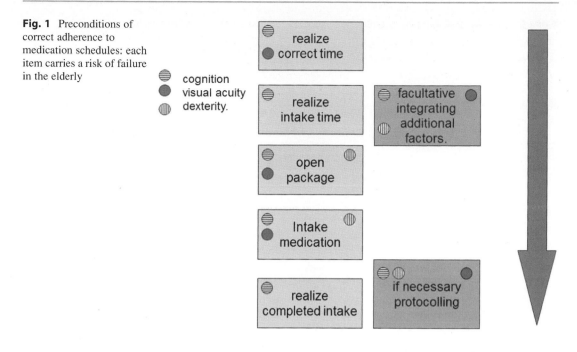

Fig. 1 Preconditions of correct adherence to medication schedules: each item carries a risk of failure in the elderly

⊜ cognition
● visual acuity
◍ dexterity.

realize correct time

realize intake time

open package

Intake medication

realize completed intake

facultative integrating additional factors.

if necessary protocolling

reduction of functionality. In particular, those patients were not diagnosed with overt dementia. Yet, a large number of patients were unable to handle standard medication packages, such as blister or flip-top containers.

In many elderly, subclinical functional impairments represent a serious barrier to adhere to the prescription schedule.

Although clearly exhibiting a critical issue determining treatment success, early detection of those problems is largely underemphasized in medical practice. Thus, self-management requirements to follow a medication schedule often are underestimated. In general, a multistep process has to be followed even if "just" oral medications are prescribed, and at every step failures may occur. For example, the intake of a tablet may be properly intended, but a little white pill may be lost, and the loss is not recognized due to reduced visual acuity; thus, its execution fails. A wide variety of failures may occur and potentially reach significance for treatment success as depicted in Fig. 1.

This is obviously more significant when treatment strategies are complex, such as insulin therapy in diabetes mellitus (see chapter "Diabetes Mellitus"). In this and other complex therapeutic situations, an assessment of self-management has to take place prior to prescription or treatment decisions. A short, but effective, assessment tool to qualify the patient's abilities to perform successful handling of drugs is the "timed test of money counting" (Burkhardt et al. 2006). If there are different treatment options in the elderly, an analysis of the complexity and self-management requirements is very helpful, maybe mandatory, to optimize the individual treatment. Table 2 provides an overview and gives some common examples and comments. If requirements for self-management capabilities belong to category 2 or above, a standardized assessment of the patient's functional capabilities is strongly recommended. Furthermore, follow-up monitoring of self-management capabilities should be performed to detect an early decline and involve caregivers or medical professionals prior to treatment failure.

The assessment of functional capabilities prior to the initiation of complex treatment strategies is strongly recommended.

Technical aids such as dosing aids or treatment schedules given in large letters or even electronic guides may be helpful on an individual basis to compensate for functional limitations.

Table 2 Analysis of the complexity of drug administration in the elderly and self-management requirements

Demand	Level of difficulty	Example	Comment
Take out a pill from a blister package	1	Aspirin	Easiest to handle, but in up to 10 % of all elderly already critical
Take out a pill from a flip-top package	2	Warfarin	In up to 45 % of all elderly critical
Take out a pill from a childproof package	3	Tilidin (some European countries, not FDA approved)	In over 60 % of all elderly critical
Intake o.d.	1	Aspirin	Easiest case, in literature nonadherence estimated from drug count (i.e., not redeemed prescriptions)
Intake > o.d. and exact timing included	2	Levodopa	Not well analyzed
Intake according to additional criteria	3	Dosage is changing day by day (e.g., warfarin)	Advanced cognitive requirements
Oral intake	1	Ramipril	Standard application, form and size of pills may influence adherence, but these aspects remain poorly analyzed
Application by technical device	3	Insulin, topical corticoid (inhaler)	Frequently analyzed, rather high rate of dosage or application errors
Transdermal system	2	Fentanyl	Problems may arise to handle package and fix the system to the skin
Monitoring, simple protocol	1	Toilet training	
Monitoring a biological quantity using a technical device	2	Blood pressure	Although rather simple to apply, infrequently used in the elderly
Monitoring a biological quantity from body fluid using a technical device	3	Blood glucose self-measurement, self-measurement INR	More demanding monitoring requires thorough patient or caregiver education

FDA Food and Drug Administration, *INR* international normalized ratio.

However, data on this topic are scarce, and—even more critical—the implementation of this issue in treatment guidelines is largely missing.

Patient Knowledge and Psychological Factors

Lack of knowledge or ignorance may also contribute to nonadherence. In the so-called brown-bag study, 19.1% of elderly patients did not know why a given medication had been prescribed (Owens et al. 1991). Although these data date back to the 1990s, no significant improvement of patient knowledge has become detectable in recent years. More recent studies also described this lack of knowledge of health-related problems and medication in the elderly and sug-gested reduced cognitive function as an explanation (Beier and Ackerman 2003; Widiger and Seidlitz 2002).

Psychological factors also determine adherence. Ried and Christensen (1988) found 29% of the adherence variability of patients to be explained by psychological constructs. Apparently, this finding is reported for all age categories and thus not exclusively seen in the elderly.

An important and widely used psychological construct to explain nonadherence is the health belief model. This model describes perception of disease severity and treatment barriers.

Health belief changes that are particular to the elderly and may explain different patterns of nonadherence compared to younger adults are not yet fully analyzed, and their existence thus is still under debate.

Another issue relevant to adherence is the style of the interaction between patients and doctors. In general, a participatory approach is seen to more favorably impact adherence and avoidance of unrecognized adherence problems (Charles et al. 1999). However, it has to be kept in mind that a participatory style is often not favored, especially by elderly patients (Beaver et al. 1996), as shown for cancer patients. Therefore, in any case an open consultation with the patient should be sought, carefully exploring if a participatory approach meets the patient's needs and attitudes (Freidson 1970). Any authoritative approach pushing certain features of the patient-doctor interaction should be avoided. The interaction style has to be developed as a dynamic approach allowing both parties to establish the appropriate interaction modus. This may also explain why a rigorous generalized approach did not produce a significant effect on adherence in a study of outpatients aiming at the improvement of hypertension control (Deinzer et al. 2009).

Interventions to Improve Adherence to Medication Schedules

Interventions to improve adherence rates to medication schedules have to cover a variety of measures. In general, all interventions have to be tailored to the individual treatment situation considering the individual patient's aspects and the environment to be successful. To achieve this, the first step is always to exclude, identify, and quantify barriers of adherence. Second, an appropriate measure to improve adherence has to be chosen. Several measures may be applied simultaneously, including supervision and assistance in medication intake by health care professionals (e.g., nursing), technical assistance (e.g., dosing aids for the visually impaired), patient education, and regular home visits by pharmacists. If the principles of individualization mentioned are not respected, the individual measures show only little effects (Higgins and Regan 2004). Another rule is to combine different measures if

possible to augment the beneficial effects (Fincham 1988; Rivers 1992).

Most successful interventions to improve adherence are individualized and multimodal.

Table 1 provides an overview of significant factors influencing adherence that should always be checked to establish an individualized approach to strengthen adherence. As there are only a few studies focusing on the elderly, a specific, evidence-based recommendation for this population cannot be given. Clearly, the single most significant element is the proper assessment of functional impairment. Further aspects frequently mentioned in that context are thorough patient education and counseling, including treatment goals, possible adverse drug reactions (ADRs), and behavioral rules. In principle, patient education is possible in the elderly even if a mild cognitive decline is present, as has been shown for patients with diabetes mellitus 2 (see chapter "Diabetes Mellitus"). Again, patients' needs and resources have to be respected not to overstrain their capabilities. Education of patients in groups is possible if group composition is not too heterogeneous. Chronological age alone is not a significant barrier for patient education. Furthermore, caregivers and relatives should be invited to attend patient education sessions as early as possible.

Owens et al. (1991) proposed a list of rules and recommendations for medication prescribers to improve adherence in the elderly. Although published 20 years ago, the following list (*modified from* Owens et al. 1991) is still up to date: *how to improve adherence in the elderly:*

1. Be aware of and respect patients' health beliefs
2. Educate the patient about health-related aspects
3. Keep medication schedules as simple as possible
4. Prioritize drugs that are most important
5. Reassure patients that care is taken to recognize beneficial effects and ADRs
6. Give information and advice concerning indication, dosage, and intake modalities
7. Find out which mnemotechnics patients use
8. Use information media to strengthen effects of counseling conversation

9. Encourage questions by the patient
10. Check the patient's knowledge and ask for the indication a patient remembers for prescribed medications (to ensure that effective information was given).

Recognizing nonadherence is an essential task for physicians and should always be followed by efforts to identify causes of nonadherence to ameliorate it in collaboration with the patient. In this context, it is important to note that the World Health Organization (WHO 2003) underlines the significance of a correct attitude of caregivers and medical professionals toward the patient: *Patients need to be supported, not blamed.*

References

Balkrishnan R (1998) Predictors of medication adherence in the elderly. Clin Ther 20:764–771

Beaver K, Luker KA, Owens RG, Leinster SJ, Degner LF, Sloan JA (1996) Treatment decision making in women newly diagnosed with breast cancer. Cancer Nurs 19:8–19

Beier ME, Ackerman PL (2003) Determinants of health knowledge: an investigation of age, gender, abilities, personality, and interests. J Pers Soc Psychol 84:439–448

Burkhardt H, Karaminejad E, Gladisch R (2006) A short performance test can help to predict adherence to self-administration of insulin in elderly patients with diabetes. Age Ageing 35:449–450

Charles C, Gafni A, Whelan T (1999) Decision-making in the physician-patient encounter: revisiting the shared treatment decision-making model. Soc Sci Med 49:651–661

Deinzer A, Veelken R, Kohnen R, Schmieder RE (2009) Is a shared decision-making approach effective in improving hypertension management? J Clin Hypertens (Greenwich) 11:266–270

Dolce JJ, Crisp C, Manzella B, Richards JM, Hardin JM, Bailey WC (1991) Medication adherence patterns in chronic obstructive pulmonary disease. Chest 99:837–841

Fincham E (1988) Patient compliance in the ambulatory elderly: a review of the literature. J Geriatr Drug Ther 2:31–52

Freidson E (1970) Professional dominance: the social structure of medical care. Atherton, New York

Haynes RB (1979) Introduction. In: Haynes RB, Taylor DW, Sackett DL (eds) Compliance in health care. Johns Hopkins University Press, Baltimore

Higgins N, Regan C (2004) A systematic review of the effectiveness of interventions to help older people adhere to medication regimes. Age Ageing 33:224–229

Hughes CM (2004) Medication non-adherence in the elderly: how big is the problem? Drugs Aging 21:793–811

Kruse WHH (1995) Comprehensive geriatric assessment and medication compliance. Z Gerontol Geriatr 28:54–61

Mallion JM, Baguet JP, Siche JP, Tremel F, de Gaudemaris R (1998) Compliance, electronic monitoring and anti-hypertensive drugs. J Hypertens Suppl 16:S75–S79

McElnay JC, McCallion CR (1998) Adherence and the elderly. In: Myers LB, Midence K (eds) Adherence to treatment in medical conditions. Harwood Academic, Amsterdam

Nikolaus T, Kruse W, Bach M, Specht-Leible N, Oster P, Schlierf G (1996) Elderly patients' problems with medication. An in-hospital and follow-up study. Eur J Clin Pharmacol 49:255–259

Owens NJ, Larrat EP, Fretwell MD (1991) Improving compliance in the older patient. In: Cramer JA, Spilker B (eds) Patient compliance in medical practice and clinical trials. Raven, New York, pp 107–119

Ried LD, Christensen DN (1988) A psychosocial perspective in the explanation of patients' drug-taking behavior. Soc Sci Med 27:277–285

Rivers PH (1992) Compliance aids—do they work? Drugs Aging 2:103–111

Spagnoli A, Ostino G, Borga AD et al (1989) Drug compliance and unreported drugs in the elderly. J Am Geriatr Soc 37:619–624

Spilker B (1991) Methods of assessing and improving patient compliance in clinical trials. In: Cramer JA, Spilker B (eds) Patient compliance in medical practice and clinical trials. Raven, New York, pp 37–56

Widiger TA, Seidlitz L (2002) Personality, psychopathology, and aging. J Res Pers 36:335–362

World Health Organization (WHO) (2003) Adherence to long-term therapies, evidence for action. http://apps.who.int/medicinedocs/pdf/s4883e/s4883e.pdf. Accessed 19 Dec 2011

Polypharmacy

Heinrich Burkhardt

Definition and Significance

Polypharmacy is a major concern in geriatrics and often categorized as a geriatric syndrome. Polypharmacy is frequently seen in the elderly mainly due to the increased prevalence of chronic diseases and impaired health conditions, and thus multimorbidity. Obviously, this is not an exclusively age-related problem but may also be seen in younger adults or even children and adolescents if multimorbidity is present.

The unfavorable effects of polypharmacy are addressed in different chapters of this book. The main negative sequelae are summarized as follows:

- Unfavorable adherence
- Incalculable interactions
- Accumulated adverse drug reaction (ADR) risk
- Increased risk of hospitalization
- Increased risk of medication errors
- Increased costs.

Therefore, polypharmacy is considered and generally accepted as an independent health risk indicator. This is particularly true for the elderly and has been implemented in recently developed screening tools to assess the general health risk (Stuck et al. 2007). In contrast to this, a remarkable paucity of studies primarily addressing the problem of polypharmacy has to be stated. The neglect of this area is furthermore characterized by a still-missing consent on the definition of polypharmacy. A recent review listed more than 15 different definitions of polypharmacy (Bushardt et al. 2008). As outlined in chapter "Adherence to Pharmacotherapy in the Elderly," five or more simultaneously prescribed drugs are considered critical in this context. Thus, we recommend accepting this number as a threshold value to define critical polypharmacy, bearing in mind that aside from the mere number of drugs, interaction patterns and cumulated ADR risk may add to the problem.

Polypharmacy—although significant and critical in every patient—is certainly more significant in the elderly due to their reduced resources and compensatory abilities. Therefore, increased occurrence of ADRs in this population is easily explained. A significant factor in this context is the total anticholinergic burden, mainly caused by several simultaneously administered centrally acting drugs (e.g., antipsychotics and antidepressants). Delirium and falls are common clinical problems that often result from increased anticholinergic burden (see related chapters "Dementia" and "Fall Risk and Pharmacotherapy").

Epidemiology

Epidemiologic data are given in chapter "Epidemiologic Aspects" in more detail. For example, a population-based German survey analyzing

H. Burkhardt (✉)
IVth Department of Medicine, Geriatrics, University Medical Centre Mannheim, Theodor-Kutzer-Ufer 1-3, Mannheim 68167, Germany
e-mail: heinrich.burkhardt@umm.de

M. Wehling (ed.), *Drug Therapy for the Elderly*,
DOI 10.1007/978-3-7091-0912-0_26, © Springer-Verlag Wien 2013

Fig. 1 Prescribing cascade. *ADR* adverse drug reaction

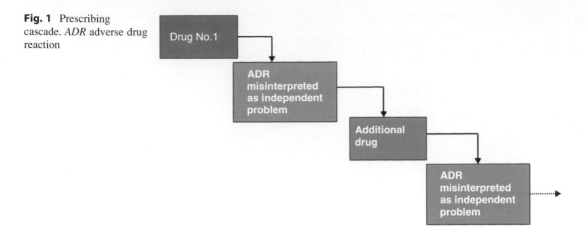

prescription patterns in an urban elderly population (BASE, Berlin Aging Study) found the prescription of five and more drugs in 53.7% of elderly patients (Steinhagen-Thiessen and Borchelt 2001). Another result from this study was a high rate of so-called OTC (over-the-counter) drugs, which add a substantial risk to the overall risk-benefit ratio. NHANES (National Health and Nutrition Examination Survey), a large-scale ongoing survey in the United States, not only performs personal interviews and assessments to identify drug problems but also provides epidemiologic data concerning prescribed medications. This study found polypharmacy in 16% of elderly over 75 years old (NHANES III; National Center for Health Statistics 1996). The quantitative discrepancy between these two studies may be explained by methodological differences and the exclusion of rural sites in BASE. Nevertheless, in Western societies in up to every second elderly person, polypharmacy may be present, a trend that will be also seen in developing countries depending on access to health care and socioeconomic conditions.

Factors Promoting Polypharmacy

As mentioned, multimorbidity mainly causes polypharmacy as physicians are educated to treat almost every disease in accordance to guidelines pharmacotherapeutically. In many circumstances, the guideline-related pressure renders it rather challenging to skip a drug from the prescription schedule although almost no guidelines are based on data if it comes to the elderly (Wehling 2011). In many instances, drugs are also given to treat symptoms caused by other drugs (ADRs), and in that case these symptoms are mistaken as primarily occurring health problems.

Polypharmacy may result from misinterpreted ADRs.

Rochon and Gurwitz addressed this phenomenon in the term *prescribing cascade* (Rochon and Gurwitz 1997). Inappropriate prescribing cascades may occur more frequently in the context of multimorbidity as ambiguous symptoms may arise, and difficulties exist in discriminating between disease-driven and medication-driven symptoms. Adding to this is the fact that in the elderly, clear symptoms are frequently missing, and an atypical presentation of disease is a well-known diagnostic problem. For example, symptoms such as dizziness and adynamy are often found in this population, pointing to a large variety of underlying health problems but may also indicate ADRs of frequently used medications (Fig. 1).

Every newly presented symptom in the elderly has to be carefully examined regarding its primary causation by concurrent medications, especially in cases of multimorbidity.

If inquiring for possible ADRs, it has to be kept in mind that nonprescribed OTC drugs may have been used. Use of OTC drugs is frequently

Table 1 Examples for significant drug-drug interactions

Interaction level	Example	Clinical significance and comments
Chemical/physical	Incompatibilities when mixing different drugs in the injection solution (e.g., tramadol and diclofenac, furosemide and morphine)	Avoid mixed injection solutions
Gastrointestinal tract	Theophylline and Mg salts, Fe preparations, milk (chelate forming)	Consider comedication, use time shift between incompatible drugs, consider interactions with nutrients
	Antibiotics may induce changes in intestinal flora, causing a decrease in vitamin K production and aggravate risk of overdosing of oral anticoagulants	Do not prolong antibiotic treatment without serious reason, in case of critical and unavoidable comedication shorter time interval of drug monitoring is warranted
Transporter systems	St. John's wort and digoxin interact at the MDR-1 transporter (P-glycoprotein), aggravating risk of digoxin overdosing	Overdosing of digoxin is frequently missed, herbal medicines may also significantly interact
CYP systems	Carbamazepine and some other drugs (e.g., serotonin reuptake inhibitors and clarithromycin) are interacting at the CYP3A4-system, carbamazepine concentrations may increase	Increased risk of falls
Pharmacodynamics	NSAID and antihypertensives (diuretics, ACE inhibitors): failure of blood pressure control	Frequent cause for hypertensive crisis or unfavorable control of hypertension after falls, trauma, or surgery

ACE angiotensin-converting enzyme, *CYP* cytochrome P, *NSAID* nonsteroidal anti-inflammatory drug

not mentioned in a patient's history and has to be asked for explicitly. Furthermore, the use of herbal medicine and similar products may also result in ADRs, an aspect often overlooked by both patients and physicians. Finally, these preparations may interact with concurrent medications. For example, St. John's wort (*Hypericum perforatum*) was promoted as depression treatment, but it was subsequently found that interaction at the site of the P-glycoprotein transporter frequently caused an increase of digoxin levels, resulting in ADRs or even intoxication. In addition, multiple interactions with drugs metabolized by cytochrome P450 species have been described for St. John's wort. Substances used and recommended in complementary or alternative medicine are not always placebo-like but may rather contain often-complex compounds (e.g., alkaloids) with a considerable risk potential for interactions and ADRs as well. If patients use herbal medicines and add them to prescribed medication, this in turn may express uncertainty and concern about the efficacy and risk-benefit ratio of marketed drugs. Physicians should actively address this problem and provide the

required education, counseling, and empathy to find the optimal solution and therapeutic answers to the patient's health problems.

Consequences of Polypharmacy

Polypharmacy further promotes the misinterpretation of ADRs and results itself in an increased risk of ADRs and prescribing cascades partly due to the fact that it impedes the correct recognition of medication problems. In addition, there is an increased risk for drug-drug interactions. Different aspects of drug-drug interactions are outlined in chapter "Age-Associated General Pharmacological Aspects." Table 1 gives some illustrative, clinically important examples.

Interactions may occur at different levels. For example, drug binding to plasma albumin is a significant interaction site for some drugs with high protein-binding characteristics, especially if the therapeutic range is narrow. Clinical significance of this interaction is found for the combination of warfarin and certain comedications (amiodarone, phenytoin, ketoconazole, itraconazole, and sulfonamides), resulting in increased anticoagulation and bleeding risk (Palareti and Legnani 1996; Podrazik and Schwartz 1999).

Uncontrolled and misdiagnosed drug-drug interactions may lead to increased drug serum levels and thereby cause adverse drug reactions.

Another important site of multiple drug-drug interactions is hepatic metabolism by the cytochrome enzyme system (cytochrome P [CYP] 450). There is a great variety of possible interactions at different subtypes of CYP enzymes, and either an increase or a decrease of plasma drug level may result, depending on inhibition or induction of the enzyme system. Prior to prescription of new drugs, possible interactions should be considered. Useful interaction lists can be found in the literature (Semla et al. 2011) or in the Internet (Flockhart 2007). Drug-drug interactions are also mentioned in chapter "Age-Associated General Pharmacological Aspects."

Strategies to Identify and to Avoid Inappropriate Polypharmacy in the Elderly

A frequently proposed strategy to optimize pharmacotherapy in the elderly is described by the catchphrase *less is more* (Chutka et al. 2004). From a geriatric point of view, this rule seems particularly plausible if vulnerable and frail elderly are concerned. Studies of the forced reduction of medication numbers in elderly residents of nursing homes showed remarkable success (Garfinkel et al. 2007). In this study, a decision algorithm was applied, resulting in a significantly reduced drug load with H2 antagonists, nitrates, diuretics, and antihypertensives most frequently stopped. Patients did not complain about any new symptoms after discontinuation of these drugs. Other studies also found that a critical reappraisal of medication schedules allows a safe reduction of drugs. However, concerns about these studies are the short follow-up period and a suboptimal analysis of clinical outcomes (Rollason and Vogt 2003). Reduction of existing polypharmacy schemes may be challenging as patients

should not be put at risk due to uncontrolled health conditions. Indeed, medication reduction without thorough analysis of a patient's history, health conditions, and indications may be risky, explaining why physicians often tend to keep on the safer side and hold to the existing schedule. Yet, exactly this may be elusive and cause more harm than benefit.

A rational analysis to assess the need for multiple drugs in a given complex treatment situation is demanding (Gurwitz 2004).

In this chapter, decision strategies to cope with this arduous task are discussed. In principle, in any given individual treatment situation the individual risk-benefit ratio needs to be estimated and drug schedules optimized accordingly. However, the prerequisite for this analysis is a thorough knowledge of all risks associated with drug therapy, all resources and individual barriers of the patient, and finally treatment preferences. Furthermore, in case of newly emerging or changing factors, these should also be recognized and dealt with immediately. These strict requirements are in contrast to common prescription situations. Especially in elderly patients with multiple health problems, a long patient history, and unapparent limitations of resources, this is even more challenging and may often be missed in everyday practice. Furthermore, risk and benefit in the elderly or at least in certain subgroups are often unknown, as repeatedly outlined in this book. Obviously, a thorough exploration of the treatment situation should take place at the beginning of drug prescription, but it may not be sufficient to realize new aspects; in vulnerable patients, organ functions may vary in short intervals, and monitoring of this is challenging or even impossible. Yet, close monitoring and reappraisal of the treatment situation, including a patient's resources and barriers, are the only way to identify hazards and pitfalls like overdosing, adherence problems, and organ or system function decline early to avoid ADRs and typical and critical incidents like falls and delirium.

Even prior to the risk-benefit ratio assessment, treatment goals have to be defined in the individual patient. What should be achieved in the given treatment situation? Will the intervention on an

Fig. 2 Prescribing algorithm to optimize pharmacotherapy in the elderly and avoid inadequate polypharmacy. *FORTA* Fit for the Aged, *PIM* potentially inappropriate medication

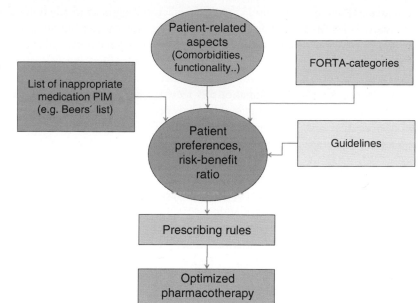

existing risk factor translate into clinical benefit (e.g., primary prevention of cardiovascular incidents)? Are symptoms to be controlled aiming at morbidity burden or prevention of further disability (e.g., pain control)? Symptom control is a must in almost every clinical situation; preventive pharmacotherapy may be secondary given an endpoint horizon of more than 1 year, often seen especially in frail and vulnerable elderly. In case of multimorbidity, treatment goals may even be conflicting, and prioritization remains difficult as recommendations and guidelines for these complex situations are mostly missing.

Particularly in the case of multimorbidity, a prioritization approach cannot be based on large-scale trials due to methodological problems, and these issues have not been sufficiently addressed in scientific literature. To reach an optimal benefit, it is certainly not helpful to add as many drugs as possible to the medication list, but rather a critical appraisal has to take place to prioritize treatment goals. This is even more true when risk is included in the reasoning, and for every new drug added, the risk increase may dominate and overrule the assumed benefit increase. Therefore, uncertainty characterizes complex treatment decisions and may explain why elderly patients are often found on inadequate medications.

An algorithm provided in Fig. 2 demonstrates how these shortcomings may be overcome and optimizing of a comprehensive appraisal of the risk-benefit ratio may take place. This algorithm tries to integrate the known and established measures supporting appropriate pharmacotherapy in the elderly. This includes guidelines based on the principle of evidence-based medicine (which are, however, rare or absent in most cases), evaluation lists of inappropriate medications, categories for appropriateness of drugs in the elderly, and patient aspects. The last covers both organ dysfunction like impaired renal function and impairment of functionality and other resources (e.g., environment and caregiver). These instruments supporting treatment decisions and risk-benefit ratio analyses in the individual situation are outlined and their strengths and weaknesses discussed in the following chapters.

Treatment Guidelines

In modern medicine, treatment guidelines summarize the best evidence available and give recommendations for a standardized treatment approach. They are widely accepted as treatment standards and form the base of modern medical treatment. However, they should not be mistaken as laws or rules for a cookbook-type approach to medicine. They have rather to be translated in the real and individual treatment situation, taking all factors into account that may govern acceptance, modification, deviance, or denial of this recommendation. An important aspect in this context is multimorbidity and polypharmacy. Treatment guidelines do not usually deal with these aspects. They rather outline the treatment options for closely defined health disorders in an exemplary way. The underlying construct concerns the ideal patient who has only this particular disease and is otherwise identical to all patients. Therefore, they do not reflect the wide variation of individual aspects in a given treatment situation, but rather focus on a few confounding conditions, if at all. Second, treatment guidelines try to summarize the best evidence available for their closely defined topic. They mainly rely on large-scale randomized studies to provide valid statements for the majority of patients with the disease. This implies shortcomings or less external validity for subjects not included or underrepresented in the underlying studies. Furthermore, for certain subpopulations risk assessment may also be missing or incomplete although principally present in the studies. As a consequence, following all treatment guidelines in case of multimorbidity simultaneously may result in a largely increased risk and often also in conflicting or inapplicable recommendations (Glaeske and Hoffmann 2009).

In their comprehensive analysis of different practice guidelines, Boyd et al. (2005) found critical issues in most of them, possibly resulting in inappropriate treatment of the individual patient. If all recommendations in a multimorbid patient are followed, the consequence may be an inapplicably complex treatment schedule. The authors provided an impressive example concerning a fictive patient with a common pattern of multimorbidity. The treatment of this 79-year-old woman with osteoarthritis, osteoporosis, hypertension, type 2 diabetes, and chronic obstructive pulmonary disease following current clinical guidelines resulted in 12 medications carrying a significant risk of adverse events and drug-drug interactions; several recommendations have to accompany this drug schedule, to which a 79-year-old lady is very unlikely to be capable of adhering. It is clearly demanding to include at least comments on limitations in usual treatment guidelines regarding defined subpopulations and multimorbidity. Among those critical subpopulations, elderly as a whole, but certainly frail elderly, have to be mentioned (Gillick 2006). Elderly represent a large, yet rapidly growing population, are often addressed by these recommendations, and are often carrying increased risks; to miss these facts in guidelines is unacceptable. Guidelines cannot be expected to provide multiple recommendations for the often-huge variety of multimorbidity patterns and conditions that potentially interact with the major recommendations in guidelines. Yet, comments on this problem are essential to avoid the impression that these guidelines claim validity for all cases. Under any circumstance, guidelines should only claim validity for the exemplary and most commonly found patients or clinical situations. Clarity on this most significant, often-misunderstood, and puzzling issue is unfortunately missing in most current guidelines.

Differentiated Evaluation of Defined Drugs

The evaluation of risk-benefit ratio differs between drug groups. It also differs between elderly and younger adults because of reduced functionality, life expectancy, and resources. However, the risk-benefit ratio cannot easily be given by standardized values such as score values or ratios in every case, although for closely defined events this can be calculated from the constructs "number needed to treat" and "number needed to harm." Unfortunately, these data are often missing (e.g., delirium), and in practice, multiple risks have to be integrated and weighed against expected treatment benefits. A differentiated risk-benefit ratio for the elderly and certain subgroups therein, like frail elderly or those with cognitive impairment, is even more difficult to describe. In reflection of these limitations, two more feasible strategies are employed in the differentiated evaluation of drugs.

Evaluation of appropriateness of drugs for the elderly is done following two principles:

- Identification of drugs that are generally inappropriate for this patient population
- Building categories from critical to beneficial with regard to prescribing in the elderly

The first strategy has been recommended and forwarded for several years by promoting the so-called Beers list (see chapters "Critical Extrapolation of Guidelines and Study Results: Risk-Benefit Assessment for Patients with Reduced Life Expectancy and a New Classification of Drugs According to Their Fitness for the Aged" and "Inappropriate medication and medication errors in the elderly"). The Beers list summarizes drugs to ban from medication schedules in the elderly. The second strategy is more complex and instrumentalized by the Fit for the Aged (FORTA) classification (see chapter "Critical Extrapolation of Guidelines and Study Results: Risk-Benefit Assessment for Patients with Reduced Life Expectancy and a New Classification of Drugs According to Their Fitness for the Aged") proposed in this book. This approach builds categories from unavoidable or "prescribe just as in younger adults" to critical or "avoid if possible due to inacceptable high risk in the elderly." Both strategies will await further developments and discussion and may complement each other.

Agreed Lists of Potentially Inappropriate Medications in the Elderly

A popular strategy is to acknowledge the risk of inappropriate medications in the elderly and build a list of most critical drugs, the so-called PIM (potentially inappropriate medication). To form such a list, usually a Delphi-type procedure is applied to bring together several experts in the field. However, these lists and the herein given consent still represent expert opinions and do not necessarily rely on evidence based on higher-ranked sources such as randomized controlled trials (RCTs). Another shortcoming is the limited scope of such lists. Only a minority of drugs is consensually regarded as inappropriate, and the majority of outcomes of the Delphi process will read "depends on." Finally, due to regional specialties of the market, the global validity and utility of these lists have to be questioned.

There are several different lists proposed and in common use. The most cited and recommended still is the Beers list from the United States, first published in 1997 (Beers 1997) and reevaluated in 2003 (Fick et al. 2003). Later, additional lists were developed and published to implement local specialties or focusing on special populations such as nursing home residents. In Western Europe (Germany), the PRISCUS list adapted this process to regional aspects and was published in 2010 (Holt et al. 2010). There are some discrepancies between these two lists explained not only by different drug availabilities but also depending on different prevalent opinions and usages (e.g., amiodarone, haloperidol). In Europe, to our current knowledge local lists were also developed in France (Laroche et al. 2007), Italy (Maio et al. 2010), and Norway (Rognstad et al. 2009), as well as in Thailand (Winit-Watjana et al. 2007) and in Canada (Rancourt et al. 2004). Gallagher et al. extended this approach to Ireland and the United Kingdom and provided not only a consensus-based list of inappropriate medication to avoid in the elderly, but also a list of essential drugs to start with; this approach is called the STOPP/START (Screening Tool of Older Persons' Prescriptions/Screening Tool to Alert Doctors to Right Treatment) concept. It is also based on physiology and provides some links to recommendations of defined diseases and related guidelines (Gallagher et al. 2008). It thus represents a hybrid approach.

Lists of inappropriate medications in the elderly have been evaluated and applied to different subpopulations to reduce drug risk and critical incidents of side effects. Most often Beers' criteria have been used to evaluate prevalence and significance of inappropriate medications. Furthermore, these lists are used to reduce polypharmacy. However, results concerning clinical endpoints are not

Table 2 Categories to stratify patients according to resources and vulnerability

Category	Criteria	Comments
"Go go" (go forward with standard treatment)	Patients without comorbidities or functional decline	Initially defined to identify patients undergoing standard chemotherapy treatment, may also applied to other forms of treatment to characterize those elderly in whom standard treatment can be applied
"Slow go" (adapt standard treatment)	Patient does not meet criteria of go go or those of no go, 1–2 comorbidities may be present or 1–2 deficits in IADL domains	Initially defined to characterize patients with some limitations in physiology in whom adaption of chemotherapy dosage has to be performed, functionally not severely impaired
"No go" (standard treatment often no longer applicable, control of symptoms remains the primary treatment goal)	Patients fulfill criteria of the frailty syndrome: they show deficits in at least 1 ADL domain or disclose 3 and more active comorbidities or they present at least 1 fully diagnosed geriatric syndrome	A rather wide range of geriatric patients will fulfill these criteria; a single ADL value does not sufficiently describe this category, a complex pattern of both comorbidities and functional limitations has to be considered instead. Initially this definition should define patients in whom a primarily palliative approach to disease management is to be preferred

ADL activity of daily living, *IADL* instrumental activity of daily living

homogeneous. Fick et al. demonstrated a beneficial effect on fall incidents and hospitalization by closely applying the Beers list (Fick et al. 2001), whereas Hanlon et al. failed to describe an additional benefit after controlling for several additional risk factors in a cohort of ambulatory elderly (Hanlon et al. 2002). In conclusion, this approach still represents an important tool to identify at least the most inappropriate drugs in the elderly, especially in frail elderly with multimorbidity, and thereby reduce total drug burden and polypharmacy. More details are given in chapter "Critical Extrapolation of Guidelines and Study Results: Risk-Benefit Assessment for Patients with Reduced Life Expectancy and a New Classification of Drugs According to Their Fitness for the Aged."

Evaluation of Patients Regarding Their Vulnerability

Drugs are not the only factors to be evaluated in the algorithm mentioned. Patients' vulnerability and patient-related aspects like special barriers and adherence problems have to be addressed as well. In this context, categories to depict vulnerability and expected risk rates of individual treatment modalities are comprehensive tools to guide treatment decisions. In this context, the frailty concept represents a powerful treatment-modifying strategy. Another quite similar strategy may be adapted from oncology in that it has been proposed to stratify patient groups according to the expected treatment risk (Balducci and Extermann 2000). The authors proposed three categories to decide if an individual patient should undergo scheduled standard chemotherapy or not (Table 2). These very simple categories may also serve as templates for groups carrying different risk burdens in the context of general pharmacotherapy. Patients classified as "no go" are carrying the highest risk for ADRs or treatment failure. Recent developments aim at integrating aspects from geriatric assessment to give more concrete and practicable instructions to identify the vulnerable patients at risk correctly (Wedding et al. 2007; Balducci et al.

Table 3 Some rules to successfully prescribe medications in elderly

Rules	Comments
Complete history of current medication (including self-purchased and self-administered medication)	Many patients use OTC drugs or herbal medicine that also may also cause ADR and interactions
Ask actively for already occurred ADR	Elderly patients often do not recognize symptoms as ADR of medication (e.g., dizziness, loss of appetite)
Carefully verify indication	If uncertain try nonpharmacological measures first
Start low, go slow (low starting dose, prolonged dosage escalation interval)	This rule respects frequently found changes in pharmacokinetics. Initially used in the context of establishing long-term pharmacotherapy it does not conflict with "hit hard and early" in case of acute crisis (e.g., infectious disease)
Check for adequate dosage	
Avoid halving of pills	Halving carries a marked risk of dosage failure and may be impossible for a majority of elderly patients due to functional limitations (as it is difficult even for younger adults)
Empower adherence (communicate clear treatment goals)	Respectful and transparent communication with patients concerning drugs and associated risks and benefits is the treatment baseline of an adequate treatment schedule
Be careful with newly developed drugs	Newly developed drugs are often not studied in elderly and may be critical especially for frail elderly
Critical reappraisal of a medication schedule after every hospital discharge or consultation of an additional physician, if necessary discuss every newly added medication	Sequential and simultaneous treatment by different physicians may cause communication problems and may also produce unnecessary polypharmacy
Regular critical reappraisal of medication schedule	Frequently missed in clinical practice
Drug monitoring and monitoring of functional state	Not only drug levels may change but also functional state may change over time and cause severe adherence problems
Discontinue medication if no longer needed	Drug therapy often is unnecessarily prolonged because discontinuation is missed (e.g., prolonged prescription of metoclopramide to control short-time nausea, no step down in PPI treatment of gastroesophageal reflux)
Avoid medication with increased ADR risk in the elderly	FORTA categories and lists of PIM help to identify critical versus beneficial drugs, ADR potential has to be considered prior to prescription

ADR adverse drug reaction, *FORTA* Fit for the Aged, *OTC* over the counter, *PIM* potentially inappropriate medication, *PPI* proton pump inhibitor

2010). These criteria are mentioned and commented in Table 2. An essential overlap with the frailty concept is found, and further developments will be expected also to integrate measures for frailty into this concept.

General Rules Concerning Pharmacotherapy in Elderly

Finally, some simple rules may help to realize comprehensive pharmacotherapy in the elderly, including the frail and vulnerable. Some of those are summarized in Table 3 (see also chapter "Critical Extrapolation of Guidelines and Study Results: Risk-Benefit Assessment for Patients with Reduced Life Expectancy and a New Classification of Drugs According to Their Fitness for the Aged"). Most of them are derived from clinical practice, where comprehensive decision making in the context of polypharmacy is often challenging. In apparent contrast, some of these rules seem primarily very simple, but they reflect major features of inappropriate drug prescriptions. Physicians need to realize that drug prescription in most cases goes far beyond an "easy-to-do" intervention and may be followed by unforesee-able cascades of unwanted effects and incidents. This is even more true for treating and managing patients with chronic rather than acute disease.

The rule most often cited, "start slow, go slow," definitively is mentioned to start treatment of a chronic disease (e.g., control of hyperten-sion). It does not contradict "hit hard and early," a rule that mostly applies to acute treatment situations (e.g., pneumonia). In the same patient, both rules may be true and applicable; it depends on the given clinical situation.

In the context of polypharmacy, the most sig-nificant rules are

- Make a regular reassessment of the patient and his or her situation
- Always try to discuss current medication with the patient
- Try to find the best solution for the individual health situation together with the patient.

In the end, both physician and patient should realize what should be achieved and how to get there. Both should be aware of the risk that may be associated with treatment and how to overcome it.

References

Balducci L, Extermann M (2000) Management of cancer in the older person: a practical approach. Oncologist 5:224–237

Balducci L, Colloca G, Cesari M, Gambassi G (2010) Assessment and treatment of elderly patients with cancer. Surg Oncol 19:117–123

Beers MH (1997) Explicit criteria for determining poten-tially inappropriate medication use by the elderly. An update. Arch Intern Med 157:1531–1536

Boyd CM, Darer J, Boult C, Fried LP, Boult L, Wu AW (2005) Clinical practice guidelines and quality of care for older patients with multiple comorbid dis-eases: implications for pay for performance. JAMA 294:716–724

Bushardt RL, Massey EB, Simpson TW, Ariail JC, Simp-son KN (2008) Polypharmacy: misleading, but man-ageable. Clin Interv Aging 3:383–389

Chutka DS, Takahashi PY, Hoel RW (2004) Inappropri-ate medications for elderly patients. Mayo Clin Proc 79:122–139

Fick DM, Waller JL, Maclean JR et al (2001) Potentially inappropriate medication use in a managed care popu-lation: association with higher costs and utilization. J Manag Care Pharm 7:407–413

Fick DM, Cooper JW, Wade WE, Waller JL, Maclean JR, Beers MH (2003) Updating the Beers criteria for potentially inappropriate medication use in older adults: results of a U.S. consensus panel of experts. Arch Intern Med 163:2716–2724

Flockhart DA (2007) Drug interactions: cytochrome P450 drug interaction table. Indiana University School of Medicine. http://medicine.iupui.edu/clinpharm/ddis/table.aspx. Accessed 7 Oct 2011

Gallagher P, Ryan C, Byrne S, Kennedy J, O'Mahony D (2008) STOPP (Screening Tool of Older Persons' Prescriptions) and START (Screening Tool to Alert Doctors to Right Treatment): consensus validation. Int J Clin Pharmacol Ther 46:72–83

Garfinkel D, Zur-Gil S, Ben-Israel J (2007) The war against polypharmacy: a new cost-effective geriatric-palliative approach for improving drug therapy in disabled elderly people. Isr Med Assoc J 9:430–434

Gillick MR (2006) The denial of aging. Harvard Univer-sity Press, Cambridge

Glaeske G, Hoffmann F (2009) Der Wettbewerb der Lei-tlinien bei älteren Menschen—Multimorbidität und Polypharmazie als Problem. Neuro Geriatrie 6:115–119, in German

Gurwitz JH (2004) Polypharmacy. A new paradigm for quality drug therapy in the elderly? Arch Intern Med 164:1957–1959

Hanlon JT, Fillenbaum GG, Kuchibhatla M et al (2002) Impact of inappropriate drug use on mortality and functional status in representative community dwell-ing elders. Med Care 40:166–176

Holt S, Schmiedl S, Thürmann PA (2010) Potentially inappropriate medications in the elderly: the PRIS-CUS list. Dtsch Arztebl Int 107:543–551

Laroche ML, Charmes JP, Merle L (2007) Potentially inappropriate medications in the elderly: a French con-sensus panel list. Eur J Clin Pharmacol 63:725–731

Maio V, Del Canale S, Abouzaid S, Investigators GAP (2010) Using explicit criteria to evaluate the quality of prescribing in elderly Italian outpatients: a cohort study. J Clin Pharm Ther 35:219–229

National Center for Health Statistics (1996) National Health and Nutrition Examination Survey (NHANES) III. http://www.cdc.gov/nchs/nhanes/nh3data.htm. Accessed 11 Jan 2010

Palareti G, Legnani C (1996) Warfarin withdrawal—pharmacokinetic-pharmacodynamic considerations. Clin Pharmacokinet 30:300–313

Podrazik PM, Schwartz JB (1999) Cardiovascular phar-macology of aging. Cardiol Clin 17:17–34

Rancourt C, Moisan J, Baillargeon L, Verreault R, Laurin D, Grégoire JP (2004) Potentially inappropriate pre-scriptions for older patients in long-term care. BMC Geriatr 4:9

Rochon PA, Gurwitz JH (1997) Optimising drug treat-ment for elderly people: the prescribing cascade. BMJ 315:1096–1099

Rognstad S, Brekke M, Fetveit A, Spigset O, Wyller TB, Straand J (2009) The Norwegian General Practice

(NORGEP) criteria for assessing potentially inappropriate prescriptions to elderly patients. A modified Delphi study. Scand J Prim Health Care 27:153–159

Rollason V, Vogt N (2003) Reduction of polypharmacy in the elderly. Drugs Aging 20:817–832

Semla TP, Beizer JL, Higbee MD (2011) Geriatric dosage handbook. LexiComp, Hudson

Steinhagen-Thiessen E, Borchelt M (2001) Morbidity, medication, and functional limitations in very old age. In: Baltes PB (ed) The Berlin aging study, aging from 70 to 100. Cambridge University Press, Cambridge, UK

Stuck A, Kharicha K, Dapp U et al (2007) Development, feasibility and performance of a health risk appraisal questionnaire for older persons. BMC Med Res Methodol 7:1

Wedding U, Honecker F, Bokemeyer C, Pientka L, Höffken K (2007) Tolerance to chemotherapy in elderly patients with cancer. Cancer Control 14:44–56

Wehling M (2011) Guideline-driven polypharmacy in elderly, multimorbid patients is basically flawed: there are almost no guidelines for these patients. J Am Geriatr Soc 59:376–377

Winit-Watjana W, Sakulrat P, Kespichayawattana J (2007) Criteria for high-risk medication use in Thai older patients. Arch Gerontol Geriatr 47:35–51

Inappropriate Prescribing in the Hospitalized Elderly Patient

Robert Lee Page 2nd and John Mark Ruscin

Defining Inappropriate Prescribing in the Hospital Setting

The medication use process is a varied and complex progression of steps that begin with *prescribing* from a health care provider to *communicating* orders to a nurse or pharmacist, *dispensing* by a pharmacist, and *administering* either by a patient's caregiver or the patient (Institute of Medicine 1999; Page et al. 2010).

Brook et al. noted that the appropriate use of a medication warrants that the potential benefit of the medication outweighs its potential risk (Brook et al. 1990). Therefore, appropriate evaluation of risk versus benefit at the point of prescribing is critical. The term *potentially inappropriate prescribing* encompasses when a medication's use introduces a significant risk of an adverse drug event (ADE) when a potentially equal or more effective medication with a possibly lower-risk profile exists (Page et al. 2010; Gallagher et al. 2011). In addition, inappropriate prescribing includes situations where a clinically indicated medication is overused at a higher dose or frequency or for a longer duration than is indicated, underused based on agist or irrational reasons, omitted in the absence of a contraindication, or prescribed in combination with other medications with documented drug-drug or drug-disease interactions (Gallagher et al. 2011). The last description raises the concern that any prescribed medication may become a potentially inappropriate medication (PIM) when used in an inappropriate manner.

When compared to younger adults, it is not surprising that inappropriate prescribing commonly occurs in older adults (e.g., ≥ 65 years of age) due to their higher prevalence of comorbidities, disability, medication burden, and dependency. A large number of studies have shown that PIM prescribing in this population occurs in the ambulatory setting, nursing home, and the emergency department (ED) leading to an increase in costly ADEs, hospitalizations, ED visits, as well as overall morbidity and mortality (Cahir et al. 2010; Dedhiya et al. 2010; Fick et al. 2008; Gallagher et al. 2011; Lund et al. 2010; Page et al. 2010). However, few data exist regarding potentially inappropriate prescribing in the inpatient setting and its impact on health outcomes. Presently, older adults account for over 35% of annual hospital admissions and are at higher risk for hospital readmission (Hanlon et al. 2004; Onder et al. 2003; Rothberg et al. 2008). In an analysis of fee-for-service Medicare beneficiaries, 19.6% of older adults who had been discharged from a hospital were

R.L. Page 2nd (✉)
Department of Clinical Pharmacy, University of Colorado Skaggs School of Pharmacy and Pharmaceutical Sciences, Mail Stop C238, 12850 E Montview Blvd. V20-4125, Aurora, CO 80045, USA
e-mail: robert.page@ucdenver.edu

J.M. Ruscin
Department of Internal Medicine, SIU School of Medicine, 701 N. 1st Street, Springfield, IL 62702, USA
e-mail: mruscin@siumed.edu

rehospitalized within 30 days and 34.0% within 90 days (Jencks et al. 2009). The hospital setting is especially perilous for the older adult as this environment has been associated with a higher incidence of adverse health outcomes, such as functional decline, delirium, infection, falls, and ADEs (Friedman et al. 2008). In a meta-analysis of 39 prospective studies from U.S. hospitals, Lazarou et al. found the overall incidence of serious and fatal ADEs in hospitalized patients was 6.7% and 0.32%, respectively, which is slightly higher that what has been documented in outpatient settings (Lazarou et al. 1998). In addition, the inpatient setting may expose older adults to new and possibly unnecessary medications, multiple providers and specialists, and restrictive hospital formularies that warrant reconciliation of home medications. Data suggest that the percentage of patients suffering medication reconciliation errors at hospital admission can be as high as 30–65% (Coleman et al. 2005; Climente-Marti et al. 2010). The overall prevalence of PIM prescribing in the inpatient setting varies dramatically from 1% to as high as 50% and is highly dependent on the tool used to define the PIM (Franceschi et al. 2008; Rothberg et al. 2008).

Risk Factors for PIM Prescribing

While no research has yet identified clear risk factors to PIM prescribing in the hospitalized older adult, it is possible to extrapolate from an evaluation of the root causes to develop a potential list.

Advanced age and changes in drug metabolism. With advanced age and acuity of illness come significant alterations in the pharmacokinetics (drug absorption, distribution, metabolism, and excretion) and pharmacodynamics (physiologic effects of the drug) of medications that alter dosing and even choice of pharmacotherapy. Lean body mass and total body water decrease with a relative increase in total body fat, leading to decreased volume of distribution for drugs with a hydrophilic, narrow therapeutic index such as digoxin. Other drugs such as

benzodiazepines have an increased volume of distribution that slows their rapid onset but could lead to dangerous accumulation with prolonged use. With a reduction in first pass through the liver, drugs such as beta-blockers, nitrates, antipsychotics, and tricyclic antidepressants (TCAs) have a higher bioavailability, warranting lower doses. Doses of drugs cleared renally that are typically used in the inpatient setting, such as aminoglycoside, digoxin, dabigatran, milrinone, and histamine type 2 receptor blockers, need to be adjusted. Other changes, such as decreased serum albumin, can effect medications that are highly protein bound and with a narrow therapeutic index, such as warfarin, digoxin, and phenytoin, leading to greater unbound drug exposure. The central nervous system becomes more vulnerable to agents that may have an impact on brain function (e.g., opioids, benzodiazepines, and psychotropic drugs). Also, decreased physiologic reserves related to aging and acute illness necessitate ongoing evaluation of medications for PIMs throughout the acute stay as condition status changes.

Complexity of medications. As a patient transitions into the hospital setting, medication reconciliation of home medications should be conducted. Based on a survey of 3,500 community-dwelling older adults, 29% took five or more prescription medications, 42% at least one or more over-the-counter medications, and 49% at least one or more nutritional supplement (Qato et al. 2008). Each of these medications will need to be reconciled and possibly switched to a formulary medication. In this process, potential prescribing or transcribing errors may occur. Discrepancies between the medications patients were taking prior to admission and their admission orders ranged up to 70% (Cornish et al. 2005; Gleason et al. 2004; Greenwald et al. 2010). Several studies have suggested that up to 60% of patients admitted to the hospital will have at least one discrepancy in their admission medication history (Lau et al. 2000; Beers et al. 1990). In a prospective evaluation of 525 admissions to a general internal medicine ward in a single institution, Cornish et al.

found that 54% of patients had at least one medication discrepancy, of which 38.6% had the potential to cause moderate-to-severe discomfort or clinical deterioration (Cornish et al. 2005). Following hospital discharge, the perpetuation of these errors may result in drug interactions, therapeutic duplication, other unintended adverse events, and additional costs. During hospitalization, additional medications may be added to the patients' medical regimen. Goldberg and colleagues found that patients taking two drugs faced a 13% risk of an adverse drug-drug interaction (Goldberg et al. 1996). This figure rises to 38% for four drugs and up to 82% if seven or more drugs are administered simultaneously.

Increased comorbidity burden. Among older adults (>65 years of age), 72% present with at least two or more chronic conditions, compared with 42% of patients between the ages of 45 and 64 years (Anderson 2007). Among adults aged 80 and older, 93% have at least one chronic condition, and 78% have two or more. Over two thirds of all U.S. Medicare spending is for older adults with five or more chronic conditions (Anderson 2007). In the hospital, the pervasiveness of comorbidity is particularly high. Sixty percent of inpatients have at least one comorbidity, and 37% have two or more (Merrill and Elixhauser 2002). With an increase in comorbidity burden comes additional exposure to a larger number of medications as well as new prescribers and specialists. In an evaluation of Medicare beneficiaries with heart failure, Page et al. found that a patient may encounter between 15 and 23 different providers within a given year in both the inpatient and outpatient settings. This scenario demands communication between providers, flawless transitions of care, and overall accurate coordination of transitions of care. Failure in any of these steps could lead to duplication of medication, prescribing of unnecessary medications, and drug-drug interactions (Page et al. 2010).

Tools for Identification and Evaluation of PIM Prescribing

Medication appropriateness can be assessed by process or outcome measures that are explicit (criterion based) or implicit (judgment based) (Spinewine et al. 2007).

– *Explicit Evaluation.* Explicit indicators are typically developed from published reviews, expert opinions, and consensus techniques. Measures are drug or disease oriented. While easy to apply and implement, these measures require little to no clinical judgment and ignore indicators of health care as defined by national guidelines for an individual patient. These measures may not address patient preference or the overall burden of the individual patient's comorbidities or acuity of illness.

– *Implicit Evaluation.* Implicit indicators take into account patient-specific information and published evidence to form judgments regarding appropriateness. The focus is placed on the patient rather than on just specific drugs or diseases. While time consuming, these measures can address patient preference and burden of comorbidities but depend highly on the user's knowledge and access to patient-specific information.

Several tools exist to evaluate PIM prescribing (Dimitrow et al. 2011).

Chapter "Inappropriate Medication Use and Medication Errors in the Elderly" reviews each of these tools as well as their advantages and disadvantages. Listed next are the more commonly used explicit and implicit tools with published data in the inpatient setting:

– *Explicit*: The Beers criteria, Improved Prescribing in the Elderly Tool (IPET), Screening Tool to Alert to Right Treatment (START)/ Screening Tool of Older Adults (STOPP), and the Health Plan Employer Data and Information Set Drugs to Be Avoided in the Elderly (HEDIS-DAE)

– *Implicit*: Medication Appropriateness Index (MAI).

Data Using Explicit and Implicit Tools in the Hospital Setting

Beers Criteria. In the United States, the Beers criteria have become the most popular and accepted explicit tool used for evaluating PIM prescribing. Many American health plans and pharmacy benefit programs have adopted these criteria, or a modification of them, to help identify and target older adults at risk of an ADE. Numerous studies have used the Beers criteria to identify and evaluate PIM prescribing in the inpatient setting. Using the Beers criteria, Gallagher et al. evaluated 597 admissions in an Irish university teaching hospital for PIMs and their impact on ADEs (Gallagher et al. 2008). These investigators found that inappropriate prescribing occurred in 32% of patients with 24%, 6%, and 2% receiving one, two, or three inappropriate medications, respectively. Compared to patients taking five or less medications, those who received six or more medications had a three-fold higher odds of receiving a medication on the Beers criteria ($p < 0.001$). Forty-nine percent of patients receiving at least one medication on the Beers criteria were admitted with an ADE, while 16% of all admissions were associated with an ADE. In a U.S. study, Rothberg et al. found that of 493,971 hospitalized older adults, 49% received at least one inappropriate medication per the Beers criteria and 6% three or more medications (Rothberg et al. 2008). In a prospective cohort study, Morandi et al. used the Beers criteria to appraise medication appropriateness in 120 critically ill older adults admitted to a medical, surgical, or cardiovascular intensive care unit (ICU) for shock or respiratory failure (Morandi et al. 2011). The investigators found that 66% of patients were prescribed at least one PIM prior to admission, which increased to 85% at hospital discharge. The number of patients with three or more PIMs increased from 16% prior to admission to 37% at discharge. At discharge, 50% of all PIMs

were first prescribed in the ICU compared to 20% on the hospital wards and 21% before admission. However, controversy exists regarding exposure to PIMs and develop of an ADE. In a study of 389 older inpatients admitted to a single university teaching hospital, Page and Ruscin found while 27.5% of inpatients were administered a PIM per the Beers criteria, only 9.2% of ADEs were attributed to a Beers criteria medication (Page and Ruscin 2006). After controlling for covariates, exposure to a Beers criteria medication was not significantly associated with ADEs, discharge to a higher level of care, or in-hospital mortality. A larger Italian study including over 5,000 patients reported similar results, failing to find an association between the use of PIMs (as defined by Beers) and risk of ADEs, length of stay, or in-hospital mortality (Onder et al. 2005).

IPET. The IPET was initially validated in a Canadian prospective study of acutely hospitalized elderly patients that identified PIM prescribing in 12.5% of patients (Naugler et al. 2000). Outside Canada, little use of this instrument exists. However, a single Irish study did demonstrate that 22% of acutely hospitalized older adults received at least one PIM at the point of admission (Barry et al. 2006).

START/STOPP. Using the STOPP and Beers criteria, Gallagher et al. evaluated for PIM prescribing and related ADEs in 715 older patients admitted to a single university teaching hospital in Ireland (Gallagher and O'Mahony D. 2008). The STOPP identified 336 PIMs affecting 35% of patients, one third of whom presented with an associated ADE, while the Beers criteria identified 226 PIMs affecting 25% of patients, of whom 43% presented with an associated ADE. Using the STOPP criteria, PIMs contributed to 11.5% of all admissions, while the Beers criteria-related PIMs contributed to significantly fewer admissions (6%). The therapeutic classes of medications identified by the STOPP criteria consisted of long-acting benzodiazepines, TCAs with clear-cut contra-indications, first-generation antihistamines, vasodilator drugs known to cause hypotension in patients with persistent postural hypotension, inappropriate use of nonsteroidal anti-inflammatory drugs (NSAIDs) and opiates, and duplicate drug class prescriptions, such as two angiotensin-converting enzyme inhibitors, two NSAIDs, two selective serotonin reuptake inhibitors, or dual antiplatelet therapy without indication. Hamilton et al. evaluated the use of the STOPP criteria in 600 older adults who were admitted with an acute illness to a university teaching hospital over a 4-month interval (Hamilton et al. 2011). The purpose of the study was to assess whether PIMs defined by the STOPP were associated with ADEs. Of the 600 patients, the STOPP criteria detected 329 ADEs in 158 patients (26.3%). Of these ADEs, 219 were considered contributory or causal to admission and either avoidable or potentially avoidable. After controlling for covariates, prescribing of a medication from the STOPP criteria was associated with a 1.87 increased risk of an ADE ($p < 0.001$). Using the Beers criteria in the same population, the investigators did find a significant association with an increased ADE risk when a Beers criteria medication was prescribed.

HEDIS-DAE. With the implementation of the Medicare Part D drug benefit in 2006, the National Committee for Quality Assurance (NCQA) announced in 2005 that it would adopt a DAE (Drugs to Avoid in the Elderly) list. Based on expert panel recommendations, the Beers criteria medications were classified and grouped into three categories: always avoid, rarely appropriate, and some indications. Of the tools discussed thus far, the HEDIS-DAE is the most recently conceived and is updated annually. While this tool is used extensively by Medicare Part D plans and national reporting by the NCQA to assess PIM prescribing, limited data exist regarding the use of this tool in the inpatient setting (Luo et al. 2011; Pugh et al. 2006, 2011).

Nonetheless, based on NCQA data between 2005 and 2008, approximately 23–24% of all U.S. Medicare beneficiaries received at least one of the HEDIS-DAE annually, and 6% received two or more DAE annually (Curtiss and Fairman 2011).

MAI. The MAI is the only implicit approach that warrants application of clinical judgment and then assesses elements of prescribing: indication, effectiveness, dose, correct directions, practical directions, drug-drug interactions, drug disease interactions, duplication, duration, and cost. In an evaluation by Hanlon et al., the investigators evaluated 11 Veterans Affairs Medical Centers involving 397 frail elderly inpatients. Ninety-two percent of subjects had received at least one drug with one or more inappropriate ratings (Hanlon et al. 2004). The most widespread problems involved expensive drugs (70%), impractical directions (55.2%), and incorrect dosages (50.9%). The most prevalent therapeutic classes with appropriateness concerns consisted of gastric (50.6%), cardiovascular (47.6%), and central nervous system (23.9%) agents. Using the MAI, Hajjar and colleagues found that 44% of frail elderly inpatients had at least one unnecessary medication at discharge (Hajjar et al. 2005). The contributing factors most commonly associated with unnecessary drug prescribing consisted of hypertension diagnosis, multiple prescribers, and nine or more medications.

The MAI has also been used in combination with other explicit tools, such as the START/STOPP criteria. In a randomized controlled trial, Gallagher et al. evaluated whether implementation of the STOPP/START criteria (intervention) improved prescribing appropriateness compared to usual pharmaceutical care (control) in 400 hospitalized older adults (Gallagher et al. 2011). The MAI and the Assessment of Underutilization (AOU) index were employed at the time of discharge and for 6 months after discharge. At the time of admission, the frequency of unnecessary polypharmacy (e.g., absence of indication, lack of efficacy, or therapeutic duplication) was similar between groups (19.0% [$n = 268$] in the control group and 20.0% [$n = 308$] in the intervention group [$p = 0.459$]), but changed to 19.8% ($n = 306$) and 5.4% ($n = 80$%), respectively ($p < 0.0001$) at discharge. Use of the STOPP/START criteria resulted in 169 improvements in these MAI criteria in the intervention group. The absolute reduction in potential drug-drug interactions from admission to discharge was 1.8% ($n = 27$) in the control and 3.3% ($n = 47$) in the intervention group. For potential drug-disease interactions, the absolute reduction was 5% ($n = 72$) in the control group and 11.2% ($n = 157$) in the intervention group. At discharge, the MAI scores had declined in 33.3% ($n = 64$) of the control group compared to only 11.5% ($n = 22$) in the intervention, which was primarily driven by domains of cost and practicality. Overall, compared to the control group, unnecessary polypharmacy, the use of drugs at incorrect doses, and potential drug-drug and drug-disease interactions were significantly lower in the intervention group (absolute risk reduction 35.7% [95% confidence interval, CI: 26.3–44.9%], number needed to screen to yield improvement in the MAI = 2.8 [95% CI: 2.2–3.8]).

Comparison of Explicit and Implicit Tools in the Hospital Setting

Presently, one study has compared the use and capability of explicit and implicit tools in assessing changes in medication appropriateness in elderly patients admitted to the hospital (Luo et al. 2011). In a retrospective observational study in two hospitals in Northern Ireland, Luo et al. evaluated the MAI, Beers criteria, IPET, and HEDIS-DAE in 192 older inpatients. Evaluations were made at three points during the patients' hospitalization: admission, during the inpatient stay, and at discharge. While time consuming, the MAI was considered to be the most comprehensive approach to assessing PIM pre-

scribing, while the HEDIS-DAE was the easiest to use as diagnosis did not have to be evaluated. Overall, in the use of the MAI, Beers criteria, and IPET, all significantly improved medication appropriateness over the three evaluation points ($p < 0.001$, $p < 0.05$, $p < 0.05$, respectively), while improvement was not demonstrated with the HEDIS-DAE. Exposure to a PIM as defined by the Beers criteria and the IPET had a positive relationship with the MAI scores.

Methods for Reducing PIM Prescribing in the Hospital Setting and Future Challenges

It seems clear that no one specific tool is optimal to identify and prevent PIMs in the acute care setting. Preventing PIM prescribing utilizing available tools in and of itself will not accomplish the ultimate objective. Disagreement among clinicians regarding what medications should be included as PIMs, along with the general lack of clear evidence to associate PIMs to definite harm, prevent the practical utilization of available tools as evidence-based clinical guidelines (Curtiss and Fairman 2011). In a recently published study utilizing adverse event data from the National Electronic Injury Surveillance System-Cooperative Adverse Event Surveillance project, annual national estimates for the frequency and rates of hospitalization following emergency department visits for adverse drug events among older adults ($\geq$65 years of age) were reported (Budnitz et al. 2011). The combination of warfarin, insulins, oral antiplatelet agents, and oral hypoglycemic agents accounted for more than two thirds of hospitalizations due to adverse drug events. In the same study using the same data set, Beers criteria medications accounted for only 6.6% of hospitalizations, and HEDIS-DAE accounted for only 1.2% of hospitalizations due to adverse drug reactions. In fact, warfarin, which is not considered a PIM, accounted for a full one third of the hospitalizations by itself. When digoxin was excluded from the Beers criteria list, only 3.2% of hospitalizations were attributed to medications appearing among the list. Similar, but smaller, studies have also implicated anticoagulants and antidiabetic medications as common causes of ADE-induced hospitalization (McDonnell and Jacobs 2002; Wu and Panteleo 2003). Studies evaluating the use of PIMs in the acute care setting have similarly not demonstrated a significant association between the use of PIMs and ADEs or other negative outcomes of hospitalization (Onder et al. 2005; Page et al. 2008). Furthermore, whether the inpatient setting is the optimal place to improve the appropriateness of chronic care medications is a question for debate. It is often difficult to convince physicians to change or discontinue chronic care medications in the acute care setting, particularly if the medication in question is not related to the reason for admission.

The use of explicit criteria as a means of screening for PIMs, along with continuous and vigilant monitoring for drug appropriateness of all prescribed medications (using the implicit principles outlined with the MAI), would seemingly do much more to prevent drug-related morbidity and mortality among older adults in the acute care setting. The utilization of electronic health records and computerized physician order entry provides additional opportunities to address appropriate prescribing. Medication-specific warning systems regarding high-risk prescribing at the point of order entry has been shown to be an effective method of reducing PIM prescribing (Mattison et al. 2010). In addition, the further development of effective and practical inpatient medication reconciliation processes will contribute significantly to medication safety, both during acute care stays and following discharge (Greenwald et al. 2010). Utilization of technology, such as with electronic personal health applications, may provide opportunities to enhance accuracy and safety in the acute care setting and as patients transition from one setting to the next (Haverhals et al. 2011).

A more comprehensive definition of PIMs is required to adequately address the problem of drug-related morbidity and mortality among older adults. Adequate development, implementation, and evaluation of practical strategies on meaningful clinical and fiscal outcomes is needed to move the science forward with this vulnerable population. Broader-based interventions with shared responsibility along the multidisciplinary continuum of care among all health care professionals will become a necessity.

References

Anderson G (2007) Chronic conditions: making the case for ongoing care. http://www.rwjf.org/files/research/50968chronic.care.chartbook.ppt. Accessed 30 Nov 2011

Barry PJ, O'Keefe N, O'Connor KA, O'Mahony D (2006) Inappropriate prescribing in the elderly: a comparison of the Beers criteria and the improved prescribing in the elderly tool (IPET) in acutely ill elderly hospitalized patients. J Clin Pharm Ther 31:617–626

Beers MH, Munekata M, Storrie M (1990) The accuracy of medication histories in the hospital medical records of elderly persons. J Am Geriatr Soc 38:1183–1187

Brook RH, Kamberg CJ, Mayer-Oaks A et al (1990) Appropriateness of acute medical care for the elderly: an analysis of the literature. Health Policy 14:225–242

Budnitz DS, Lovegrove MC, Shehab N, Richards CL (2011) Emergency hospitalizations for adverse drug events in older Americans. N Engl J Med 365:2002–2012

Cahir C, Fahey T, Teeling M et al (2010) Potentially inappropriate prescribing and cost outcomes for older people: a national population study. Br J Clin Pharmacol 69:543–552

Climente-Marti M, Garcia-Manon ERG, Artero-Mora A, Jimenez-Torres NV (2010) Potential risk of medication discrepancies and reconciliation errors at admission and discharge from an inpatient medical service. Ann Pharmacother 44:1747–1754

Coleman EA, Smith JD, Raha D, Min SJ (2005) Posthospital medication discrepancies: prevalence and contributing factors. Arch Intern Med 165:1842–1847

Cornish PL, Knowles SR, Marchesano R et al (2005) Unintended medication discrepancies at the time of hospital admission. Arch Intern Med 165:424–429

Curtiss FR, Fairman KA (2011) Protecting patients from adverse drug events: propoxyphene, PIMs, and drugs to avoid in older adults. J Manag Care Pharm 17:60–68

Dedhiya SD, Hancock E, Craig BA et al (2010) Incident use and outcomes associated with potentially inappropriate medication use in older adults. Am J Geriatr Pharmacother 8:562–570

Dimitrow MS, Airaksinen MSA, Kivela SL et al (2011) Comparison of prescribing criteria to evaluate the appropriateness of drug treatment in individuals aged 65 and older: a systematic review. J Am Geriatr Soc 59:1521–1530

Fick DM, Mion LC, Beers MH, Waller JL (2008) Health outcomes associated with potentially inappropriate medication use in older adults. Res Nurs Health 31:42–51

Franceschi M, Scarcelli C, Niro V et al (2008) Prevalence, clinical features and avoidability of adverse drug reactions as cause of admission to a geriatric unit: a prospective study of 1756 patients. Drug Saf 31:545–556

Friedman SM, Mendelson DA, Bingham KW, et al (2008) Hazards of hospitalization: residence prior to admission predicts outcome. The Gerontologist 48:537–541

Gallagher P, O'Mahony D (2008) STOPP (Screening Tool of Older Persons' potentially inappropriate prescriptions): application to acutely ill elderly patients and comparison with Beers' criteria. Age Ageing 37:673–679

Gallagher PF, Barry PJ, Ryan C et al (2008) Inappropriate prescribing in an acutely ill population of elderly patients as determined by Beers' criteria. Age Ageing 37:96–101

Gallagher PF, O'Connor MN, O'Mahony D (2011) Prevention of potentially inappropriate prescribing for elder patients: a randomized controlled trial using STOPP/START criteria. Clin Pharmacol Ther 89: 845–854

Gleason KM, Groszek JM, Sullivan C, Rooney D, Barnard C, Noskin GA (2004) Reconciliation of discrepancies in medication histories and admission orders of newly hospitalized patients. Am J Health Syst Pharm 61:1689–1695

Goldberg RM, Mabee J, Chan L, Wong S (1996) Drug-drug and drug-disease interactions in the ED: analysis of a high-risk population. Am J Emerg Med 14:447–450

Greenwald JL, Halasyamani L, Greene J et al (2010) Making inpatient medication reconciliation patient centered, clinically relevant and implementable: a consensus statement on key principles and necessary first steps. J Hosp Med 5:477–485

Hajjar ER, Hanlon JT, Sloane RJ et al (2005) Unnecessary drug use in frail older people at hospital discharge. J Am Geriatr Soc 53:1518–1523

Hamilton H, Gallagher P, Ryan C et al (2011) Potentially inappropriate medications defined by STOPP criteria and the risk of adverse drug events in older hospitalized patients. Arch Intern Med 171:1013–1019

Hanlon JT, Artz MB, Pieper CF et al (2004) Inappropriate medication use among frail elderly inpatients. Ann Pharmacother 38:9–14

Haverhals LM, Lee CA, Siek KA, et al (2011) Older adults with multi-morbidity: medication management processes and design implications for personal health applications. J Med Internet Res 12:e44

Institute of Medicine (1999) To err is human: building a safer health system. National Academies Press, Washington, DC

Jencks SF, Williams MV, Coleman EA (2009) Rehospitalization among patients in Medicare fee-for service programs. N Engl J Med 360:1418–1428

Lau HS, Florax C, Porsius AJ, De Boer A (2000) The completeness of medication histories in hospital medical records of patients admitted to general internal medicine wards. Br J Clin Pharmacol 49:597–603

Lazarou J, Pomeranz BH, Corey PN (1998) Incidence of adverse drug reactions in hospitalized patients: a meta-analysis of prospective studies. JAMA 279: 1200–1205

Lund BC, Carnahan RM, Egge JA et al (2010) Inappropriate prescribing predicts adverse drug events in older adults. Ann Pharmacother 44:957–963

Luo R, Scullin C, Mullan AMP et al (2011) Comparison of tools for the assessment of inappropriate prescribing in hospitalized older people. J Eval Clin Practice. http://onlinelibrary.wiley.com/doi/10.1111/j.1365-2753.2011.01758.x/pdf. Accessed 29 Nov 2011

Mattison ML, Afonso KA, Ngo LH, Mukamal KJ (2010) Preventing potentially inappropriate medication use in hospitalized older patients with a computerized provider order entry warning system. Arch Intern Med 170:1331–1336

McDonnell PJ, Jacobs MR (2002) Hospital admissions resulting from preventable adverse drug reactions. Ann Pharmacother 36:1331–1336

Merrill CT, Elixhauser A (2002) Hospitalization in the United States, HCUP fact book no 6. Agency for Health Care Research and Quality, Rockville

Morandi A, Vasilevskis EE, Pandharipande PP et al (2011) Inappropriate medications in the elderly IUC survivors: where to intervene? Arch Intern Med 171:1032–1034

Naugler CT, Brymer C, Stolee P, Arcese ZA (2000) Development and validation of an improving prescribing in the elderly tool. Can J Clin Pharmacol 7:103–107

Onder G, Landi F, Cesari M et al (2003) Inappropriate medication use among hospital older adults in Italy: results from the Italian Group of Pharmacoepidemiology in the Elderly. Eur J Clin Pharmacol 59:157–162

Onder G, Landi F, Liperoti R et al (2005) Impact of inappropriate drug use among hospitalized older adults. Eur J Clin Pharmacol 61:453–459

Page RL 2nd, Ruscin JM (2006) The risk of adverse drug events and hospital-related morbidity and mortality among older adults with potentially inappropriate medication use. Am J Geriatr Pharmacother 4: 297–305

Page RL 2nd, Strongin K, Millis R et al (2008) Medicare beneficiaries with mild to moderate heart failure see 15–23 different providers annually (abstract 5922). Circulation 118:S1030

Page RL 2nd, Linnebur SA, Ruscin JM (2010) Inappropriate prescribing in the hospitalized elderly patient: defining the problem, evaluation, tools, and possible solutions. Clin Interv Aging 5:75–87

Pugh MJ, Hanlon JT, Zeber JE et al (2006) Assessing potentially inappropriate prescribing in the elderly veterans affairs population using the HEDIS 2006 quality measure. J Manag Care Pharm 12:537–545

Pugh MJ, Hanlon JT, Wang CP et al (2011) Trends in use of high-risk medications for older veterans: 2004 to 2006. J Am Geriatr Soc 59:1891–1898

Qato DM, Alexander GC, Conti RM et al (2008) Use of prescription and over-the-counter medications and dietary supplements among older adults in the United States. JAMA 300:2867–2878

Rothberg MB, Pekow PS, Liu F et al (2008) Potentially inappropriate medication use in hospitalized elders. J Hosp Med 3:91–92

Spinewine A, Schader KE, Barber N et al (2007) Inappropriate prescribing in elderly people: how well can it be measured and optimized? Lancet 370:173–184

Wu WK, Panteleo N (2003) Evaluation of outpatient adverse drug reactions leading to hospitalization. Am J Health Syst Pharm 60:253–259

Index

M. Wehling (ed.), *Drug Therapy for the Elderly*,
DOI 10.1007/978-3-7091-0912-0, © Springer-Verlag Wien 2013

Printed by Printforce, the Netherlands